Dietetics
Practice and Future Trends

Esther A. Winterfeldt, PhD, RD
Professor Emeritus
Department of Nutritional Sciences
College of Human Environmental Sciences
Oklahoma State University
Stillwater, Oklahoma

Margaret L. Bogle, PhD, RD, LD
Executive Director
Lower Mississippi Delta Nutrition Intervention Research Initiative
Agricultural Research Service
U.S. Department of Agriculture
Little Rock, Arkansas

Lea L. Ebro, PhD, RD, LD
Professor and Director
Dietetic Internship Program
Department of Nutritional Sciences
College of Human Environmental Sciences
Oklahoma State University
Stillwater, Oklahoma

AN ASPEN PUBLICATION®
Aspen Publishers, Inc.
Gaithersburg, Maryland
1998

Aspen Publishers, Inc., is not affiliated with the American Society of Parenteral and Enteral Nutrition.

Library of Congress Cataloging-in-Publication Data

Dietetics : practice and future trends/edited by Esther A. Winterfeldt,
Lea L. Ebro, Margaret L. Bogle.
p. cm.
Includes bibliographical references and index.
ISBN 0-8342-0888-1
1. Dietetics—Vocational guidance. 2. Dietetics—Practice.
I. Winterfeldt, Esther A. II. Ebro, Lea L. III. Bogle, Margaret L.
RM218.5.D54 1998
613.2'023—dc21
97-42006
CIP

Orders: (800) 638-8437
Customer Service: (800) 234-1660

About Aspen Publishers • For more than 35 years, Aspen has been a leading professional publisher in a variety of disciplines. Aspen's vast information resources are available in both print and electronic formats. We are committed to providing the highest quality information available in the most appropriate format for our customers. Visit Aspen's Internet site for more information resources, directories, articles, and a searchable version of Aspen's full catalog, including the most recent publications: **http://www.aspenpub.com**
Aspen Publishers, Inc. • The hallmark of quality in publishing
Member of the worldwide Wolters Kluwer group.

Editorial Services: Ruth Bloom
Library of Congress Catalog Card Number: 97-42006
ISBN: 0-8342-0888-1

Printed in the United States of America

1 2 3 4 5

CONTENTS

iii

CONTRIBUTORS

Donna Alexander-Israel, PhD, RD, LD, LPC
President
Preferred Nutrition Therapists, Inc.
Richardson, Texas

Margaret L. Bogle, PhD, RD, LD
Executive Director
Lower Mississippi Delta Nutrition
  Intervention Research Initiative
Agricultural Research Service
U.S. Department of Agriculture
Little Rock, Arkansas

Lea L. Ebro, PhD, RD, LD
Professor and Director
Dietetic Internship Program
Department of Nutritional
  Sciences
College of Human Environmental
  Sciences
Oklahoma State University
Stillwater, Oklahoma

Robin B. Fellers, PhD, RD, LD
Assistant Professor
Director of Didactic Program in
  Dietetics
Department of Nutrition and Food
  Science
Auburn University
Auburn, Alabama

Susan Calvert Finn, PhD, RD, FADA
Director
Nutrition Services
Ross Products Division
Abbott Laboratories
Columbus, Ohio

Helene M. Kent, RD, MPH
Director
Women's Health Section
Colorado Department of Public
  Health and Environment
Denver, Colorado

Carolyn Moore, PhD, RD
Assistant Manager
Clinical Nutrition
The Methodist Hospital
Houston, Texas

Phyllis Nichols, RD, LD
Consultant Dietitian
Private Practice
McAlester, Oklahoma

L. Charnette Norton, MS, RD, LD, FADA, FCSI
President
The Norton Group, Inc.
Missouri City, Texas

Sara C. Parks, RD, MBA, PhD
Associate Professor
Associate Dean
School of Hotel, Restaurant &
    Recreation Management
College of Health & Human
    Development
The Pennsylvania State University
University Park, Pennsylvania

Carmen Roman-Shriver, PhD, RD, LD
Assistant Professor
Food & Nutrition Program
Education, Nutrition & Restaurant/
    Hotel Management
Texas Tech University
Lubbock, Texas

Wendy M. Sandoval, PhD, RD
Associate Professor, Emeritus
University of New Mexico
College of Education
Nutrition/Dietetics Program
Albuquerque, New Mexico

M. Rosita Schiller, RSM, PhD, RD, LD, FADA
Professor and Director
Medical Dietetics Division
School of Allied Medical
    Professions
The Ohio State University
Columbus, Ohio

Kathy Stone, MBA, RD, FADA, CDE
Owner
Strictly Nutrition
Boca Raton, Florida

Esther A. Winterfeldt, PhD, RD
Professor Emeritus
Department of Nutritional
    Sciences
College of Human Environmental
    Sciences
Oklahoma State University
Stillwater, Oklahoma

Martin M. Yadrick, MS, MBA, RD, FADA
Senior Implementation Consultant
Computrition, Inc.
Chatsworth, California

INTRODUCTION

Dietitians, through their unique knowledge of both the science and art of nutrition, are the professionals taking the lead in the promotion of nutritional health of the public (or as some would say the "promotion of public nutrition"). Because of this blend of scientific knowledge and social and cultural factors that influence what people eat, dietitians are able to use their skills to help individuals in illness and disease prevention as well as those who are healthy and active. Dietitians also interact with professionals of other disciplines that affect nutrition and are able to blend their assorted expertise for the benefit of clients. Their participation in basic research and in integrating new scientific concepts into practice of both clinical nutrition and public/community nutrition adds an invaluable dimension to the practice of dietetics.

Dietitians are prepared to be versatile through their educational preparation in the biologic and physical sciences including nutrition, in foods and food preparation and service, in management, and in sociology and psychology. This versatility of expertise of dietitians is especially critical as the "global village" emerges, opening many opportunities in international nutrition, management, and food service.

The purpose of the authors and the many contributors to this book about the profession of dietetics is to present an overview of the many career directions and opportunities open to dietitians. The real-life stories of dietitians who are practicing in a broad spectrum of positions will, we think, help show the many choices that may be made and introduce students to the creative and futuristic side of the profession. This is truly a time when the profession will be what the students of tomorrow make it. It is hoped that we have opened a few windows for students to glimpse real people taking charge of their career.

The reader will find this is not a "how-to" book; rather it is about dietitians, what they do, and where they practice. It is primarily a book for students, those in dietetics as well as those who are undecided and looking for career possibilities. Dietitians or others considering a career change may find that the accounts of dietitians who have taken new directions and in so doing created exciting careers will be an inspiration. Along with careers, we have included information about education and experience requirements as well as credentialing and continued education. The historical development of the profession, The American Dietetic Association as the governing body, and the future outlook are included.

We hope that students, teachers, advisors, and counselors will find the book informative, perhaps even eye-opening, in regard to career decisions. The authors believe this profession has much to offer students of the future. We remain excited about and pleased with the fulfilling careers that we have enjoyed. We further hope that many who read this book will be inspired to become the dietitians of the twenty-first century and help create additional innovative career options.

Esther A. Winterfeldt
Margaret L. Bogle
Lea L. Ebro

PART I

Dietetic Education

CHAPTER 1

Introduction to the Profession of Dietetics

Esther A. Winterfeldt

"An honorable past lies behind us, a developing present is with us, and a promising future lies before us." Mary I. Barber, ADA President 1940–41.[1]

Outline—Chapter 1

- Introduction

- Early Practice of Dietetics
  - Cooking schools
  - Hospital dietetics
  - Clinics

- Founding of The American Dietetic Association
  - Structure of the association
  - Influential leaders

- Dietetics as a Profession
  - Specialized knowledge
  - Continuing education
  - Code of ethics
  - Service to others

- Growth of the Profession and Historical Milestones
  - Membership
  - Registration and licensure
  - American Dietetic Association Foundation

INTRODUCTION

"What is a dietitian?" "What does a dietitian do?"

Recognition of the dietitian as a food and nutrition expert became official in 1917. This, however, was not the actual beginning of the practice of dietetics. The use of diet in the treatment of disease was already an ancient practice, even though it was based more on trial and error than on scientific knowledge. Besides physicians, others including home economists, nurses, and cooks were practicing and teaching about good dietary practices, and researchers were uncovering the secrets of nutrients in foods and their health-promoting effects.[2]

What the dietitian did in 1917 could easily be described in one of four areas (dieto-therapy, teaching, administration, social welfare), with by far the majority working in hospitals. In the 1990s, the roles for dietitians are many and varied. In the descriptions of these roles, we show what the dietitian does as well as the opportunities available in a broad spectrum of areas. We also show that the future looks very promising and that roles for dietitians are predicted to continue to grow and expand well into the twenty-first century.

Dietetics has been practiced as long as people have been eating. The term itself derives from *dieto* meaning diet or food. According to earliest historical evidence, our ancestors were forced to concentrate on simply finding food, with little concern about the variety or composition of that food. Today, however, food is plentiful. At least in the developed countries of the world, being able to choose and eat too much from an abundant food supply has become a great problem for many. The prevalence of obesity and nutrition-related diseases in many countries of the world is evidence that not only is food available but too much food is eaten or the wrong kinds of food are chosen by many.

Recommendations about eating and food choices have come from biblical admonitions as well as from early physicians and scientists who advocated specific practices about eating and diet. Early physicians in Europe and China, including Hippocrates, formed theories about the relationship between food and the state of a person's health.[3] Many of these early physicians and scientists emphasized adding or eliminating certain foods from the diet according to disease symptoms although there was no knowledge at that time about nutrients and recommendations were based largely on trial and error. Until the discovery of the major nutrients in foods during the nineteenth and twentieth centuries, a scientific basis for many of the eating recommendations was tenuous at best.

During the eighteenth century, research by chemists and physicists began to yield information about digestion, respiration, and other metabolic functions.[4] These studies were forerunners of the twentieth century scientific discoveries that identified the elusive substances in foods (i.e., the nutrients that were responsible for many of the effects described much earlier in the etiology of disease). Fats, carbohydrates, and amines (or albuminoids) were known by the mid-1800s, but vitamins and minerals were discovered only during the early 1900s.

One of the most fascinating accounts of the relationship between specific foods and illness is Lind's *Treatise on Scurvy,* written in 1753.[5] When it was discovered that lemons and limes or their juice would prevent the dreaded scurvy among sailors at sea for long periods of time, it was a life-saving piece of knowledge. Vitamin C from citrus fruits was later termed the *antiscorbutic* vitamin for this property. Other breakthroughs came when vitamin A was found to be a factor in the prevention of skin lesions and blindness in both animals and humans and when niacin, one of the B vitamin group, was found to prevent pellagra in humans and "black tongue" in dogs.[6] There are equally vivid accounts of scientific discoveries involving the other nutrients.[7-9]

EARLY PRACTICE OF DIETETICS

Cooking Schools

Early cooking schools in America, following their emergence in Europe in the early 1800s, were forerunners of the education of dietitians in the United States.[10] One of the first was the New York Cooking Academy founded in 1876. It was soon followed by schools in Boston and Philadelphia as well as other major cities.[3] Many of the schools offered not only cooking instructions but laboratories in chemistry and special classes on diet for the sick.[11] The schools trained many of the men and women who were put in charge of food services in hospitals as well as serving in the armed services and Red Cross during World War I.

Hospital Dietetics

Among the first persons who practiced dietetics were those who fed the sick in hospitals. Because little was known about nutritional needs either in health or during illness, feeding was not a major concern. Menus were monotonous and featured only a few foods, sometimes served with beer. One account of menus in the New York Hospital in the late eighteenth century indicated that mush, molasses, and beer were served for breakfast and supper several days of the week. Fruits and vegetables were not added to the menu until much later and then usually only as a garnish.[12] More hospitals opened during the 1800s and gradually food service improved.

Florence Nightingale is credited not only with improving nursing and care of the sick during the Crimean War in the mid-1880s but also with greatly improving the food supply and sanitary conditions in hospitals.[13]

Clinics

The Frances Stern Clinic in Boston, originally called the Boston Dispensary, was one of the leading food clinics established in the late 1900s to help provide better diets for the sick poor. This clinic, still a leading treatment center, has served as a model for similar clinics throughout the United States.

Dietitians have played important roles during times of war including the Civil War and later World Wars I and II. Many served during World War I in hospitals for the armed forces both overseas and in the United States.[12] Later in World War II in the 1940s, hundreds of dietitians volunteered for active service. Dietitians also worked closely with the Office of the Surgeon General and the Red Cross during this period to help train more individuals in nutrition. The fast pace of education was greatly increased to help the war effort.

FOUNDING OF THE AMERICAN DIETETIC ASSOCIATION

The history of the profession of dietetics in the United States is also the history of The American Dietetic Association (ADA), as they grew together in increasingly important ways. The profession flourished because the association took early steps to establish and administer requirements for the education and practice of dietetics. In turn, dietitians supported the association and its activities. The author is unaware of any other professional organization that has as successfully combined the requirements for a career with affiliation with the professional organization. The strength of both has thus been reinforced.

Before the founding of the ADA, persons who worked in food and nutrition could join the American Home Economics Association (AHEA) in order to associate with and communicate with others of like interests. Dietitians were few in number at that time, and although they had somewhat similar educational backgrounds, there was no common way to identify persons who were professionally qualified.

In 1917, the AHEA did not hold its annual meeting because of World War I. Instead, a group of about 100 dietitians met in Cleveland. The purpose of the meeting was "to provide an opportunity for the dietitians of the country to come together and meet with the scientific research workers and that the feeding of as many people as possible be placed in the hands of women who are trained and especially fitted to feed them in the best possible manner."[12] Because this was wartime, the government had extensive food conservation programs in effect involving home economists, dietitians, and volunteers.

At the first meeting of the association, officers were elected and a constitution and bylaws drawn up overnight. Dues were one dollar a year, and there were 39 charter members. Lulu Grace Graves was the first president and Lenna Frances Cooper was the first vice president.

World War I was, in great part, the impetus that brought early dietitians together to discuss feeding needs. But it was also recognized that the services of dietitians in hospitals were rapidly assuming even greater importance, both in food service and in treating illness. Researchers were making great strides in nutrition science, and as more became known about individual nutrients, maintaining good nutrition and treating certain illness through diet became more precise.

Structure of the Association

Dietitians at this time were primarily working in four general areas, and to share and communicate, it was decided that these would be designated as interest areas in the new association.[3] The vision of these early leaders is evident in that the same four areas of practice have continued up to the present time, although terminology as well as actual practice in each area has varied and developed. *Dietotherapy*, the area having to do with the treatment of disease by diet, was later named diet therapy, then clinical dietetics, and is currently referred to as medical nutrition therapy. From quite restricted diets for a few disease conditions, this area of practice is now characterized by more liberal diets and much more emphasis on overall nutritional status of patients.

The *teaching* section dealt with the education of dietetics students, nurses, physicians, and patients. Later called the education section, this group established the first set of standards for the education of the dietitian. By 1924, dietetic education included a four-year course of academic study plus an internship. The internship experiences were further refined by 1927. At that time, 62 hospitals offered training for student dietitians that followed ADA guidelines. The chairman of the education section personally visited all hospitals with internships yearly to ensure that standards were being met. Eligibility for membership in the ADA has always included education and experience requirements. Although specific requirements have changed over the years, the education/experience pattern was set in 1924 and has never changed.

The *social welfare* section was later renamed the community nutrition section. Public health nutrition programs had been established as early as 1906 in New York and 1908 in Chicago, where the Red Cross dietetic service began programs to improve nutrition services in that city.[12] The fourth section, named *administration,* included dietitians working in business, school food service, hospital food service, and industrial cafeterias. Many of the first cafeterias that served the public, as well as providing food service in hospitals, hired persons trained in home economics and/or dietetics as the manager. The term *institution administration* was later used to describe this area of practice, and today it is termed *food service systems management.*

The young association continued to grow. By 1927, the ADA had 1,200 members. There was a headquarters office in Chicago, and the association had been legally incorporated in the State of Illinois. The first edition of the *Journal of The American Dietetic Association (JADA)* was published in 1925 with four issues a year. The first editor was Eleanor Smith; she later also served as president of the association. The early issues of the *JADA* featured many subject areas similar to those published today. For instance, articles on hospital food service, personnel issues, and special diets—especially the diabetic diet—were included.

Influential Leaders

Sarah Tyson Rorer was one of the first instructors in the cooking schools of the late 1800s and she educated both dietitians and physicians in hospital dietetics. She also published widely on food preparation and gave cooking demonstrations for the general public.[14] She worked with physicians in setting up a diet kitchen where special diets were prepared and patients educated about how to use them. She has been credited with being the first American dietitian.

The Massachusetts Institute of Technology was the first university to accept women in this country, and Ellen H. Richards was the first woman graduate in 1876. Mrs. Richards was one of the first leaders to be concerned with food purity and the proper preparation of food. She is credited as the founder and leader of the modern home economics movement, which later led to the founding of the AHEA in 1909. Because dietetics and home economics have always been closely related, Mrs. Richards is also claimed as one of the early leaders in dietetics.

The first president and cofounder of ADA, Lulu Graves, served in that office from 1917 to 1920. She was on the faculty of Iowa State College and later on the faculty at Cornell University, where she set up a training course for hospital dietitians. She was also a dietitian at hospitals in Chicago, Cleveland, and New York and helped plan kitchens and dietary departments of many hospitals in the United States, Sweden, Switzerland, and Australia.[15]

Lenna Frances Cooper, a cofounder and first vice president of ADA, later served as president in 1937–1938. She was the first head dietitian and director of the School of Home Economics at the Seventh-Day Adventist Health Care Institution in Battle Creek, Michigan. In her career, she was later appointed as dietitian on the staff of the Surgeon General of the United States in Washington, D.C. Mrs. Cooper published widely and was coauthor of a popular nutrition textbook with 17 editions. A lecture is presented each year at the annual meeting of ADA in her honor by a chosen current leader in the profession.

Ruth Wheeler, president of ADA in 1924, prepared the first detailed outlines of a course for student dietitians. Although at first they were only recommendations, these outlines were the beginning of education requirements for dietetics practice.[16] Dr. Wheeler was also a great "idea" person, and one of her ambitions was to establish a professional journal in dietetics. This ambition became a reality in 1925 with the publication of *JADA*. She taught for many years at the University of Iowa Medical School and is said to have been the first to teach that the therapeutic diet should be based on the normal needs of the individual.

Mary E. Barber, president in 1941, was the director of home economics for the Kellogg Company, Battle Creek, Michigan, for several years. In 1941, she was appointed as a food consultant to the Secretary of War to assist with menus, confer with food authorities, and give talks throughout the country on the problems of feeding 1.5 million soldiers. She was the editor of the first official history of the association, *The History of The American Dietetic Association (1917–1959)*.

Mary Schwartz Rose was a leader in nutrition research and a pioneer in both teaching and developing nutrition education for the general public. She was perhaps the leading contributor to the advancement of every aspect of nutrition in this century.[15] She established the Department of Nutrition at Columbia University. Dr. Rose was closely associated with ADA from its beginning and was a frequent speaker at annual meetings. She was made an honorary member in 1939.[12] The Mary Schwartz Rose Fellowship for graduate study is awarded each year by ADA to honor this outstanding scientist, teacher, and scholar.

Mary P. Huddleson became the second editor of *JADA* in 1927 and remained editor until 1946. She increased the number of issues from 4 to 12 per year and introduced many innovations and features, leading to the respected journal it is today. She also helped write the first history of the association. Each year, a Mary

P. Huddleson award is presented by ADA to the author of an outstanding article published in the journal.

Anna Boller Beach was the first executive secretary of ADA, having been appointed in 1923. The first office was located in her home. She served as executive secretary until 1927 and continued to serve in other capacities in ADA, including a term as president in 1928–1930. She was the historian of the association for many years.

Lydia J. Roberts was a pioneer nutritionist on the faculty of the University of Chicago and, later, the University of Puerto Rico. She initiated nutrition education programs designed to better the nutritional status of children in Puerto Rico and was recognized by the American government for her efforts. She was world renowned for her expertise in the feeding of infants and children.[17] Dr. Roberts was a member of the first committee to develop recommended dietary allowances in 1941 and served on the committee making the first revision in 1944. She gives a fascinating account of this historical event and the background for the recommendations in a 1958 article published in *JADA*.[18] An essay contest in her name was conducted by ADA for several years, and a fellowship in public health nutrition is awarded by ADA in her honor.

Mary de Garmo Bryan, the second president of ADA, 1920–1922, had an early career serving overseas with the Red Cross during World War I. In 1931, she became the first "inspector" to travel yearly to all hospital training courses for dietitians in the United States.[12] After a year, inspection every two years was deemed sufficient. Mrs. Bryan was chair of the first joint committee with AHEA to develop a training course and sponsor regional conferences for directors of school lunch programs in 1938. She also published a popular textbook for school food service. On the faculty of Columbia University for several years, she was regarded as one of the foremost teachers in institution administration.

There are scores of other influential leaders in dietetics. The reader is referred to the most recent and very comprehensive history of the association, *Carry the Flame,*[12] and to the *JADA* for more information. Many are referred to throughout this book. This brief listing highlights those leaders who played key roles in laying the foundations of the association and thus were influential in establishing the profession of dietetics.

DIETETICS AS A PROFESSION

A profession is characterized as being different from a business or a trade. A profession has specific characteristics, including *specialized preparation or knowledge, continuing education, a code of ethics, and service to others* (versus individual gain or profit). Plato first defined a profession as "the occupation . . . to which one devotes himself, a calling in which one professes to have acquired some special knowledge used by way of instruction, guiding, or advising others, or of servicing them in some art."[16] Dietetics, like other professions that fit Plato's description, fulfills all these requirements.

The dietetics profession, from 1917 to the present, has organized around the above four principles.

Specialized Knowledge

Educational standards for members and for dietetic training programs were considered important from the beginning, and the ADA recommended standards of education as early as 1919. The association first recommended two years of college for dietitians, but by 1921, a four-year degree was required for dietitians or a two-year course for institutional managers. The courses for the degree were designated in a detailed course outline for student dietitians. The plan included a bachelor's degree with a major in food and nutrition and hospital training of at least six months. Later, this recommendation became a requirement for membership in ADA as well. "The Standardization of Courses for Student Dietitians in Hospitals" was approved by ADA in 1927, and by 1928, the first list of hospitals offering the courses was published.[12] Sixty-two hospitals were soon offering the program.

Hospital training programs varied in length, the average being six months. By 1930, 400 students were enrolled in 65 student dietitian courses. It was decided in 1930 that a person should be designated to inspect all dietetic education programs yearly to determine if they met standards and Mary de Garmo Bryan was the person appointed to make these inspections. Gradually, both colleges and hospitals offering dietetics training would meet the association's education standards, thus ensuring uniform preparation of dietitians.

By the 1940s, internships were located in hospitals, including Veterans Administration and Army hospitals; in administrative programs such as college food services; and in food clinics. Shortages of dietitians during the 1940s also gave rise to training of dietetic aides who could assume some of the routine duties of the dietitian.

Because it was thought that ADA needed to assume more responsibility for training of dietitians, not just the recommendation of educational standards, a dietetic internship board was appointed in 1949 to assume some of the former responsibilities of the professional education section. The purpose of the new board was to develop standards for approval of new internships and reapproval of established ones. Much more direct assistance to the internships was also a goal. In 1954, "Generalizations for the Curriculum Guide for the Dietetic Intern and Evaluation Scales Form" for interns and staff dietitians was developed and used in approving programs.[12] In 1966, a dietetic internship council was appointed, and in 1970, the association established a department of education in the headquarters office. The department had three priorities: nutrition education of the public, nutrition education of personnel in other allied fields, and education of dietetic professionals. Dietetics education had three components: undergraduate education, internship, and continuing education. Minimum standards of education continued to be reviewed and, in 1970, were revised again. The progression of educational plans is discussed further in Chapter 2.

A master plan for education and practice was developed, and a key report was issued in 1983 titled "Promoting Quality Dietetic Education: A Report of The American Dietetic Association Task Force on Education." In this report, a series of recommendations was made that changed some of the association's education-related activities and led to the development of the standards of education.

The standards of education were published in 1987 and continue to be the educational requirements followed by all programs, both undergraduate and practice-based. The new standards were designed to align education closely with professional practice.

It is obvious that the association has taken steps over the years to continually review and update educational requirements as the profession grew and matured. Dietitians and employers alike acknowledge the well-recognized body of specialized knowledge required to practice in dietetics.

Continuing Education

Lifelong learning is a hallmark of the professional. In dietetics, as early as the 1930s, attention was given to the continuing education needs of dietitians after five years of experience.

In 1957, a continuing education services director was appointed by ADA to coordinate efforts among states, but there was, as yet, no centralized planning for continuing education. Professional registration for dietitians became a reality in 1969, and for dietetic technicians in 1988, and included a requirement for continuing education during each five-year period.

A committee in 1978 studied further continuing education needs and recommended that a headquarters staffperson be hired to coordinate these activities. The committee also recommended that the association offer specific continuing education conferences and workshops for the benefit of members. Continuing education events are now a well-established activity of ADA, offering a large variety and number of educational events for dietitians. Dietitians may also participate in many state and district activities as well as in academic course work for continuing education (see Chapter 4).

Code of Ethics

Members of a profession are bound by a code of ethics that guides practice. The first code was written for dietitians in 1924.[12] A comprehensive code was accepted in 1942 and revised in 1953. The document produced was entitled "Code of Ethics for Members of The American Dietetic Association" and was widely distributed. In 1962, a "Dietitian's Oath" was added to the code of ethics as well as a further revision of the code itself.

In 1970, a new "Code of Professional Conduct" and guidelines for professional practice were accepted. The word *ethics* was replaced in the new document because it was considered a somewhat intangible term. However, the statements regarding practice were much the same in both documents. One further update occurred in the late 1970s (see Appendix A).

Service to Others

The dietetics profession performs its services for the benefit of people. Indeed, the seal of the association carries the motto of the association: "Quam Plurimis Prodesse"—to benefit as many as possible. Dietitians are employed in many work settings in which they work with the public: in hospitals, clinics, and extended care facilities; in food services; in community nutrition programs; in education; and in private practice. Their expertise in the knowledge of foods and nutrition places dietitians in the forefront of professionals concerned with health and wellness. Dietitians are well educated, and they have been imbued early in their education with the idea that they have a "cause"—to help the public attain better health and longevity through the use of good nutrition practices.

GROWTH OF THE PROFESSION AND HISTORICAL MILESTONES

Membership

From the beginning, membership in the association meant meeting education and experience requirements. In 1917, the first requirements for membership were fairly lenient. The association tried to be inclusive. Stricter requirements ensued over the years. For instance, many of the first dietitians were graduates of a two-year course in home economics or a one-year course before 1917 plus one year of experience, or they were research workers or practicing physicians and some were practicing in allied areas to dietetics. By 1926, a BS degree in home economics from an "institution of high rank," with a major in food and nutrition was required, plus at least six months training in a hospital under the supervision of a dietitian.[16] Although the experience component was later expanded to allow working experience as well as internships, the requirements for active membership remained education and experience.

Eventually, other categories of membership in ADA were added, such as life membership and associate. Later, honorary, retired, student, and returning student categories were added.[19] Membership was extended to dietetic technicians in 1975, along with specific education and experience requirements. An outline of the current membership categories and requirements is shown in Appendix F.

The number of members in ADA has risen steadily over the years. Figure 1–1 shows the growth from its inception to the present. It is noteworthy that while the membership grew by about 1,000–1,500 each decade until 1970, there was a huge growth spurt beginning in the late 1960s and resulting in a growth of almost 15,000 members between 1968 and 1978 and 18,600 new members between 1978 and 1990. Another 15,930 members were added from 1990 to 1996. Membership in 1996 totals 68,075, indicating a continuing healthy growth rate.

Registration and Licensure

In 1969, the association established a system of national professional registration by which a dietitian who met certain requirements could be designated a registered dietitian (RD). The title now had legal status.

Employers soon became familiar with the RD credential and began specifying it as a condition of employment. Between 70 and 80 percent of dietitians today are registered.

Licensure for dietitians was first proposed by the states of California and Minnesota. The association did not actively assist states in obtaining licensure before 1980, although a Model Licensure Law was later produced to assist states that were interested in pursuing this legislation. California was the first state to pass licensure laws for dietitians (1982), and many other states followed in the 1980s and 1990s. At present, 38 states have state licensure laws for dietitians.

American Dietetic Association Foundation

The foundation (ADAF) was established in 1966 with a tax status as an educational and scientific organization. This status enabled tax-free monies to be donated to the foundation that could, in turn, award scholarships and set up programs to further educational and scientific activities in the profession and the public. Several major studies have been funded by the foundation; programs and lectureships at the annual meeting have been made possible through gifts and donations to the foundation.

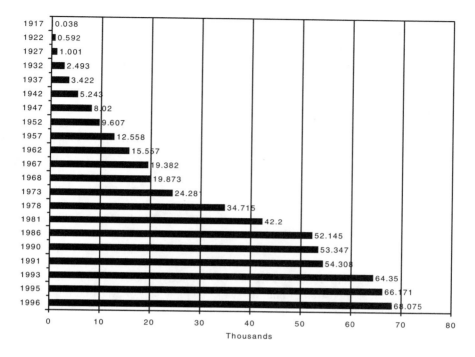

Figure 1–1 ADA Membership. *Source:* References: 12, 13, 20–25.

The largest project undertaken by the foundation was to raise funds in the 1980s to purchase a building to house the association and to establish the National Center for Nutrition and Dietetics. The center, created for the purpose of developing and providing programs in food, nutrition, and health for the general public, was staffed in 1986 and has continued to grow. Both individuals and corporations contributed money to establish the center. By 1987, ADAF had raised more than $2 million for the center, provided about $170,000 in awards and scholarships, supported dietetics research, and underwritten countless continuing education programs for practitioners. More than 1,500 dietetic interns, undergraduate, and graduate students and dietitians have been recipients of ADAF awards over the years.

Dietetic Technicians and Managers

The Hospital, Institution and Educational Food Service Society (HIEFSS) was formed in 1960 in Cleveland as an organization for food service supervisors. It was an independent society but closely tied to ADA through setting of membership standards and through advice and support from ADA. State associations were formed and a correspondence course offered through ADA to train supervisors, who, in turn, became eligible for membership in HIEFSS. In 1967, guidelines were developed for a two-year post–high school program that later became the basis for membership in ADA as a technician member. In 1983, the name of the organization was changed to the Association for Managers of Food Operations (AMFO) and titles of members changed to "food manager." Persons completing a voluntary certification program were called "certified food managers."

Legislation

Dietitians were active in legislation that affected dietetic practice and interests as early as 1921 when a committee was appointed to promote passage of a bill to grant military status to dietitians. In 1931, the women's joint congressional committee joined ADA in efforts to promote favorable legislation. In the early 1940s, there was extensive legislative activity related to food and nutrition. The legislative interest was so high that, in 1944, the president of ADA commented that the association "needed to be actively concerned with all bills pertaining to the interests of members, and to nutrition, education, health and welfare."

A change in legislative policy came in 1966 when the tax status of the association was changed to allow active participation in legislative affairs. The change in tax status meant that other activities also changed: educational activities for the public and the acceptance of donated funds. A Washington legislative consultant was employed by ADA in 1969, and an ADA member became a part-time liaison for legislation and public policy for the association.[12] The association began taking positions on national issues and the association legislative committee became quite active, working closely with the association's Washington representatives. By 1970, state associations were also becoming more active in legislation actions at both the state level and national level. Five legislative workshops were held around the nation in 1971 in collaboration with AHEA and in 1973, the first national ADA legislative conference was held in Washington. A similar conference has been held yearly since 1973 and is an event that has grown in importance as a way of informing members about current legislation and the legislative process. The conference also gives members an opportunity to meet face to face with congressmen and other Washington agency representatives.

The National Nutrition Consortium was formed during the 1970s with ADA as one of the four associations represented. Its purpose was to provide a common voice to legislators and the public on good nutrition and food practices. A Senate Select Committee on Nutrition, chaired by Senator George McGovern, issued the first "Dietary Goals for the United States" at about the same time.[26] Although these goals were controversial at the time, coming from a congressional committee rather than a professional group, they helped focus national attention on nutrition and health issues and led to guidelines issued later by the US Department of Agriculture, Health and Human Services, and the National Academy of Sciences.

Each year, pending legislative issues are identified by ADA as those the association wishes to promote through the ADA headquarters office, the ADA Washington office, and the state coordinators. This coordination allows exertion of a strong presence and an influence on issues important to dietitians.

Areas of Practice

The employment settings for dietitians have traditionally been varied. The sections into which the organization was structured (administration, clinical, community, and education) more or less defined the dietetic practice areas. Little information was available on the actual areas of practice by dietitians until periodic membership surveys were begun in the early 1980s. In the first of these, a grouping of the reported places of employment into seven categories was used in the report (Table 1–1). In 1986, 1990, and 1991, the groupings were still being used, with some further collapsing of categories; then in 1993, the areas of practice were changed to those adopted by the ADA Council on Practice (COP).[27]

As shown in Table 1–1, clinical dietetics has been the area in which most dietitians practice. The number of dietitians practicing in the food and nutrition

Table 1–1 Primary Areas of Practice by Dietitians

Practice Area	(Percent of RDs reporting on membership surveys)					
	1981	1986	1990	1991	1993	1995
Clinical dietetics	39	37	37	42	45(1)	45
Food service administration	26	25(2)	25	24	20(3)	26
Community dietetics	10	12	11	11	14(4)	15
Consultation/private practice	4(5)	18	18	14	13(6)	7
Education/research	4	8	9	9	8	7
Generalist	9(7)					
Other	8(7)					

Note: (1) Changed to clinical nutrition.
        (2) Changed to management practice.
        (3) Changed to food and nutrition management.
        (4) Changed to community nutrition.
        (5) Consultation only.
        (6) Changed to consultation and business practice.
        (7) Not reported after 1981.

Source: Data from ref. 20–25.

management area has remained about the same, whereas a definite increase in the number of dietitians practicing in consultation and private practice began in 1986. The decreased percentage of practitioners in this area in 1995 may be due to renaming the categories.

Dietetic Practice Groups

Dietetic practice groups (DPG) were formed in 1978 and, as a group, within a short period of time became one of the strongest and most influential entities within the association. An outgrowth of, and logical progression from, the earlier sections (administration, clinical, community, and education) by which interests of members were met, DPGs provided visibility for dietitians practicing in a wide variety of areas and settings and allowed them to join forces. So popular were these practice groups that from an original 9 groups in 1978, there were 22 groups in 1981 and 28 groups by 1996.

Role Delineation Studies

As the profession grew in the 1970s and 1980s, there was a need to continually assess the quality of both dietetic education and practice. To this end, a task force on competencies was appointed in the mid-1970s to develop the first stage of a conceptual framework for the profession. The task was completed with the acceptance of a document in 1982, "Conceptual Framework for the Profession of Dietetics," which set forth a philosophy, mission statement, and definition of practice for the profession and the association.[12]

In 1979, a study was begun to determine the actual and appropriate roles and responsibilities of the entry-level clinical dietitian. This was followed by similar studies of food service systems management dietetics and community dietetics. These "role delineation" studies were valuable to the profession because they provided the first comprehensive look at dietetic practice and produced data used, with further updates, until the present time in the setting of standards for dietetic practice. The studies are discussed in more detail in Chapters 6 and 7.

Long-Range Planning

Leaders in dietetics have consistently taken steps to position the profession to meet present as well as future needs. This positioning has been achieved through planning groups, task forces, specially appointed committees, and outside consultants as well as governing groups within the Association.

Long-range planning became a major thrust in the Association with a committee in 1959 that suggested active recruitment, educational opportunities, work with other professional groups, and emphasis on research for continued growth and development of the profession. These goals continued to be emphasized throughout the 1960s and were expanded in the 1970s through the appointment of a Task Force for the Seventies and a Study Commission on Dietetics. Funded by the W.K. Kellogg Company, the study commission issued a report in 1972 that dealt with the roles of dietitians and their educational needs for the future. Titled *The Profession of Dietetics: The Report of the Study Commission on Dietetics,*[28] the report influenced Association direction for many years. A second in-depth report on the status of the Association in 1984,[3] again funded by the W.K. Kellogg Company, became a major reference source for futures-oriented planning from that time to the present.

In 1969 a Task Force for the Seventies[12] reviewed goals of the Association and looked at future needs. Later, the Conceptual Framework for the Profession of Dietetics outlined a philosophy, mission, and definition of practice. A marketing plan was also developed for the Association, which targeted the public, the media, physicians, and dietitians as the audiences to be reached.[29]

Many activities were initiated in the 1980s, the effects of which moved the profession forward in significant ways. For instance, the first of a series of long-range planning conferences convened in 1981 and a second in 1984. In the conferences, invited leaders in the profession discussed goals and needs in the profession and made far-reaching recommendations for dietetics. The future was also explored in a Strategic Planning Conference in 1995.[30] Throughout the 1980s and 1990s, the Association moved decisively toward both outreach to the public and increased involvement in the policy arena, although much attention continued to be directed toward members and their welfare.

Further landmark studies looked at the education of dietitians, practice in dietetics, registration and licensure, and advanced practice. Dietetic education has always been closely tied to dietetic practice and as the roles for dietitians grew and expanded, so too did the need to assess and update education. A Master Plan for Education and Practice in the 1970s and a Task Force on Competencies[31] at about the same time outlined major steps toward moving the emphasis in education from content of learning to the outcomes of learning based on the attainment of competencies. Another task force in 1981[32] made recommendations toward assuring quality education based on Standards to be achieved and, in 1993, the emphasis on quality was continued through the accreditation process. Education, practice, and credentialing were the topics at a Futures Search Conference in 1994 that explored future trends, consumer and professional needs, and future practice roles.[33]

Concurrent with these important studies, other studies were also undertaken, such as a Manpower Study in the 1970s[34] that identified trends affecting the demand for dietitians and estimated future numbers of people that might be needed. Among the most significant of planning efforts at this time were the studies that, for the first time, began an indepth look at the actual and the appropriate roles and responsibilities of dietitians: the Role Delineation Studies of 1979 and 1980,[35–37] updated in 1989.[38] The 1989 study was broader in scope in that it also included dietetic technicians and measured what dietetic practitioners actually did in a variety of settings. These, and other studies in the 1990s, such as the Task Force on Critical Issues: Registration Eligibility and Licensure,[39] continued to discuss opportunities to enhance all aspects of both education and practice.

These long-range planning activities, especially those in education, credentialing, and practice are referred to in some detail throughout several chapters of this book. They were events and actions that met needs and led to continued advances in the profession.

WORKING WITH OTHER PROFESSIONAL GROUPS

Since its beginning in 1917, the dietetics profession has worked closely with professionals in allied areas. Mutual interests have thus been advanced, and many programs and activities have been made possible through these associations.

Dietitians were initially organized as an interest section in the AHEA; the first joint committee of ADA was created with the AHEA in 1919 to develop a course in dietetics. In 1941, a joint committee between the two associations was formed to determine professional qualifications for persons in health and welfare programs. Beginning in 1971, legislative workshops were conducted with AHEA for several years, and in 1985, the two groups, along with several other associations, sponsored a two-day national conference for nutrition education. The close relationship between the two professions is evident in undergraduate education, in which traditionally most dietetics education programs have been located in home economics divisions or departments in universities. Many members of each group hold membership in both associations.

Another organization with which ADA has been closely allied is the American Public Health Association (APHA) and its members serving in the US Public Health Service (USPHS) and national, state, and district public health departments. The first joint project with the APHA was the development of diabetic exchange lists in 1950, with the American Diabetes Association participating as the third collaborator. Grants from the USPHS also allowed ADA to sponsor workshops on programmed learning in the 1960s. Many dietitians are employed in departments of public health where nutrition is an integral part of the programs provided for the public. The USPHS first established a nutrition section or division in 1945, and this section continues to administer programs critical to health care in the United States. Dietetic internships are also offered in some of the USPHS schools and hospitals.

The American Hospital Association (AHA) was another organization important in the creation and development of ADA. Many early members of ADA were members of AHA first and participated in section and committee work in that association. The ADA provided a session at the AHA annual meeting for many years, and on occasion, joint annual meetings were held. Because many dietitians have traditionally worked in hospitals, there is good reason to promote common interests and goals of the two groups. In 1947, a joint committee between ADA and AHA was formed to develop professional standards in hospital dietetics. Because of the close ties already established, this committe produced several important publications pertaining to hospital dietary practice and led to the recognition and title of a new category of dietitian's aide, the food service supervisor.

The American Diabetes Association has been a close ally of ADA in the development of the diabetes exchange lists as noted earlier. The two associations also collaborated to write *The Whole Family Diabetic Cookbook.*

In 1992,[27] the Food and Nutrition Science Alliance (FANSA) was formed with the Institute of Food Technologists, the American Society for Clinical Nutrition, and the American Society for Nutritional Sciences. This linkage brings together a combined membership of more than 100,000 food, nutrition, and medical scientists. Its members have joined forces to speak with one voice on food and nutrition science issues and to translate scientific information into practical advice for consumers.

The first International Congress of Dietetics was held in Amsterdam in 1952 and the second in Rome in 1956, with ADA as one of the founding groups. Twelve national dietetic associations were represented at the first congress. Organized for the purpose of sharing information about nutrition and dietetics, an international bulletin was begun in 1956 as a means of communication. Congresses are held approximately every five years, the most recent in Manila in 1996.

The ADA has actively participated in many programs with governmental agencies such as the US Department of Agriculture, Health and Human Services, the National Institutes of Health, the National Research Council, and Congress. In the 1980s, some 40 associations and groups were listed as having allied interests and programs with ADA. Alliances had been established with 147 other professional groups by 1995, and ADA maintained a liaison with each of the groups.[40]

REACHING OUT TO THE PUBLIC

ADA has initiated several programs over the years directed to the general public. As was indicated earlier, the creation of the National Center for Nutrition and Dietetics in 1990 provided a central focus and a headquarters structure enabling a much more comprehensive outreach. Donated funds were used to set up a "hotline for consumers" that provided answers to consumer questions. Many educational materials, database searches, and library facilities were made available to both members and the public through the center.

Before 1990, periodic projects have been initiated by ADA to provide nutrition education for the public and expand the outreach of the profession. One very effective undertaking that began as a small effort in three states was the declaration and observance of a "dietitian's week" in 1957. The effort was so well received by the public as well as dietitians that the week became a month in 1978 and is now a significant March event in the profession. During the month, national, state, and district dietetic associations organize media events, provide advertising and educational programs and materials, and encourage hospitals, schools, and businesses to promote good nutrition.

Another activity designed for consumers also started on a small scale in Detroit in 1961 on a trial basis. This was the dial-a-dietitian program initiated through a grant from the Nutrition Foundation.[12] Within a few years, other states started similar programs, and by 1977 there were 31 dial-a-dietitian programs in existence. The programs generally provided information about foods, food safety, food preparation, normal nutrition, and nutrition information related to special diets. Because these programs were so successful, one of the first services established in the National Center for Nutrition and Dietetics was the nutrition hotline, patterned after the state programs but administered from the national office and accessed through an 800 number. The services of the dial-a-dietitian and hotline programs have grown every year, greatly enhancing the role of the dietitians in the eyes of the public through the provision of timely and authoritative information.

In 1982, a program was initiated to use selected and specially trained professional dietitians as media spokespersons. Termed the *ADA ambassadors,* the first group of 15 persons appeared nationwide in print and on television. They immediately established themselves as nutrition experts. The program was expanded in 1985 when state media spokespersons were also selected and trained. These dietitians networked with the national group and established state and local media contacts. This program, now called the *spokesperson network,* continues as a highly successful program reaching the public with current and reliable information.[40]

Position papers are another way ADA and the dietetics profession take a stand on issues and provide direction for the public. First issued in 1970, a position paper represents the official position of the association on a stated issue and is therefore considered an authoritative document. The papers are distributed widely and are often quoted in the media and used in legislation. Each paper has a designated lifetime after which it is withdrawn or reissued to accurately portray a valid position based on the most current information.

Participation in national projects and campaigns is another way the association and the profession affects the public. During the 1980s and 1990s, many of these opportunities arose. Among them were the Nutrition and Health Campaign for Women in 1992,[27] the Physician's Initiative Education Project in 1992, the Food Labeling Workshop in 1992, the Child Nutrition and Health Campaign in 1995,[41] the National Osteoporosis Action Campaign in 1996,[42] and Healthy People 2000 in 1990.[43] These are far-reaching programs with great impact on the public health because of the participation of the health-related professional groups and government agencies.

PERCEPTIONS OF DIETETICS

Several studies have been conducted over the years to determine how dietitians are perceived or identify their "image."

The 1984 study commission[3] made the following observations about the dietitian's image: "The profession of dietetics should grow to encompass new areas, through more intensive education and training, so that the services of dietitians are recognized as crucial components in the care and treatment of patients with special problems. Dietitians should also look for new ways to apply their expertise for the good of society. The profession should not try to delimit its boundaries, nor to erect barriers to prevent others from entering, but should expand its activities into new areas where knowledge of foods and nutrition is valuable."

During the 1980s and early 1990s, many events occurred in the association that served to bring the dietitian into much greater public visibility and, in turn, to enhance the image of the profession. The success of national nutrition month, the ambassadors program, the greatly expanded role of the foundation and creation of the National Center for Nutrition and Dietetics, the dial-a-dietitian programs, and others added greatly to the perception of dietetics and dietetics professionals as experts in food and nutrition.

Leadership training is vital in any professional area as it is one of the important ways by which practitioners advance in their career and gain professional competence. ADA has strongly promoted leadership training and, by continuing to look at how the profession affects the public and their needs and taking steps to meet those needs, is providing the means for dietitians to succeed and to be viewed positively.

Salaries

Salary levels of dietitians have risen over the years, more in some areas of practice than others. The extent of these changes, when viewed over many years, no doubt reflects changes in the economy of the country as a whole but also growing awareness of the roles played by dietitians. The first reference to salaries in the history of the association was in 1938,[3] when it was reported that the hospital dietitian usually earned $1,080 to $7,000, the higher figure being less common. Other services such as room, board, and laundry were commonly provided by the hospital. In other than hospitals, the average salaries were $1,200 to $4,000 per year. In 1946, the average salary was $3,000, not a significant improvement. In 1952, salaries were reported to be slightly higher in the Midwest than the East.

Beginning in 1981, the association began regular surveys of members that included salary information. In 1981, the average yearly salary was reported as $16,414,[23] although the study did not equate all salaries with full-time practice so the actual average was probably higher. Also, in 1981, 71.3 percent of dietitians surveyed reported incomes less than $20,000 (of this number, 17.7 percent were less than $10,000) and 28.9 percent greater than $20,000. Only 10.9 percent reported salaries greater than $25,000.

In 1986, the ADA membership surveys began including data on areas of practice and years of work experience in dietetics, although salary levels were reported only by income categories. All studies since that time have reported income by both area of practice and years of experience, thus yielding useful data. In 1986, the largest percentage of dietitians (55.2 percent) were earning between $20,000 and $30,000 per year (Table 1–2). In 1990, 49 percent earned in the $20,000 to $30,000 category, the highest percentage, but an almost equal percentage was making higher salaries. In 1991, 41 percent were making $30,000 to $40,000 per year, the highest level, and this trend continued in the 1993 study with 43 percent of dietitians earning this amount. The percentage of dietitians making $40,000 to $50,000 per year and more amounted to slightly more than 29 percent in 1993 compared with 5 percent in 1986.

In comparing salaries by areas of employment in dietetics, there are definite differences. The highest salaries are reported by dietitians working in food and nutrition management, consultation and private practice, and education/research. In these three areas, median incomes were greater than $40,000 while median incomes in the other two areas of practice were between $30,000 to $35,000 per year (Table 1–3).

In 1995, the level of earning for the highest percentage of dietitians in clinical nutrition and community nutrition was $30,000 to $35,000 per year. By contrast, the highest percentage of those in management, in consultation and private practice, and in education/research were at $50,000 or more.

Salaries also vary by years of experience. In clinical dietetics and management dietetics, the highest salary levels are reached at 16 to 20 years of experience; in consultation and private practice and education/research, highest salary levels are reached at 11 to 15 years and in community nutrition after 20 years. In comparing salaries of dietitians to other salaries in related professions, there are differences.

Table 1–2 Salary Levels of Dietitians per Year
(all employment areas and length of time-employed periods)

Salary Range	Average Percentage				
	1986	*1990*	*1991*	*1993*	*1995*
$20,000 or less	21.9	2.7	1.8	1.5	0.9
$20,001–30,000	55.2	49.0	33.0	26.0	19.3
$30,001–40,000	17.4	33.7	41.4	43.3	42.6
$40,001–50,000	4.2	10.4	15.7	18.8	22.5
$50,001 and more	1.3	4.6	8.2	10.5	14.5

Source: Data from ref. 20, 21, 22, 24, 25.

Dwyer[44] points out salaries in clinical dietetics have lagged behind salaries in nursing, pharmacy, physical therapy, and other specialties over the past 30 years. Salaries are lower than for most physicians or persons with MBA degrees, and this is true even for dietitians with doctorates and extensive management experiences. She attributes this in part to a lack of specialized skills among dietitians and a lack in reimbursement skills especially needed in the clinical setting. Multiskilled training may be one answer to this dilemma.

In a 1992 study,[45] salaries for male food service directors were significantly higher than for women even when controlling for experience, size of hospital, academic preparation, and professional certification. In another study in 1996,[46] it was reported that male food service directors received higher salaries when compared with females, but this was ascribed to the fact the men had more experience.

Table 1–3 Comparison of 1993 and 1995 Estimated Median Incomes for Registered Dietitians by Area of Practice

Practice Area	1993	1995	% Increase
Clinical nutrition	$32,116	$34,131	6.30
Food and nutrition management	$40,441	$42,964	6.20
Community nutrition	$31,810	$33,902	6.60
Consultation and business practice	$40,365	$43,374	7.50
Education and research	$39,427	$42,784	8.50
All areas of practice	$34,578	$36,919	6.80

Source: Data from J.A. Bryk and T.K. Soto, Report on the 1993 Membership Database of The American Dietetic Association, *Journal of The American Dietetic Association*, Vol. 94, pp. 1433–1438, © 1994, The American Dietetic Association and J.A. Bryk and T.H. Kornblum, Report on the 1995 Membership Database of The American Dietetic Association, *Journal of The American Dietetic Association*, Vol. 97, pp. 197–203, © 1997, The American Dietetic Association.

THE FUTURE

If the life of a profession is viewed as a continuum, then it is important and appropriate to plan for the future through forecasting trends and attempting to determine how the profession will be affected by those trends. Dietetics has done this. At the Future Search Conference in 1994,[33] several speakers referred to areas of changes and trends that will affect dietetics practice. Future practice roles, technology trends, credentialing and licensing issues, research in nutrition and dietetics, and education for future dietetics practice were highlighted. Communications technology, international interconnectedness, and continually expanding research needs are said by many futurists to be among the important trends that will affect dietetics.

Bezold[47] and Parks[48] emphasize the importance of forecasting trends as a way of predicting how the profession will be affected and the way dietitians will be judged and regulated. Both stress that changes are occurring rapidly in the health field and that the demand for practitioners who are prepared to fit into new roles will increase. The final chapter in this book looks closely at some of the changes likely to occur in the future and the implications for the practice of dietetics.

CONCLUSION

If the past is prologue to the future, as the philosophers believe, then the dietetics profession has been on a path since the early 1900s toward both meeting the needs of today and planning for tomorrow. Standards have been set for both education and practice, a code of ethics has been adopted, registration and licensure to ensure the accountability and competency of practitioners have been established, long-range planning and goal setting have become a consistent formalized process, and progress has been shown at every stage in ADA's history toward the goal of meeting societal and public needs. The profession has grown in membership and outreach and has its rightful place among forward-planning professions concerned with the health and well-being of all individuals and groups.

DEFINITIONS

The American Dietetic Association (ADA) Professional organization for dietitians.

The American Dietetic Association Foundation (ADAF) Arm of the association with a tax status enabling acceptance of funds for designated purposes of benefit to the association and the public.

Dietetic Practice Group (DPG) Organized groups of dietitians with similar interests in an area of practice or a particular subject area.

Dietetic Technician Graduate of an approved dietetic technician program.

Dietetics Practitioner Person who qualifies to practice the profession of dietetics/ nutrition as recognized by The American Dietetic Association.

Dietitian Professional who translates the science of food and nutrition to enhance the health and well-being of individuals and groups.

Licensed Dietitian (LD) Dietitian meeting the credentialing requirement of a state to engage in a given occupation.

Nutritionist Professional with academic credentials in nutrition; may also be an RD.

Position Paper Policy stand on an issue by the association that is used in legislation, public outreach, and nutrition education.

Professional Person in a career, such as dietetics, who required specialized knowledge, intensive academic preparation, high standards of achievement and conduct, and commitment to continued study and renders service to the public.

Quality Assurance Certification of the continuous, optimal, effective, and efficient outcomes of a service or program.

Registered Dietitian (RD) Dietitian meeting eligibility requirements (education, experience, and a credentialing examination) of the commission on dietetic registration.

Role Configuration of major and specific responsibilities for which a practitioner is accountable.

Role Delineation Study Empirical research resulting in levels of involvement in activities performed and specific roles of doing and policy setting for a profession.

Standards of Practice Statements of the dietetic practitioner's responsibility for providing quality nutrition care or other designated responsibilities according to the area of practice.

REFERENCES

1. Barber MI. *History of The American Dietetic Association (1917–1959)*. Philadelphia: JB Lippincott Co; 1959.

2. Corbett FR. The training of dietitians for hospitals. *J Home Econ*. 1909;1:62.

3. ADA. *A New Look at the Profession of Dietetics. Report of the 1984 Study Commission on Dietetics*. Chicago: The American Dietetic Association; 1985.

4. Todhunter EN. Development of knowledge in nutrition. I. Animal experiments. *J Am Diet Assoc*. 1962;41:328–334.

5. Beeuwkes AM. The prevalence of scurvy among voyageurs to America 1493–1600. *J Am Diet Assoc*. 1948;24:300–303.

6. Goldberger J. Pellagra. *J Am Diet Assoc*. 1929;4:221–227.
7. Todhunter EN. Development of knowledge in nutrition. II. Human experiments. *J Am Diet Assoc*. 1962;41:335–340.
8. Todhunter EN. Some classics of nutrition and dietetics. *J Am Diet Assoc*. 1964;44:100–108.
9. McCoy CM. Seven centuries of scientific nutrition. *J Am Diet Assoc*. 1939;15:648–658.
10. Shircliffe A. American schools of cookery. *J Am Diet Assoc*. 1947;23:776–777.
11. Rorer ST. Early dietetics. *J Am Diet Assoc*. 1934;10:289–295.
12. Cassell J. *Carry the Flame: The History of The American Dietetic Association*. Chicago: The American Dietetic Association; 1990.
13. Cooper LF. Florence Nightingale's contribution to dietetics. *J Am Diet Assoc*. 1954;30:121–127.
14. Huddleson MP. Sarah Tyson Rorer—pioneer in applied nutrition. *J Am Diet Assoc*. 1950;26:321–324.
15. The Cleveland Connection. *The American Dietetic Association. 1917–1992. A Factbook*. Cleveland ADA Founders Fund; 1992.
16. Beeuwkes AM. Organization and growth of dietetics as a profession in the US. *Nutrition*. 1958;12:3–8.
17. Doyle MD, Wilson ED. *Lydia Jane Roberts: Nutrition Scientist, Educator, and Humanitarian*. Chicago: The American Dietetic Association; 1989.
18. Roberts LJ. Beginnings of the recommended dietary allowances. *J Am Diet Assoc*. 1958;34:903–908.
19. ADA. *Directory of Dietetics Programs*. Chicago: 1997–1998. The American Dietetic Association.
20. Bryk JA, Kornblum TH. Report on the 1990 membership database of The American Dietetic Association. *J Am Diet Assoc*. 1991;91:1136–1141.
21. Bryk JA, Kornblum TH. Report on the 1991 membership database of The American Dietetic Association. *J Am Diet Assoc*. 1993;93:211–215.
22. Bryk JA, Soto TK. Report on the 1993 membership database of The American Dietetic Association. *J Am Diet Assoc*. 1994;94:1433–1438.
23. Baldyga WW. Results from the 1981 census of The American Dietetic Association. *J Am Diet Assoc*. 1983;83:343–348.
24. Bryk JA. Report on the 1986 census of The American Dietetic Association. *J Am Diet. Assoc*. 1987;87:1080–1085.
25. Bryk JA, Kornblum TH. Report on the 1995 membership database of The American Dietetic Association. *J Am Diet Assoc*. 1997;97:197–203.
26. Truswell AS. Dietary goals and guidelines: national and international perspectives. In: Shils ME, Olson JA, Shike M, eds. *Modern Nutrition in Health and Disease*. 8th ed., Vol. 2. Philadelphia: Lea & Febiger; 1994.

27. ADA. *ADA Annual Report, 1992–93*. Chicago: The American Dietetic Association; 1993.

28. ADA. *The Profession of Dietetics: The Report of the Study Commission on Dietetics.* Chicago: The American Dietetic Association; 1972.

29. Parks SC, Moody DL. A marketing model: Applications for dietetic professionals. *J Am Diet Assoc.* 1986;86:33–43.

30. ADA. *ADA Annual Report, 1994–95*. Chicago: The American Dietetic Association; 1995.

31. Council on Educational Preparation. Report of the Task Force on Competencies. *J Am Diet Assoc.* 1978;73:281.

32. Report of the Task Force on Education. *Promoting Quality Dietetic Education.* Chicago: The American Dietetic Association; 1983.

33. The American Dietetic Association and Commission on Dietetic Registration. *Challenging the Future of Dietetic Education and Credentialing. Dialogue, Discovery, Directions;* 1994.

34. Fitz PA, Baldyga WW. Estimates for the future demand for dietetic services: results of the Dietetic Manpower Demand Study. *J Am Diet Assoc.* 1983;83:186–189.

35. Baird SC, Armstrong RVL. *Role Delineation for Entry-Level Clinical Dietetians.* Chicago: The American Dietetic Association; 1980.

36. Baird SC, Burrelli JS. *Role Delineation and Verification for Entry-Level Positions in Foodservice Systems Management.* Chicago: The American Dietetic Association; 1983.

37. Baird SC, Burrelli JS. *Role Delineation and Verification for Entry-Level Positions in Community Dietetics.* Chicago: The American Dietetic Association; 1983.

38. Kane MT, Estes CA, Colton DA, Eltoft CS. Role Delineation for Dietetic Practitioners; Empirical Results. *J Am Diet Assoc.* 1990;90:1124–1133.

39. ADA. *Report of the Critical Issues: Registration Eligibility and Licensure Task Force.* Chicago: The American Dietetic Association; 1992.

40. *1994–1995 Annual Report.* The American Dietetic Association, p. 3.

41. Child nutrition and health campaign kicks off at annual meeting. *ADA Courier.* 1995;34(10):1.

42. American Dietetic Association Supports National Osteoporosis Action Campaign. *ADA Courier.* 1996;35(1).

43. Browner Y. Healthy People 2000: a call to action for ADA members. *J Am Diet Assoc.* 1991;91:1520–1521.

44. Dwyer JT. Scientific underpinnings for the profession. Dietetians in research. In: *Challenging the Future of Dietetic Education and Credentialing. Dialogue, Discovery, Directions.* The American Dietetic Association and Commission on Dietetic Registration; 1994:57–75.

45. Barrett EB, Nagy CM, Maize RS. Salary discrepancies between male and female foodservice directors in JCAHO-accredited hospitals. *J Am Diet Assoc.* 1992;92:1079–1082.

46. Barrett EB, Shanklin CW. Sex-role orientation and career importance factors do not explain salary inequities between male and female foodservice directors. *J Am Diet Assoc.* 1996;96:181–183.

47. Bezold C. Future practice roles. In: *Challenging the Future of Dietetic Education and Credentialing. Dialogue, Discovery, Directions.* The American Dietetic Association and Commission on Dietetic Registration; 1994:26–32.

48. Parks S. Anticipating the future by identifying and tracking today's trends. *J Am Diet Assoc.* 1994;94:843–845.

Educational Preparation in Dietetics

Esther A. Winterfeldt

"As a profession, the one thing that we can predict is that the greatest change in our practice will be the change in knowledge and how we integrate new science into our daily practice."[1]

Outline—Chapter 2

- Introduction
- Undergraduate Education
  - Educational standards
  - Standards of education
  - Current educational requirements
- Types of Dietetic Education Programs
  - Didactic program in dietetics
  - Coordinated program
  - Dietetic Technician Program
  - Program choice
- Education Planning in The American Dietetic Assocation
- Dietetic Education in the Future
- Conclusion

INTRODUCTION

Dietetics education is the key to dietetic practice and to the future of the profession. As is true of all professions, a specialized body of knowledge is required of practitioners in dietetics. Because of the importance of education to the profession, the early leaders in dietetics set standards for the education of dietitians. The educational standards have been revised at intervals over the years as practice evolved and the needs of those being served also changed.

To be eligible to practice in dietetics, a combination of didactic and experiential learning through supervised practice is required as it is accepted by educators that classroom learning is retained best when it is immediately applied.

UNDERGRADUATE EDUCATION

The educational preparation of the dietitian begins in the undergraduate program. The course of study is based in the sciences (i.e., biologic, physical, and social sciences) and includes both theoretical and applied courses. The college or university offering a dietetics degree program plans a series of courses in a curriculum that meets both the university requirements and the educational standards of The American Dietetic Association (ADA). A baccalaureate degree from an accredited college or university is a requirement to practice. To complete the educational process, professional experience is attained either concurrently with the course work in a coordinated program or following the degree program. The Council on Professional Issues of the ADA establishes the educational requirements. The Commission on Accreditation/Approval for Dietetic Education (CAADE) monitors quality and implements the educational standards.

The dietetics major is offered in colleges and universities throughout the United States including Hawaii and Puerto Rico. A complete listing of programs is available in the "Directory of Programs,"[2] which is published yearly by the ADA.

At times, students may change their major or decide to study dietetics after having completed a degree in another subject area. The director of the dietetic program will then designate the courses needed to meet all requirements for the dietetics major. A second degree is generally not required if basic foundation courses were met earlier. In similar circumstances, some students complete the required undergraduate courses while working toward the master's degree.

Educational Standards

Dietitians

The first educational requirements for dietitians were developed in 1927 and described in the "Standard Course for Student Dietitians."[3] Students were required to have a bachelor's degree with a major in home economics from an institution of "recognized high rank" for membership in ADA and for hospital training. The hospital providing the training was required to be a member of the American Hospital Association, have an accredited nurse's training school, and employ staff dietitians eligible for ADA membership. The training was under the supervision of a dietitian.

In 1931, a list of recommended requirements in college course work was issued, although only two institutions offered a curriculum that met the recommendations at the time. Further changes were made in the ensuing years, and in 1947, academic standards for entering internships were published as Plan I. This was followed in 1955 by Plan II, which included four subject areas and a range of credit hours. Plan III, in 1958, required courses grouped under core, emphasis, and concentration, with choices in the latter two. Departing from a list of courses, the next set, or Plan IV in 1977, set competency-based minimum academic requirements that allowed greater flexibility for colleges and universities in determining courses. The last of the series, Plan V, was introduced in 1987 as knowledge requirements. These were part of the newly developed standards of education (SOE). The knowledge requirements were statements of competencies or outcomes of the learning process. Competencies are defined as statements of the performance expected of the beginning practitioners.[4] In 1991, the numbering system for the various plans was discontinued.[5] The progression of education plans is shown in Figure 2–1.

In 1996, the knowledge requirements were replaced by "foundation knowledge and skills for the didactic component of entry-level dietitian education programs" and the standards of education also underwent revisions.[5]

Each college or university offering the dietetics major indicates their plan for meeting the knowledge requirements through courses required of students. Programs will differ in the specific courses required, but each program meets the competencies and each must be approved or accredited by ADA.

Dietetic Technicians

The education requirements for the dietetic technician are also established by ADA. They have undergone revisions since the first set of requirements in the 1960s. The current requirements are discussed further in this chapter.

Standards of Education

A major shift in dietetic education occurred when the SOEs were introduced in 1987. This was because they applied to both didactic and experiential programs and they diverged from earlier plans that were much more specific in terms of requirements. The standards provided for a common body of knowledge, skills, and values in dietetic education.[6,7] They encompass the goals and philosophy of

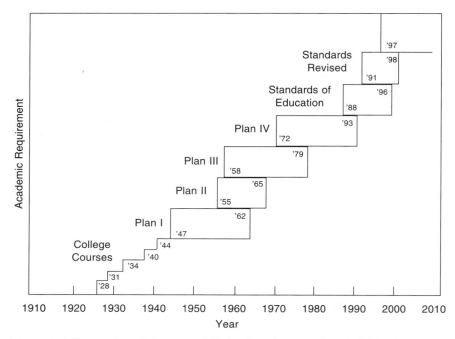

Figure 2–1 Progression of Programs Offering Requirements for Eligibility for Active Membership in The American Dietetic Association. *Source:* Reprinted with permission from B. Wenberg, Dietetics Education: Past, Present and Future, in *Proceedings of Future Search Conference, Challenging the Future of Dietetic Education and Credentialing—Dialogue, Discovery, and Directions*, © 1994, The American Dietetic Association and Commission on Registration.

the program, the students, the curriculum, the program resources, and evaluation. In stating broad standards for the education of dietitians, there is flexibility in the way they are applied and evaluated. And just as competencies represent the outcomes of learning, the final product is a dietitian prepared for the first job.

The five standards are the following:[5]

1. The mission statement of philosophy and measurable goals for the program shall provide guidance to the program.
2. A program should be accountable to its students.
3. Resources available to the program shall be identified and their contribution to the program described.
4. The curriculum shall provide for attainment of expected competence of the program graduate.
5. A systematic approach shall be used in managing and evaluating the program.

An abbreviated text of the standards is shown in Appendix B, and the complete text is found in the *Accreditation/Approval Manual for Dietetics Education Programs*.[5]

Each department or program providing dietetic education initially prepares a self-study document showing how the SOE are met in the program. This document is submitted to the ADA and is the basis for approval (didactic program in dietetics [DPD]) or accreditation (coordinated program in dietetics [CP]) by the CAADE program. (See definition of terms for *approved* and *accredited*.) The approval period may be for a period of 1 to 10 years. Yearly reports are submitted to ADA showing that the program continues to offer optimal education for the dietetics students.

The SOE are reevaluated and revised at intervals by the council on professional issues of ADA to ensure they remain valid and continue to provide for quality education. The impetus for the latest revision and updating of the standards occurred in 1994 at the Futures Planning Conference of ADA.[8] As an outcome of the deliberations, revised standards were approved in 1996 and implemented in 1997.[9,10]

Current Educational Requirements

A schematic of dietitian and dietetic technician education is shown in Figure 2–2. Both the didactic and the experience portion of dietetic education are shown. Together, these result in competencies expected to be attained in order to perform in an entry-level position.

The complete listing of the educational program components is found in the Accreditation/Approval Manual for Dietetics Education Programs[5] and in Appendix C. An expanded discussion of the supervised practice component of education is in Chapter 3. The knowledge and skills required in the didactic portion of education programs are grouped under eight areas: communications, physical and biological sciences, social sciences, research, food, nutrition, management, and health care systems. The same areas are required for the dietetic technician although the specific knowledge and skills differ. Foundation learning is further divided into basic knowledge of a topic, working or in-depth knowledge, and ability to demonstrate the skill at a level that can be developed further. To achieve the foundation knowledge and skills, graduates must have demonstrated the ability to communicate and collaborate, solve problems, and apply critical thinking skills.

In developing the 1997 requirements, the planning committee was guided by a model of lifelong learning showing the stages in professional growth (Figure 2–3). The model shows the professional growth and mastery of a discipline begins with the novice who cannot perform, but with education and experience, over time becomes competent.[9]

DIETITIAN EDUCATION

Didactic Program in Dietetics

- General Education: Required by Institution
  —Courses that meet DPD requirements may be applied to general education requirements, at the discretion of the institution
- Professional Program
  —Courses that incorporate the foundation knowledge and skills for entry to the supervised practice component

Dietetic Internship Program

- Core professional competencies for entry-level dietetics practice
- Emphasis: One or more *in addition* to the core professional competencies

| Nutrition Therapy | Community | Food Service Systems Management | Business/ Entrepreneur | General | Program Designed |

Coordinated Program in Dietetics

- General Education: Required by Institution
  —Courses that meet CP requirements may be applied to general education requirements, at the discretion of the institution
- Professional Program
  —Courses that incorporate the foundation knowledge and skills for entry to the supervised practice component
- Supervised Practice Component
  —Core professional competencies for entry-level dietetics practice
  —Emphasis: One or more *in addition* to the core professional competencies

| Nutrition Therapy | Community | Food Service Systems Management | Business/ Entrepreneur | General | Program Designed |

Option 1

Option 2

DIETETIC TECHNICIAN EDUCATION

Dietetic Technician Program

- General Education: Required by Institution
  —Courses that meet DT requirements may be applied to general education requirements for the associate degree, at the discretion of the institution
- Professional Program
  —Courses that incorporate the foundation knowledge and skills for entry to the supervised practice component
- Supervised Practice Component
  —Competencies for entry-level practice as a dietetic technician

Figure 2–2 Schematic for Dietetics Education. *Source:* Reprinted with permission from *Accreditation Manual for Dietetics Education Programs,* © 1994, American Dietetic Association.

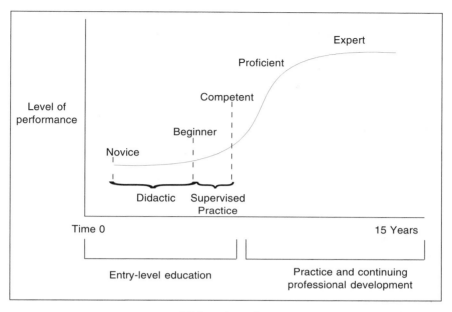

Lifelong Learning

Figure 2–3 Competency-Based Education: Schematic Representation of the Stages in Professional Growth: Mastery of Discipline and Professional Development along a Continuum from Novice to Expert. *Source:* Reprinted with permission from Educational Competencies Steering Committee, Final Report, © 1996, The American Dietetic Association.

The current plan for dietetic education is believed to be designed to meet the future needs of the profession for several reasons:[6]

1. They are based on national practice and employer data.
2. They build on assumptions that educational programs are responsive to market changes by being flexible in curricula, methods, and collaboration; emphasize critical thinking, problem solving, and communications; and provide the basis for lifelong learning.
3. They increase focus on areas of need such as food, public policy, and outcomes research.
4. They strengthen communication and management skills.
5. They increase expected performance level of entry-level practitioners in areas where dietetics professionals can assume leadership.
6. They specify breadth and depth in curriculum and course planning.
7. They identify the technician role in promoting team work and career laddering.
8. They address other higher education issues.

TYPES OF DIETETIC EDUCATION PROGRAMS

The two types of undergraduate programs are the DPD and the CP. The curriculum for either undergraduate program is based on course work to meet the foundation knowledge skills in eight areas of education: communications, physical and biological sciences, social sciences, research, food, nutrition, management, and health care systems.

The titles and the number of courses in a curriculum will vary from one university to another, yet all meet the required educational standards. An example is demonstrated in a survey showing that the number of chemistry courses ranged from one to six and the credit hours from 4 to 24 among several programs.[11] All required general and organic chemistry but not all required biochemistry; instead it was being taught in nutrition courses. Knowledge of computers and computer usage is universally required. Each university will have general education as well as departmental requirements that round out the curriculum. Information on specific courses and degree requirements will be found in each school's catalogue or from the director of the dietetic education program.

Didactic Program in Dietetics

In the DPD, the didactic portion of the educational requirements is completed during the degree program (either undergraduate or graduate). Following the degree, the student completes a supervised practice program (see Chapter 3).

The traditional DPD is a four-year undergraduate BS degree. Many of the courses required in the program are a combination of classroom and laboratory work, especially those in professional areas such as food production service or clinical nutrition, and in science courses such as chemistry and microbiology.

During this later part of the program, usually the senior year, the DPD student applies to a dietetic internship or AP4 program through a computerized matching program. Notification is given in April or November about a "match" or acceptance to the student's program of choice.

Coordinated Program

In the coordinated program, the didactic portion of a program is completed plus supervised practice during the degree program. The student graduating from this program is thus prepared for entry-level practice upon completion of the degree. As in the DPD, this program may also be at the undergraduate or graduate level.

In most universities, students enter the CP for the junior and senior year. The programs are sometimes referred to as "two by two," meaning the first two years are general study and may be at a community or junior college and the last two include the integrated courses leading to the degree. Some programs may be longer than the traditional four years depending on the specific program require-ments.

A university will designate the criteria for admission to the CP to ensure that students will be able to successfully complete the concentrated program. The selection criteria commonly include grade point average, writing skill, work experience, letters of recommendation and, sometimes, an interview. Personal characteristics considered important in success include communication skill, both oral and written, leadership ability, and professionalism.[12,13]

A minimum of 900 clock hours in supervised practice is required in the CP. The practice is primarily in hospitals, foodservices, and in community nutrition programs. The CP is intense in terms of time requirements and experiences, but when completed, the student is ready to practice.

Dietetic Technician Program

The dietetic technician (DT) program is similar to the coordinated program in that both didactic knowledge and skills and supervised practice are required in the program. These are specified. The requirements are specified by the council on professional issues and the programs are approved or accredited by CAADE.

The curriculum in dietetic technology is usually two years in length and, according to the educational institution, leads to an associate degree. Graduates of the program are eligible to take the registration examination for dietetic techni-cians and for entry-level practice.

Examples of a typical, or generic, curriculum and an actual curriculum for three different dietetic programs (DPD, CP, DT) are shown in Appendix E.

Program Choice

As shown in Table 2–1, there are more DPD than CP programs. The two reasons that primarily account for this are location and cost. Many universities are not located in areas where linkages can easily be formed with health care and other institutions and programs for the necessary student experiences. The DPD is also generally less costly in terms of number of faculty needed and because of larger class sizes.

The advantages of the CP are in less time to complete the dietetic education experience and because of the integration of learning. In fact, these were the reasons the CP was first developed and they continue as very positive aspects of the program. In the DPD, many students find it is helpful to have more time to absorb classwork at a somewhat slower pace and that there is time for more elective courses. Students who work part time may also choose the DPD. The programs provide an equally good experience and they meet the same standards. Prospective students are advised to contact their university of choice or an advisor for information on program options. The Directory of Programs,[2] published yearly by ADA, also lists all programs with contact information.

EDUCATION PLANNING IN THE AMERICAN DIETETIC ASSOCIATION

The responsibility for setting standards and providing direction to dietetic education programs is with the house of delegates, specifically, the council on professional issues. Three members of the council represent dietetics programs and one represents dietetic technician programs. Their functions include the following: (1) to address issues related to education practice and research, (2) to advocate and provide direction for entry level, advanced, and continuing education and professional development, and (3) to develop, approve, maintain, and evaluate standards for education in collaboration with the commission on accreditation/approval for dietetic education.

DIETETIC EDUCATION IN THE FUTURE

The education of the dietitian must be focused on the future practice roles of dietitians. It is generally accepted that traditional roles of dietitians are changing and that the future is anything but clear.[14] Several environmental and practice trends were identified by the ADA in 1995 as among those that are or will influence dietetic practice.[15] These were:

Table 2–1 Dietetic Education Programs and Enrollment Data

Program Type	Number of Programs		Number Enrolled		Number Graduates	
	1995	1996	1995	1996	1995	1996
DPD	234	231	11,383	11,975	3,309	3,783
CP	51	49	1,354	1,350	623	622
Diet. Tech.	72	72	3,318	2,981	732	714

Source: Reprinted with permission from *CAADE Newsletter,* © 1997, The American Dietetic Association.

- increasing emphasis on outcomes and revenue
- changing demographics
- increasing awareness of the relationship of diet to health
- changing governmental influence over health care
- changing role of technology
- increased emphasis on environmental issues
- changing vehicles of nutrition information
- converging industries restructuring the US national economy
- restructuring of the health care industry
- consumer-driven economy
- changing food and food service industry
- changing education system
- rapidly changing food and nutrition knowledge base
- moving to a world economy

What are the implications for students in dietetics? One is that it is crucial to be well prepared by acquiring the knowledge and skills needed in the profession and to anticipate that continuing education will be vital in one's future planning. "Future-oriented continuing professional education" is described as essential for keeping abreast of new development, in anticipating change and planning for what is to come.[16] The concept of multiskilling or cross-training has implications for educators as well as students as they progress through an educational program.[17,18] This concept is gaining attention because of predictions that cross-trained health professionals will be needed in health care both to reduce health care costs and for a more efficient health care system. For students, multiskilling may increase employment opportunities through being prepared to provide a wider range of services.

Skills such as leadership, communication, use of technology, ethical practice, counseling, and marketing are all part of dietetics training, and they also define the competent dietitian and dietetic technician.

CONCLUSION

Dietetics education has evolved over time but has always been based on the physiological, psychological, and sociological skills that prepare the student for practice in the profession. ADA designates educational standards that are met by all dietetic programs, thus assuring competent practitioners. With a background of academic knowledge and practical skills, dietitians are prepared for a wide variety of careers, which are described in other chapters in this book.

Traditional roles of dietitians are changing as the population itself and the health care industry change. Education that includes skills that will allow the dietitian to innovate and even cross practice boundaries has become increasingly important by enlarging the range of services the dietitian is prepared to offer. The ability of the dietitian to shape the nutritional health of all begins with education.

DEFINITIONS

Accreditation Process whereby a private nongovernmental agency or association grants public recognition to an institution that meets qualifications and periodic evaluation. In dietetics, the process includes a self-study by the institution and a site visit by the council on accreditation/approval for dietetic education.

Approval Recognition given to a dietetic education program (DPD, AP4, DT) that is substantially in compliance with the standards of education. Includes a self-study but not a site visit.

Basic Requirement Fundamental requirements for dietetics education programs.

Competency-Based Education Learning that is functionally adequate in performing the tasks and assuming the role of a specified position.

Coordinated Program Degree program combining didactic and experiential learning.

Council on Accreditation/Approval for Dietetic Education (CAADE) Group in ADA with responsibility to accredit or approve all dietetics education programs.

Council on Professional Issues Elected members in the house of delegates with the responsibility for policy direction in education, research, and practice in dietetics.

Didactic Instruction Knowledge acquired through classroom instruction.

Didactic Program in Dietetics (DPD) An educational program providing the standards of education.

Experiential Learning Learning attained through actual experiences.

Standards of Education (SOE) Authoritative model or example in education to be followed.

Support Courses Courses outside of professional required courses in dietetics that contribute to the total educational experience and lead to competence in dietetics practice.

REFERENCES

1. Parks SC, Schiller MR, Bryk J. President's page: investment in our future—the role of science and scholarship in developing knowledge for dietetics practice. *J Am Diet Assoc.* 1994;94:1159–1161.

2. ADA. *Directory of Dietetics Programs. 1997–1998.* Chicago: The American Dietetic Association; 1997.

3. Wenberg B. Dietetics education: past, present and future. In: *Proceedings of Future Search Conference Challenging the Future of Dietetic Education and Credentialing—Dialogue, Discovery, and Directions.* Chicago, IL.: The American Dietetic Association and Commission on Registration; 1994:3–12.

4. Chambers DW, Gilmore CJ, Maillet JO, Mitchell BE, et al. Another look at competency-based education in dietetics. *J Am Diet Assoc.* 1996;96:614–617.

5. ADA. *Accreditation/Approval Manual for Dietetics Education Programs.* Chicago: The American Dietetics Association; 1997, 4th ed.

6. Smitherman AL, Anderson CR. President's page: Standards of Education—ADA's foundation for the future. *J Am Diet Assoc.* 1987;87:1221.

7. Owen AL, Rinke W. President's page: changes in dietetic education to maximize our contribution to society. *J Am Diet Assoc.* 1986;86:375.

8. Parks SC, Fitz PA, Maillet JO, Babjak PA, et al. Challenging the future of dietetics education and credentialing—dialogue, discovery, and directions: a summary of the 1994 Future Search Conference. *J Am Diet Assoc.* 1995;95:598–606.

9. Gilmore CJ, Maillet JO, Mitchell BE. Determining education preparation based on job competencies of entry-level dietetics practitioners. *J Am Diet Assoc.* 1997;97:306–316.

10. Education Competencies Steering Committee. Final Report. ADA. 1996.

11. Shetler A. Chemistry requirements in didactic programs. *DEP Line.* 1995;(3):13.

12. Dittus KL. Criteria that predict dietetics success: how to prepare students for coordinated undergraduate programs. *J Am Diet Assoc.* 1994;94:150.

13. Barrett EB, Shanklin CW, Canter DD. Graduate and supervisor evaluation of the coordinated program at Kansas State University determines criteria deemed critical for success in entry-level practice. *J Am Diet Assoc.* 1993;93(suppl):A-79. Abstract.

14. Wenberg BG. Dietetic practice—what next. *DEP Line.* 1996;14(2):1–4.

15. Nutrition leadership. *ADA Courier.* 1995;34(11):4–8.

16. Berenbaum S. Future-oriented continuing professional education. *Top Clin Nutr.* 1995;10:66–70.

17. Sandoval WM. Multiskilling and dietetics education. *DEP Line.* 1996;14(2):5–8.

18. Braverman S. Focusing dietetic education in a challenging health care environment. *Top Clin Nutr.* 1995;10:8–13.

Preprofessional Practice in Dietetics

Wendy M. Sandoval

"We can empower young dietitians to reach their full potential by mentoring them during training and encouraging the development of the nontraditional qualities needed to succeed in the contemporary market place."[1]

Outline—Chapter 3

- Introduction

- Supervised Practice

- Supervised Practice Programs
  - Early programs
  - Dietetic internship—accredited
  - Preprofessional practice program—approved
  - Coordinated programs—accredited
  - Dietetic technician programs—accredited/approved

- Recent Changes to Supervised Practice Programs
  - Common questions about supervised practice programs

- Applying to Supervised Practice Programs

- Conclusion

INTRODUCTION

Preprofessional or supervised practice is an essential step in the path to becoming a registered dietitian (RD) or dietetic technician registered (DTR).

Supervised practice takes place in the work setting as opposed to the classroom. In the classroom, students learn knowledge and reasoning skills; in supervised practice, they learn to apply their knowledge and build the skills to be competent entry-level practitioners.[2] Successful completion of a supervised practice program is required for students to establish eligibility to take the registration examination for dietitians or dietetic technicians and/or apply for membership in The American Dietetic Association (ADA). This chapter provides an overview of supervised practice, describes types of supervised practice programs, and answers common questions that students ask about these programs.

SUPERVISED PRACTICE

RDs, dietetic technicians, and other professionals serve as preceptors or supervisors for students in supervised practice programs. Students learn to do what preceptors do on a day-to-day basis; how to identify problems, collect data, interpret and synthesize the findings, formulate plans and alternatives, and evaluate the outcomes. Preceptors in supervised practice teach students the steps in acquiring skills and becoming skilled enough to take over the job of the preceptor. It is not expected that students will do the job at the same level or at the same pace as the preceptor, but it is expected that they can do the job. In fact, by the end of the supervised practice experience, staff relief is often an expectation. When students substitute for their preceptors, it gives them the opportunity to practice as a professional while still having support. Students often report that the supervised practice part of their training was the best component of their academic training.[2]

Competency in dietetics practice is the goal of supervised practice. Competency is the ability to carry out tasks within certain expected standards or parameters. By using a three-stage approach of students observing preceptors, preceptors observing students, and students practicing independently, students become competent.[3] A model, entitled DR FIRM (demonstrations, rehearsal, feedback, independent practice, review, and motivation[4]) describes one approach that may be used to teach students the skills that they need. Each of these components is important in developing and refining professional skills. For example, through *demonstrations,* students observe preceptors as they practice. They learn the rationale for various steps and the assumptions behind what the preceptor is doing. *Rehearsal,* via role playing, simulations, scenarios, or video tapes, allows the student to practice the skills and provides the opportunity for the preceptor to observe the student. The preceptor then provides open and constructive *feedback* on the student's performance, with specific suggestions on what to do next or do differently the next time. The next step is *independent practice,* in which the student practices on his or her own and completes tasks in a specific amount of time. The student then reports back to the preceptor, and the preceptor *reviews* the student's work. The student may need more rehearsal and feedback or be judged competent. Positive encouragement and praise for a job well done will help provide *motivation* to continue to improve.

SUPERVISED PRACTICE PROGRAMS

Supervised practice programs are based on the standards of education (SOE) of the ADA and the competencies for entry-level practice as a dietitian and the competencies for entry-level practice as a dietetic technician.[5] Each supervised practice program is required to provide the core competencies plus at least one area of emphasis. The competency statements are shown in Appendix D. All supervised practice programs are provided through an accredited/approved dietetics education program and must provide 450 hours or 900 hours of experiences for DTR and RD programs, respectively. A current listing of supervised practice programs is available in the *Directory of Dietetics Programs. 1997–1998* from the ADA.[6] The directory provides information on the length of program, number of students per class, estimated tuition, availability of financial aid and stipends, and the date for the next accreditation/approval. More detailed information on supervised practice programs can be obtained in the *Applicant Guide to Supervised Practice Experience. 1997–1998.*[7]

The Council on Education (COE) of the ADA carried out the functions of accreditation/approval of dietetics education programs from 1987 to 1994. The 1987 performance requirements were based on the role delineation studies completed in 1984 by the COE of the ADA.[8] These studies identified the knowledge and skills necessary for competent dietetics practice.

In 1994, the commission on accreditation/approval for dietetics education (CAADE) was established to create an independent administrative body of the association responsible for accreditation/approval. CAADE is recognized as the official accrediting body of the ADA by the US Department of Education.

Although all supervised practice programs use the same standards, there is a great deal of flexibility in how programs meet these standards. Although CAADE approves/accredits programs, it does not mandate a list of experiences or amount of time in different areas of supervised practice. Each program sets the curriculum and experiences that meet the goals of the program and needs of the students. All programs must demonstrate how they meet the SOE and the performance requirements. All programs provide experiences in clinical nutrition, food service systems management, and community dietetics. Some programs may provide staff relief, in which students function independently in one or more settings. Other programs may have an "enrichment rotation" in which students design their own culminating experiences.

Early Programs

Supervised or preprofessional practice experiences have been a part of the professional training of dietitians since the early days of the profession. The first standards approved by the ADA for a "student dietitian" in 1927 included at least a six months' training period under the supervision of a dietitian in a hospital. In 1928, a list of hospitals with approved courses was published, and by 1929 the association announced that each hospital would be visited by a three-member team to ensure the quality of the program. Thus, the dietetic internships began and were the only route to membership for dietitians until 1962.[5]

Over time, several different routes leading toward eligibility to take the registration examination for dietitians were approved by ADA. All individualized experiential pathways, such as traineeships, were discontinued in 1988. Since 1988, the supervised practice component of training of dietitians and dietetic technicians can only be obtained from accredited or approved programs. The following discussion presents the definition of all approved/accredited programs with supervised practice components.

Dietetic Internship—Accredited

The academic requirements for entry into a dietetic internship (DI) were first published in 1947 and are revised periodically to continually update the academic and practice components of the training of dietitians. Currently, there are 201 accredited DIs throughout the United States. As an accredited program, a DI is required to have a site visit from CAADE. Students in DI programs are eligible for federal loans and deferment of loans, such as guaranteed student loans. The definition of a DI is

- supervised practice program sponsored by a health care facility, college or university, federal or state agency, business, or corporation
- provision of a minimum of 900 hours of supervised practice experiences to meet the competencies for the supervised practice component of entry-level dietitian programs
- follows completion of ADA-approved didactic program in dietetics (DPD) and a baccalaureate degree[5]

Preprofessional Practice Program—Approved

In 1988, approved preprofessional practice programs (AP4) became an alternative to DIs with the implementation of the SOE. There are currently 54 AP4s throughout the United States. The only difference between these two types of programs is that an AP4 is approved and a DI is accredited. The definition for an AP4 is the same as for a DI. Both AP4s and DIs must be based on the SOE, provide for a minimum of 900 hours of supervised practice designed to meet the performance requirements for entry-level dietitians, and follow the completion of the knowledge requirements and a baccalaureate program. As an approved program, a site visit by CAADE is not required, and students may or may not be eligible for student loans or loan deferments. Students are advised to discuss financial aid options with the program director of AP4s and DIs before applying to the programs.

Data about the number of programs, students, and graduates are shown in Table 3–1.

Coordinated Programs—Accredited

Coordinated programs in dietetics (CP) began in 1962. CPs integrate the classroom learning and supervised practice components in one curriculum. Originally, CPs were undergraduate programs. Now, CPs can be either undergraduate or graduate level programs, although they are predominantly undergraduate. Currently, there are 49 accredited CPs. (See Chapter 2 for further data about programs and enrollments.) The current definition of a CP is

- academic program in a regionally accredited college or university culminating in a minimum of a baccalaureate degree
- provision of didactic instruction and a minimum of 900 hours of supervised practice experiences to meet the foundation knowledge and skills for the diatetic component of entry-level dietitian education programs and the competencies for the supervised practice component of entry-level dietitian programs (Appendices C and D)
- supervised practice experiences planned concurrently with or following the didactic component[5]

Table 3–1 Practice Program Data

Program Type	Number of Programs			Number Enrolled		Number Graduates	
	1995	1996	1997	1995	1996	1995	1996
Diet. Internship	163	190*	201	1,557	1,795*	1,326	1,546*
AP4	83	64	54	688	604	511	504

*Increase in dietetic internships and decrease in AP4s reflect accreditation and reclassification of AP4s and internships.

Source: Reprinted with permission from *CAADE Newsletter,* © 1997, The American Dietetic Association.

Dietetic Technician Programs—Accredited/Approved

In the early 1970s, the ADA membership identified a need for support personnel at the associate degree level trained in food service management and nutrition care. In 1974, the COE published the guidelines for dietetic technician programs that would lead to eligibility to take the registration examination for DTR.[5] Dietetic technician programs (DT) are defined as

- academic programs in a regionally accredited college or university culminating in an associate degree
- provision of didactic instruction and a minimum of 450 hours of supervised practice to meet the foundation knowledge and skills for didactic component of entry-level dietetic technician education programs and the competencies for the supervised practice component of entry-level dietetic technician programs (Appendices C and D).

RECENT CHANGES TO SUPERVISED PRACTICE PROGRAMS

The dietetics education task force, established in 1992 by the ADA and commission on dietetic registration (CDR), responded to a variety of diverse issues and concerns about the multiple pathways to registration eligibility and quality and availability of dietetics education programs. As a result of the task force report, several changes in supervised practice programs are currently under way.[9] The major change is that all dietetics education programs with a supervised practice component will fall under the accreditation process. Currently, CAADE has a plan to accredit DIs and AP4s, and all currently approved programs are expected to be accredited by 2004. As AP4s are phased into the accreditation process, they will be designated as a DI. Thus, all programs leading to registration eligibility will be accredited. Using one process will simplify the recruitment of students into programs and provide for a mechanism for quality assurance of all programs.

Common Questions about Supervised Practice Programs

Being a successful applicant to a supervised practice program begins long before the actual process of filling out the application forms. Two surveys identified the importance of different selection criteria for admission used by DI program directors[10] and by AP4 program directors.[11] The selection criteria rated highly by DI program directors included academically strong students, with good references and either paid or volunteer dietetics-related work experience. Similar results were found for AP4 programs; however, the AP4 program directors also identified scores on the Graduate Record Examination as an important selection criteria. Many of the supervised practice programs are affiliated with university programs and carry graduate credit.

To obtain additional information on successful candidates, the COE conducted a survey of 1,129 graduates of dietetics programs who received a supervised practice program appointment in 1993.[12] The survey provided answers to some commonly asked questions related to supervised practice programs, such as the following:

- *What did students want to know before applying to supervised practice?* The survey respondents indicated that students should know that a supervised practice program is required to establish eligibility for the RD examination and that acceptance into a program is competitive. Also, students need to know that good grades, relevant work experience, and volunteer activities are also important.

- *What are characteristics of successful applicants?* Although programs have varying selection criteria, successful applicants had the following characteristics: 79 percent had over 3.0 grade point average (GPA) for all courses; 89 percent had over 3.0 GPA for food, nutrition, and management courses; and 56 percent had over a 3.0 GPA for biologic and physical science courses. Related to work experience, 85 percent had more than one year of paid work experience, 54 percent had dietetics-related volunteer experience, and 53 percent worked with a registered dietitian.

- *What advice did these students have?* In addition to maintaining good grades and getting relevant dietetics work experience, the students recommended that applicants investigate programs early to identify the specific admission criteria, apply to more than one program (successful applicants applied to an average of three programs), and be flexible and willing to relocate.

APPLYING TO SUPERVISED PRACTICE PROGRAMS

Students interested in applying to a DT or CP should contact the program director for specific information on when and how to submit an application. For students interested in applying to supervised practice programs after completion of the requirements of a DPD and a baccalaureate degree, a two-step process is involved. First, information and an application must be requested from the director of the program(s) that the student is interested in. Second, students applying to all DIs and most AP4s must participate in computer matching. For students currently enrolled in a dietetics program, information on the computer matching process can be obtained from college or university didactic program directors. If a student is not currently enrolled in a program, they can contact the ADA to obtain information on computer matching.

Students can apply to as many supervised practice programs as they want and also can apply to both DIs and AP4s at the same time. As part of the computer matching process, students must rank all programs applied to in rank preference. Each supervised practice program reviews their own applications and submits a rank order preference list of applicants to the computer matching process, along with the number of available positions to be filled. The computer matching process does not change the applicant's or program's selection process. Students will not be "matched" to a program not on their ranked list. If a program does not rank an applicant, the program is removed from the applicant's list. The student is notified regarding her or his status. If a student is matched to a program, the student then must notify the program of acceptance or rejection of the appointment.[13]

Once a student has successfully completed the supervised practice program, the program director issues a *verification of completion* form. This form, with an original signature of the program director, is a legal document and must be presented along with other required material to establish eligibility to take the registration examination.

CONCLUSION

Supervised practice is the culminating experience in the process of becoming an RD or a DTR. It cannot be replaced by classroom learning. The supervised practice experience prepares students for current and future practice. The ADA and the CAADE continually review trends in the profession and identify the impact on dietetic education programs. Education must provide students with the traditional skills they need today but must also incorporate skills needed to succeed in tomorrow's nontraditional careers. In this way, students will be prepared not only for the challenges of today's practice as RDs and DTRs but for future practice as well.

DEFINITIONS

Academic Training The totality of didactic and experiential learning.

Experiential Learning Practice-related knowledge and skill primarily acquired through supervised experience in real-life situations; may be augmented by role playing, simulations, etc.

Preceptor Person that guides, mentors, and evaluates a student during the supervised practice experience.

Preprofessional Practice Experiences in real-life situations prior to an entry-level position.

Program Director Individual who meets the criteria for program director as stated in the standards of education and who is designated to ensure program account-ability and communication with ADA.

Standards of Practice Statements of dietetic practitioner's responsibility for providing nutrition care.

Supervised Practice Learning experiences associated with activities in selected situations that enable the student to apply knowledge, develop and retain skills, and develop professionally.

REFERENCES

1. Moore KK. Criteria for acceptance to preprofessional dietetics programs vs. desired qualities of professionals: an analysis. *J Am Diet Assoc.* 1995;95:77–81.

2. Rengers BD, Gary J, Kimbel K, Schvaneveldt N. *Developing Clinical Preceptors.* Workshop background paper. Chicago: Council on Education, The American Dietetic Association; 1994.

3. Gates GE, Cutts M. Characteristics of effective preceptors: a review of allied health literature. *J Am Diet Assoc.* 1995;95:225–227.

4. Pitchert JW. Teaching strategies for effective nutrition instruction. In: Powers MA, ed. *Handbook of Diabetes Management.* Rockville, MD: Aspen Publishers;1987:465–479.

5. Commission on Accreditation/Approval for Dietetics Education. *Accreditation/Approval Manual for Dietetics Education Programs.* 4th ed. Chicago: The American Dietetic Association; 1997.

6. ADA. *Directory of Dietetics Programs. 1997–1998.* Chicago: The American Dietetic Association; 1997.

7. Dietetic Educators of Practitioners. *Applicant Guide to Supervised Practice Experience. 1997–1998.* Chicago: The American Dietetic Association; 1997.

8. Smitherman AL, Anderson CR. President's page: standards of education—ADA's foundation for the future. *J Am Diet Assoc.* 1987;87:1221–1222.

9. ADA. *Report of the Task Force on Dietetic Education.* Chicago: The American Dietetic Association; 1993.

10. Carruth BR, Sneed J. Selection criteria for dietetic internship admission: what do internship directors consider most important? *J Am Diet Assoc.* 1990;90:999–1001.

11. Sneed J, Carruth BR. Selection criteria for approved preprofessional practice programs: are they different from those for dietetic internships? *J Am Diet Assoc.* 1991;91:950–953.

12. Thinking of becoming a registered dietitian? *Affiliate News ADA Members.* 1994;6(2):2.

13. Supervised practice (DI/AP4) appointments and computer matching fact sheet. *Affiliate News ADA Members.* 1993;5(2):1–3.

CHAPTER 4

Graduate and Continuing Education

Lea L. Ebro

"Nothing is ever completed, least of all, education." Victor A. Rice[1]

Outline—Chapter 4

Part 1— Continuing Education

- Introduction

- Assessment Surveys

- Meeting Continuing Education Needs

- Delivery Methods

- Continued Certification

- The Future

Part 2—Graduate Education

- Defining Graduate Education
  - Types of programs
- Benefits of Graduate Study

- The Graduate Experience
  - Plan of study
  - Special opportunities

- Research experience
- Innovative Graduate Programs

• Research in Dietetics

• Conclusion

Part 1—CONTINUING EDUCATION

INTRODUCTION

The term *continuing education* (CE), used interchangeably with *continuing professional education* (CPE), implies learning that advances from a previously established level of accomplishment to extend and amplify knowledge, sensitivity, or skill.[2] The ultimate goal of CPE is the improvement of the ongoing performance of the practitioner.[3] Although not specifically required by many professions until the 1960s,[4] CPE has been a priority of The American Dietetic Association (ADA) since the 1950s and was mandated when professional registration was established in 1969.[5-8] To maintain registration status, the Commission on Dietetic Registration (CDR) mandated that registered dietitians (RD) must participate in a minimum of 75 clock hours of approved CPE each five years. Most dietitians meet this eligibility requirement in CE, as evidenced by the fact that most dietitians are registered. In addition, many states now license dietitians and some require CPE for yearly renewal of the license.

Many professions recognize that basic academic education is inadequate for lifelong professional practice. The necessity of lifelong learning through CE has steadily increased as knowledge and practice skills have expanded. CE for various professions is one of the fastest growing as well as profitable areas in the learning industry.[9] It reflects the mandatory requirements for licensure, the pressure from employers in the competitive world, and the growing interest in specialization, in dietetics as in other professions. A high proportion of career professionals will pursue graduate education, and demographics indicate that two-thirds of the people who will be working in the year 2000 are already in the work force. For this reason, educators must consider tailoring programs to meet the needs of professionals who desire programs or materials for self-study that are offered at the individual's convenience and by varied formats. Many universities are providing programs of study specifically for the working adult and are using innovative means of providing the education.

Students graduating from universities today are often surprised to discover that within a decade, 90 percent of what they initially learned has become obsolete.[3] Entry-level dietitians must keep pace with new developments, monitor change as it occurs, know how to predict or forecast change, and make plans to manage what the future brings.[10,11] CPE is acknowledged as critical to ensure the competence of health care professionals[12] and indeed, for this reason, was made mandatory for registered dietitians (75 clock hours each five years) and for registered dietetic technicians (DTR) (50 clock hours each five years) in 1988.[8]

ASSESSMENT SURVEYS

Several assessment surveys were conducted during the 1970s to the 1990s to explore the CE needs and concerns of dietitians. Vanderveen and Hubbard[13] found that Ohio dietitians needed updates in managerial sciences, nutritional care sciences, and technical and human relations skills. Burkholder and Eisele[14] reported that dietitians in the upper Midwest region expressed moderate-to-high needs for all topics in managerial science, specifically in managerial effectiveness and performance appraisals. In nutritional care, topics of interest were drug–nutrient interactions and progress in heart disease research.

RDs in the Chicago area accepted responsibilities for CPE but did not necessarily seek learning activities for credentialing purposes.[15] Partlow et al.[16] concluded in a study that "dietitians are less satisfied with continuing education that requires independent study or self-planning." Pennsylvania dietitians' CE needs were in clinical procedures, professional development, and managerial skills.[17]

Studies in Ohio and Oklahoma[18,19] found that CE topics of interest varied from quality assessment and nutrition care, organization and management, to computers and cost control measures. In almost all these studies, the preferred format for CE was local and district dietetic association meetings and one-day workshops for small groups.

A national study was conducted by the ADA in 1990 to determine the CPE needs of RDs and DTRs. Dietitians surveyed indicated that they needed updates in cardiovascular disease, diabetes, nutritional assessment, obesity and weight control, grantsmanship, and computer applications. Preferred formats for delivery were workshops and lectures, whereas the least preferred formats were computer-assisted instruction and use of audiotapes.[20] Similarly, diabetes educators preferred meetings, symposia, and workshops.[21]

Bobeng[22] reported in 1986 that dietetic technicians, before registration, were highly in favor of credentialing and its concomitant CPE requirements. Topics most often mentioned for CPE activities were clinical nutrition updates, community nutrition, food service management techniques, and food service systems. Technicians also preferred meetings and workshops, journal clubs, and self-study with videocassettes. The 1990 study of DTRs indicated that DTRs were becoming more skilled and that CPE needs were in grantsmanship, conducting research, computer applications, and media skills. Advanced-level CPE needs were in obesity and weight control, food service equipment and production, nutritional assessment, and diabetes.[20] Almost half the respondents preferred not to use study groups, journal clubs, and computer-assisted instruction.

A 1989 study of DTRs in the Chicago area indicated that their CPE needs were in laboratory tests and nutritional implications, geriatric nutrition, weight reduction and diets, and nutrition assessment and screening.[23] DTRs in the study of Miller, et al. in 1996[24] indicated that workshops and lecture were preferred over other delivery formats for CE activities. Eighty percent of the 194 respondents' choice of CPE topics were diabetes, nutritional assessment and screening, cardiovascular diseases, and cancer. About two-thirds also expressed a need for education methods and behavioral modification techniques. Choices of CPE topics were highly influenced by area of work and employment facility, as in previous studies.

CE needs of school-level managers in child nutrition programs included study of state and federal regulations, laws affecting personnel, health and safety laws, inspections, and reinforcement. Others were work simplification, employee motivation, transmitting child nutrition mission and values, professionalism, time management, teamwork, and employee relations.[25]

MEETING CONTINUING EDUCATION NEEDS

How well are CPE needs being met for dietitians and dietetic technicians in the 1990s and beyond? The ADA, state and district associations, and dietetic practice groups offer a great variety of CPE actitivies. The CDR approves a wide range of educational activities for CPE credit, including

1. Self-assessment modules. Hypothetical practice scenarios are provided in dietetic practice by which members may determine their performance in responding to questions about the materials. Modules are available from CDR in management, research, nutrition education, nutrition care plans and nutrition counseling, and clinical dietetics.
2. Self-study programs. These include audiocassettes, study kits, and study guides. CPE credit is given after successful completion of the study program.
3. Video and audio tapes of prior-approved education sessions. Audio tapes of sessions presented at the annual ADA meeting are available each year during and after the meeting.
4. Exhibits at trade and educational shows. A limited number of credit hours are given for viewing exhibits on the basis that they provide new information on products and services.
5. Research presentations of original research at national and state meetings. Persons presenting the research as well as those attending the display or verbal sessions may receive credit.

6. Presentations to professional audiences. Professional presentations involve time and expertise, and RDs who make such presentations are given CPE for this activity.
7. Demonstrations related to nutrition and dietetics such as grocery store tours, meal preparation techniques, and use of special diet foods are examples of approved activities.
8. Academic course work. CPE credit of 15 clock hours per semester credit is given for completion of a college course. For the completion of an advanced degree, 50 credits are given. In addition, 12 CPE hours are awarded for thesis research and 25 CPE hours for dissertation research.
9. Writing for publication. Articles, books, monographs, or similar written materials published in professional journals or by publishing companies may be presented for credit.
10. Study groups and journal clubs. Popular among busy practitioners, RDs participating in in-depth studies and reports from professional publications may receive credit for the study time.
11. Conferences and professional meetings. The hours that have been preapproved by CDR as offering important CE may be used for credit.
12. Seminars and workshops. ADA offers CE workshops each year at the annual meeting and throughout the country. Many of the dietetic practice groups also offer workshops and conferences. These provide in-depth information plus hands-on experiences and are an important means of ensuring that dietitians and dietetic technicians are kept abreast of new developments.

Credit for seminars and workshops offered by educational institutions or by other professional groups may also be used if preapproved by CDR.

DELIVERY METHODS

In planning CE, educators need to be aware of the types of delivery formats available to offer the material most effectively. As discussed earlier, some professionals continue to prefer an interactive format with small group discussions and group presentations.[26] Preferences are often based on relevance and timeliness, cost, accessibility, and practicality.[27] But with the need for more workplace programs and programs offered by different timelines, innovative programming such as distance education can address many of these criteria. Further, several studies support the effectiveness of distance education when the teaching is carefully planned, uses visuals and graphics, is highly interactive, and when the teacher has a good understanding of the equipment and its use. It is shown to be as effective as traditional methods under these circumstances.[28–32]

Distance education has been defined as education that takes place when a teacher and student are separated by physical distance and when communication technologies are used.[33,34] The types of media used vary from correspondence courses using printed materials to fully interactive video, audio, and integrated delivery means.

Distance education represents a fast-growing segment of education. Dietetic educators, in and beyond the classroom, are being increasingly challenged to use technologies such as computers for electronic mail and the Internet, the telephone, and television for teleconferences. Other interactive methods may use videotapes, voice mail, and fax machines. Whatever the medium of delivery, rapid feedback is critical in motivating learners, as is the provision of course materials ahead of sessions.

A summary of various delivery system technologies and their characteristics is shown in Exhibit 4–1.[28]

Distance education is not new to dietetic professionals. In the 1970s, CE via telelectures, satellite television broadcasts, and one-way–two-way video were pioneered by ADA.[35] Many dietetic education programs currently use some form of interactive video by distance. In a 1995–96 study by the council on education and the ADA education and accrediting staff, they found that 37 educational program directors indicated that distance education was available in their program. The four common delivery formats were correspondence course, audioconferencing, video teleconferencing, and televised classes.[28]

The use of information and communication technologies is being increasingly used in adult education and CE by universities. Some universities are developing statewide consortia that will allow several universities to share resources. Networks are also being developed to link US universities with their international campuses overseas and with universities internationally. Many challenges and opportunities are available to dietetic professionals who can design and deliver distance programs nationally and internationally. They may well be the entrepreneurs of the future.

CONTINUED CERTIFICATION

The CDR is developing a new process that will involve the RD in designing a plan for professional development best suited to his or her own needs. Six steps will be involved in the process: (1) self-assessment based on the individual's professional needs, (2) development of a learning plan based on the needs, (3) submission of the learning plan to CDR for verification, (4) implementation of the plan through participation in professional development, (5) evaluation of the plan outcomes and application to practice, and (6) submission of the portfolio to CDR for verification. A final plan was submitted by CDR at the ADA annual meeting in 1997 and, after acceptance and pilot testing, will be implemented in 2001.[36]

Exhibit 4–1 Characteristics of Available Delivery System Technologies (key: ITFS = instructional television fixed services; DBS = direct broadcast satellite)

Broadcast television
- Any television set can receive the signal
- Programming times are limited; public television audience
- Programming is costly and time is needed to develop
- Communication is one way (usually no access to instructor)

Cable television
- Designed for educational access; thus, more programming time is available
- Audience is smaller; i.e., students must be subscribers
- Programming may be less costly to develop
- Existing cable companies do not serve all geographic areas

Narrowcast television (e.g., ITFS, microwave)
- Features live real-time instruction, interactive medium
- Programming times and locations are fixed
- Design can be directional or omnidirectional
- Reach can extend for a 25-mile radius
- Reception equipment and technical support are needed

Videocassette
- Students can determine viewing location and pace of learning
- Students need learning skills and independence
- Usually there is no access to the instructor at viewing time

Radio/broadcast (e.g., audiocassettes, subcarrier service)
- Features easy to access, convenient, flexible format
- Specialized audiences may be served

Telephone (e.g., wired networks or dial-up services)
- Is inexpensive, easy to access, interactive, and flexible
- Audiographics can add visual support

Computer conferencing, bulletin boards, electronic campus
- Communications are asynchronous; the reach is worldwide
- Medium is compatible with available equipment/software

Interactive videodisc
- Learning stations are portable, e.g., school, worksite
- Flexible: students determine time/pace of learning
- Individualized instruction, multiple applications are possible
- Computer tools for instructional management

Satellite technology (e.g., C-Band, Ku-Band, DBS)
- Can be designed for point to multi-point transmission
- C-Band and Ku-Band use 10 to 12 foot dish/more powerful satellites allow smaller dish size
- Interference can occur from microwave or weather

continues

Exhibit 4–1 continued

Fiber optics
- Interactive medium has two-way full-motion video/audio
- Signal transmission is reliable and of superior quality
- Channels are leased on dedicated basis/equipment standards affect system capability

Digital compression/multimedia communications
- Digital video may be merged with other media
- Capable of desktop video conferencing, video production
- Technology is newer and may require new equipment, software, and applications
- Equipment standards affect system compatibility

Virtual reality
- Learning is experiential, interactive, computer-generated
- 3-D environments and simulations are featured

Source: A.A. Spangler, B. Spear, and P.A. Plavcan, Dietetics Education by Distance: Current Endeavors in CAADE–Accredited/Approval Programs. Copyright The American Dietetic Association. Reprinted by permission from *Journal of The American Dietetic Association*, Vol. 95, pp. 925–929, © 1995.

Professional development includes the attainment of formal education and, for most RDs and DTRs, CE activities. The proposal expands the kinds of professional education activities that may be used and increases the flexibility of options each person has to meet his or her personal objectives. CE will continue to be a cornerstone of dietetics practice, and dietitians will have the opportunity to design the kind of CPE of most benefit to them under the new plan.

THE FUTURE

Dietitians must keep abreast of ever-increasing knowledge and new technologies while maintaining a perspective that meets present needs as well as anticipates the acquisition of newer ones for future multiple roles. To broaden one's practice, new skills throughout a career are needed.[37] Role expansion will be a reality for many, and multiskilling and cross-training are being discussed as ways of preparing dietitians for new roles and for mobility.[11,37–39] Depending on the career area, dietitians may also be expected to be proficient in areas such as the use of low literacy skills, in partnering and mentoring others, in effective public education, and in dietetic practice in a health care environment that is changing. For most, the attainment of new knowledge and skills will come through CE.

Part 2—GRADUATE EDUCATION

Current trends indicate that in the new millennium, there will be increased demands for food and nutrition services throughout both the private and public sectors. Unparalleled opportunities for dietitians to expand dietetics creatively in new situations may not only require CPE but graduate education as well.[40,41]

Interest in graduate education increased during the 1990s. More baccalaureate students are pursuing graduate degrees, more employers are requiring advanced degrees or training for employees, and more disciplines are becoming specialized, requiring advanced study in the discipline.[11,42]

DEFINING GRADUATE EDUCATION

Graduate education is formal study beyond a baccalaureate degree that leads to an advanced degree. Graduate study involves specialized knowledge and concentrated study in a specific area. One of the most important purposes of graduate education is to provide opportunities for individuals to explore new ideas and gain the higher level of knowledge and understanding required to recognize and discharge personal, social, and professional responsibilities to the fullest extent possible.[1,43] There are other practical benefits such as advancement in a career, a career change, and financial advantages.

Types of Programs

The Master of Science (MS) degree usually requires one to two years of full-time study and may be longer depending on the major area of study, the type of research for the degree, and whether the student is employed while working toward the degree. In some universities, the MS will be offered with the option of a thesis or nonthesis. The thesis is based on an original research study. In the nonthesis option, either additional course work or a creative project may be required instead.

The Doctor of Philosophy (PhD) degree requires at least three to five years of full-time study. The PhD or the EdD (Doctor of Education) may be offered. Original research is required for either degree, the type depending on the field of study. The doctoral degree is considered the "terminal degree" and is also the primary credential for college teaching or research.

In some professions, a professional degree may be awarded at either the master's or doctoral level. This degree will generally have a title descriptive of the profession (i.e., MD for medical practice, JD for law, DDS for dental practice, and MBA for business administration).

Dietitians who obtain advanced degrees usually have the MS and/or the PhD, as both are science based.

BENEFITS OF GRADUATE STUDY

Although a graduate degree is not required to take the registration examination in dietetics, there are valid reasons why dietitians pursue advanced study. In the 1995 membership database of the ADA, it was reported that 51 percent of RDs have received or are working toward the master's or doctoral degree. Among DTRs, 30 percent have received or are working toward the BS degree and slightly more than 4 percent are working toward a graduate degree.[40]

What are the benefits? There are personal benefits such as the development of intellectual skills including the ability to master complex information, to problem-solve, and to explore new ideas. There are career benefits such as the development of advanced practice skills, the in-depth exploration of subjects in one's area of practice, and the acquisition of new perspectives.[44]

Career advancement and preparation for a career change are often reasons dietitians pursue graduate study. Dietitians who are prepared to perform in multiskilled or cross-trained positions will usually rely on graduate education to increase both knowledge and practice skills.[45] The types of positions dietitians assume as they progress up the career ladder are usually those with increasing responsibility and autonomy, and they require managerial and leadership skills. In addition, competition for jobs may increase the demand for an advanced degree. New and expanding career options, and the job market in general, affect demand and availability of persons prepared to enter the new job markets and, in turn, influence dietitians in their education choices. Graduate education provides an opportunity for students to develop expertise that will allow them to assume leadership roles throughout dietetics practice and beyond.

With career advancement, higher pay is often a benefit. The 1995 ADA membership database revealed that the highest salaries are earned by those working in food and nutrition management ($42,964), consultation and business ($43,374), and in education and research ($42,784).[41] Salaries of $50,000 or more are reported by those with the most experience in the three areas cited. These three areas of practice are the ones most often requiring advanced degrees. The financial advantage of an advanced degree, regardless of career choice, is demonstrated in Figure 4–1, in which monthly earnings are shown to progress the higher the degree.

Another reason for the RD to pursue graduate study is for CE credit to maintain the credential. As noted earlier, CPE credit may be obtained for graduate level

Thousands

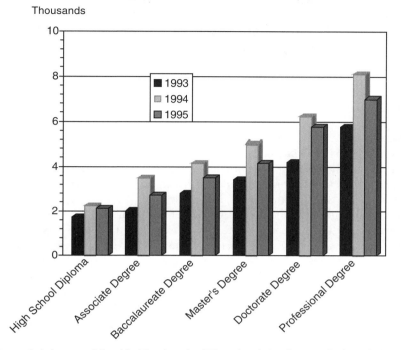

Figure 4–1 Average Monthly Earnings by Educational Attainment Spring 1993, 1994, and 1995. *Source:* Reprinted from US Bureau of the Census, unpublished data.

academic work and research. ADA has established board certification for specialists in metabolic support, pediatric nutrition, and renal nutrition. The certified dietitian (CD) in one of these areas meets eligibility requirements of the CDR, including a specialized examination. Although a graduate degree is not a specific requirement for a CD, the person who is a specialist often holds an advanced degree. A further credential as fellow of the ADA (FADA) may also be awarded when a dietitian meets qualifying criteria including the MS or PhD degree.

Active membership in ADA is now available to persons with an advanced degree who have met the academic requirements or who holds one degree in a specified area (dietetics, food and nutrition, nutrition, community/public health nutrition, food science, food service systems management).[46] This pathway to active membership does not qualify a person for RD status; however, for persons in allied professional areas, affiliation with ADA may be of professional benefit.

A further benefit of graduate study is in gaining research skills and knowledge of research methodology. All dietitians must apply research findings in the practice of dietetics. The foundation knowledge and skill requirements state that graduates will have demonstrated the ability to interpret current research and basic statistics. The basics of research are included in the undergraduate dietetics curriculum; however, designing research and participating in research usually occur at the graduate level.

THE GRADUATE EXPERIENCE

Information about graduate programs, their location, areas of emphasis, and contact person is available in the ADA *Directory of Programs* as well as via the Internet.[46] Many other universities also offer graduate degrees and may be contacted. Prospective students will find it helpful to talk with faculty and to request college catalogs and departmental information before applying. No two programs are alike, and the best fit between the student and a program will be important once the student is admitted to the program. Universities that give students an active role in departmental activities and who give individual time and attention in a mentoring and supportive atmosphere will greatly enhance the graduate experience.[47,48] The faculty, the departmental research, and the availability of financial aid through graduate assistantships or from other sources should all be explored. Assistantships not only provide financial help but give the student teaching, research, and administrative experience according to the assignment.

Plan of Study

A graduate course of study will include some core courses, but most courses will, in most cases, be individually planned according to the student's interests and goals. The plan of study will be developed with an advisor who is usually the thesis advisor. The major is usually in a specific academic area such as nutrition, community nutrition, food service management, or food science. The research is planned and conducted with guidance from an advisor and graduate faculty committee.

Special Opportunities

Dietitians, as members of a predominantly female profession, may have access to assistance because many universities have incentive programs for women. The opportunities for acceptance into programs and successful completion of graduate degrees by women is also shown in that the number of women obtaining advanced degrees has been increasing. Four in 10 of all doctoral degrees awarded in 1995 were earned by women, an increase from 34 percent in 1985. Women earned more than one-third of all doctorates in the sciences in 1995 and slightly more than half of doctorates awarded in other fields (health, education, and the humanities).[49]

Attracting minority students into graduate study is also a priority in many colleges and universities. Minority students (Asian-American, African-American, Hispanic, and Native American) account for only 17 percent of the doctoral degrees awarded in the social sciences. Because colleges would like to increase this number, incentives may be available for these students.[50]

Research Experience

The selection of a research study by the student and advisor is based on the area of interest, the need as determined by literature search, and the feasibility (cost, time involvement, availability of equipment and/or subjects) and is a mutual selection process at most universities. Ongoing departmental faculty research may provide a way for the student to assume a part of the research for his or her thesis.

The process of defending a problem, reviewing the literature to support the need for the study, planning and implementing the project, collecting and analyzing data, and writing a clear and well-developed document that is accepted by a graduate faculty committee is a significant effort. It is one that serves all graduates who have had this experience at the master's or doctoral level very well regardless of the position that the individual wishes to pursue. The research experience involves initiative, resourcefulness, creativity, written and verbal communication, skills, critical thinking, problem solving, and ethics. These are aspects of professional function that are vital to success in life, as well as a career. Research is not appropriate for all but greatly enhances the expertise of those who pursue and complete a successful research project.

The successful completion of a research study often launches a student into publishing the results and into further research, thus making an important contribution to scholarship as well.

Overall, the graduate experience is one that is individualized and flexible, that allows the student to become more specialized, and that leads to career advancement and personal growth.[51]

INNOVATIVE GRADUATE PROGRAMS

One of the first graduate programs providing a practicum with graduate course work was the program offered at the Massachusetts General Hospital Institute of Health Professions.[52] A specialty in management combined with course work in clinical dietetics allowed students to enhance their clinical knowledge and expertise while also developing management skills through applied practice in real-world settings.

At the University of Arkansas for Medical Sciences, the department of nutrition and dietetics in the College of Health Related Professions offers a graduate program leading to a master's degree in clinical nutrition for RDs. The program targets those dietetians who wish to update their skills and knowledge in clinical nutrition and who wish to specialize through graduate education. Three areas of specialization are available: pediatrics, geriatrics, and health and wellness promotion. A research project and thesis in the area of specialization is required. Clinical practices are available in a variety of settings and are encouraged.

A practice doctorate in clinical dietetics has been proposed by Christie and Kight.[53] The program would be a professional degree aligned academically with the MD degree and provide indepth experiences in clinical practice. Advanced practice, as in a residency, was proposed as a part of the degree.

Practicum or residency requirements, as in the programs just described, can increase the versatility and employability of graduates. Settings for such experiences may be in business and industry, health care institutions, community organizations, government, and communications companies. Competence in practice can only increase as the student is exposed to new environments and indepth experiences that serve to enhance the total educational experience.

Another innovative graduate program is offered by the department of nutrition and food management at Oregon State University.[54] This is a Master of Science degree with a concentration in dietetic management. Distance learning technologies are utilized in the program, which provides students with the potential to combine technical expertise with management skills.

RESEARCH IN DIETETICS

Research is important to the dietetic professional both in undertaking and interpreting research findings and in using research methods to improve practice. Dietetic leaders have affirmed and strongly supported the need for research in the profession.[55–58] Chernoff[59(p. 1049)] emphasized the need as follows: "Research strengthens the credibility of the dietetic profession; it makes it on par with other health professions that base practice advances on the discovery of new knowledge. Advances in the science of all aspects of food and nutrition should be made by dietitians."

The intregration of education, practice, and research was an objective in establishing the Council on Research in ADA. When the Council was formed in the 1980s, broad research focus areas were initially identified. They reflected concerns and priorities of members of the Association at the time and included research into cost-benefit data, a research base for provision of food and nutrition services, research to support the dietetic practitioner, and identification of management processes to better deliver food and nutrition services. These priorities were further evaluated and expanded in a 1992 national consensus conference at which papers were prepared in advance and discussed. This led to mutual agreement for research priorities in 12 major areas of practice. Though not inclusive of all practice areas in dietetics, the research agenda for action that resulted from the conference was a significant step in moving forward in research as well as providing a model for continuing review and priority setting among research needs in the profession.

At a 1994 conference "Challenging the Future of Dietetic Education and Credentialing," Dwyer[60] skillfully outlined reasons why dietitians need to be involved in research. She also pointed out both the opportunities and barriers to broader involvement in research. Three imperatives for dietitians being involved in research were (1) to ensure that new developments improving human food and nutritional health are incorporated into dietetic practice, (2) dietitians need to be leaders as well as followers in research, and (3) research competence to develop new knowledge must be included in dietetic practice because dietetics is a field that focuses on speedily applying the best of food and nutrition knowledge to solve human needs. What better rationale could be given?

CONCLUSION

More than half of practicing dietitians today hold or are working toward a graduate degree. There are benefits in doing so, among them the attainment of research competence, CE for personal and professional growth, and career enhancement. If the trend continues, ever larger numbers of dietitians will seek an advanced degree in the next millennium and will thereby bring expertise to bear on practical problems. The outcome will be a healthy and informed public and heightened recognition of the dietitian as the expert in food and nutrition.

DEFINITIONS

Assistantship Paid position in which graduate students may be appointed to perform academic functions such as teaching, research, and administration.

Communications Technology Electronic and automatic working channels that lead to interaction between the source and the receiver.

Cross-Training Process of learning how to perform in two or more occupations.

Dissertation Paper reporting original research required for the doctoral degree.

Distance Education Learning that takes place in a location other than the classroom and that is usually conducted using communications technology.

Multiskilling Process of becoming proficient in more than one procedure or skill.
Self-Assessment Self-examination of a person's status or needs.
Thesis Paper reporting original research required for the master's degree.

REFERENCES

1. Campbell JR. *Reclaiming a Lost Heritage, Land-Grant and Other Higher Education Initiatives for the Twenty-First Century.* Ames: Iowa State University Press; 1995.
2. Houle CO. *Continuing Learning in the Professions.* San Francisco: Jossey-Bass Publishers; 1980.
3. Berenbaum S. Futures-oriented continuing professional education. *Top Clin Nutr.* 1995;10:66–70.
4. Scanlan CL. Practicing with purpose: goals of continuing professional education. In: Cervero RM, Scanlan CL, eds. *Problems and Prospects in Continuing Professional Education.* San Francisco: Jossey-Bass Publishers; 1985.
5. Kirk RB. Continuing education. *J Am Diet Assoc.* 1959;35:66–70.
6. Hunscher HA. Continuing education: an antidote to obsolescence. *J Am Diet Assoc.* 1963;43:115–119.
7. Committee on Goals of Education for Dietitians, Dietetic Internship Council. Goals of the lifetime education of the dietitian. *J Am Diet Assoc.* 1969;54:91–93.
8. Commission on Dietetic Registration. *Continuing Professional Education: Guidelines for the Registered Dietitian.* Chicago: The American Dietetic Association; 1991.
9. Miller DA, Rose PB. Communication professionals: a new market for continuing higher education. *J Continuing Higher Educ.* Winter 1995;43:32–43.
10. Casebeer L. Updating the theoretical constructs of change. *J Continuing Educ Health Professions.* 1992;12:105–110.
11. Balch GI. Employers' perception of the roles of dietetics practitioners: challenges to survive and opportunities to thrive. *J Am Diet Assoc.* 1996;96:1301–1305.
12. Mote JR. Continuing education enhancing the quality of patient care. *Hosp J Am Hosp Assoc.* 1976;50:175–180.
13. Vanderveen E, Hubbard RM. Continuing education needs as perceived by dietetic practitioners. *J Am Diet Assoc.* 1979;75:429–433.
14. Burkholder VR, Eisele JE. An assessment of continuing education needs of dietitians. *J Nutr Educ.* 1984;16:132–136.
15. Holli BB. Continuing professional learning: involvement and opinions of dietitians. *J Am Diet Assoc.* 1982;81:53–57.
16. Partlow CG, Spears MC, Oakleif CR. Noneconomic and economic benefits of continuing education for dietitians. *J Am Diet Assoc.* 1989;89:1321–1324.
17. Klevans DR, Parrett JL. Continuing professional education needs of clinical dietitians in Pennsylvania. *J Am Diet Assoc.* 1990;90:282–286.

18. Crenshaw B. *Continuing Education Needs of Registered Dietitians in Oklahoma.* Stillwater: Oklahoma State University; 1984. Unpublished master's thesis.

19. Fisher RR. *Analysis of the Role Functions and Continuing Education Needs of Ohio, as Compared to Oklahoma Consultant Dietitians in Health Care Facilities.* Stillwater: Oklahoma State University; 1984. Unpublished master's thesis.

20. Flynn C, Bryk JA, Neal ML. Perceived continuing education needs of RDs and DTRs. *J Am Diet Assoc.* 1991;91:933–939.

21. Anderson RM, Arnold MS, Donnelly MB, Frennell MM, et al. Continuing education needs of dietitians who are diabetic educators. *J Am Diet Assoc.* 1992;92:607–609.

22. Bobeng BJ. Results of the 1985 dietetic technician needs assessment survey. *J Am Diet Assoc.* 1986;86:672–673.

23. Wisner P, Lucas JA. *Continuing Education Needs Assessment Study of Dietary Technicians.* Vol. 18. Office of Planning and Research. Chicago: William Rainey Harper College, Palatine University; 1989.

24. Miller AK, Sleezer CM, Ebro LL. Dietetic technicians—historical perspectives and modern trends. *J Health Occupations Educ.* 1997;11:1–21.

25. Sneed J, White KT. Continuing education needs of school-level managers in child nutrition programs. *School Food Serv Res Rev.* 1993;17:103–108.

26. Smith DH. Developing a more interactive classroom: a continuing odyssey. *Teaching Sociol.* 1996;24:64–75.

27. Hess AN, Haughton B. Continuing education needs for public health nutritionists. *J Am Diet Assoc.* 1996;96:716–718.

28. Spangler AA, Spear B, Plavcan PA. Dietetics education by distance: current endeavors in CAADE-accredited/approved programs. *J Am Diet Assoc.* 1995;95:925–929.

29. Abusatha R, Kiel ML, Achterberg C. Evaluation of a mixed-model teleconference approach for distance education in nutrition and dietetics. *Top Clin Nutr.* 1997;12:27–37.

30. Cohen NL, Parnell W, Amick TL. Distance teaching as a method of postgraduate continuing education in community nutrition. *Ecology Food and Nutrition.* 1994;33:37–43.

31. Cohen NL, Beffa-Negrini PA, Sternheim MM, et al. The internet as a method of continuing education. *Top Clin Nutr.* 1997;12:21–26.

32. Kipp, D. Developing interactive computerized modules accessible on the World Wide Web for medical students. *Top Clin Nutr.* 1997;12:38–44.

33. Willis BD. *Effective Distance Education: A Primer for Faculty and Administrators.* Fairbanks: University of Alaska; 1992.

34. Moore MG, Kearsley G. *Distance Education: A Systems View.* Belmont, California: Wadsworth Publishing; 1996.

35. O'Connell W, Hubbard RM, McCormick AR, et al. Stardate I. Continuing education via communications satellite; II. Workshops on financial management for nutritional care, III. Workshop on patient nutritional assessment. *J Am Diet Assoc* 1978;73:270–280.

36. CDR: Progress report on Professional development 2001. Draft 3. *ADA Courier.* 1997;36:3.
37. Mataarese LE. Expanded skills: fad or future. *Support Line.* 1996;18:17.
38. Sandoval WM. Multiskilling and dietetics education. *DEP Line.* 1996;14(2):5–9.
39. Dowling R. Role expansion for dietetics professionals. *J Am Diet Assoc.* 1996;96:1001–1002.
40. Bryk JA, Soto TK. Report on the 1995 membership database of The American Dietetic Association. *J Am Diet Assoc.* 1997;97:197–203.
41. Chernoff R. President's page: future shock. *J Am Diet Assoc.* 1997;97:195.
42. Khahil EM. *Organization and Administration of Graduate Education.* Washington, DC: Council on Graduate Schools; 1990.
43. Brooks P. Point of view. Graduate learning as apprenticeship. *Chron Higher Educ.* 1996;XLIII:A52. Abstract.
44. Gaffney NA. *Graduate School and You: A Guide for Prospective Graduate Students.* 4th ed. Washington, DC: Council on Graduate Schools; 1996.
45. Dowling R. Role expansion for dietetics professionals. *J Am Diet Assoc.* 1996; 96:1001–1002.
46. ADA. *Directory of Dietetics Programs.* Chicago: The American Dietetic Association; 1997.
47. Anderson MS. Collaboration, the doctoral experience and the departmental environment. *Rev Higher Educ.* 1996;19:305–326.
48. Austin AE, Baldwin RG. *Faculty Collaboration: Enhancing the Quality of Scholarship and Teaching.* ASHE-ERIC Higher Education Report 7. Washington, DC: George Washington University; 1997.
49. Knopp L. *More Young Adults Combine Education and Employment.* Vol. 3. Higher Education and National Affairs. Washington, DC: American Council on Education; 1996:3.
50. Crawford I, Suarez-Balcazar Y, Figert A, Nyden P. The use of research participation for mentoring prospective minority graduate students. *Teaching Sociol.* 1996;24:256–263.
51. Rhoades PK, Franz M. Market research to recruit graduate students in dietetics. *J Am Diet Assoc.* 1993;93:920–922.
52. Carey M, Manola JB. A strategy for developing a graduate program to prepare managers in dietetics. *J Am Diet Assoc.* 1994;94:722–724.
53. Christie BW, Kight MA. Educational empowerment of the clinical dietitian: a proposed practice doctorate curriculum. *J Am Diet Assoc.* 1993;93:173–176.
54. Messersmith AM. Distance learning at Oregon State University. *FSMEC Newsletter.* 1997;12:4.
55. South ML. The president's page. *J Am Diet Assoc.* 1981;78:267.
56. Parks SC, Schiller MR, Bryk J. President's page: investment in our future—the role of science and scholarship in developing knowledge for dietetics practice. *J Am Diet Assoc.* 1994;94:1159–1161.

57. Gould R, Shanklin CW, Canter DP, Miller JL. Stimulating research among dietetics students. *J Am Diet Assoc.* 1994;94:1103.

58. Monsen ER. Answering opportunity's knock. *J Am Diet Assoc.* 1994;94:240.

59. Chernoff R. Research agenda conference discussion papers: a summary. *J Am Diet Assoc.* 1993;93:1045–1049.

60. Dwyer JT. Scientific underpinnings for the profession: dietitians in research. In: *Challenging the Future of Dietetic Education and Credentialing Proceedings.* Chicago: The American Dietetic Association; 1994:57–75.

PART II

About The American Dietetic Association

Credentialing of Dietetic Practitioners

Margaret L. Bogle

"Experts at curing diseases are inferior to specialists who warn against disease. Experts in the use of medicines are inferior to those who recommend proper diet." 11th Century Chinese Physician[1]

Outline—Chapter 5

- Introduction

- Development of Certification/Registration
  - Implementation
  - CDR and eligibility requirements
- Specialty Certification
  - Role delineation studies
  - Certification and designation of board certified specialists
- Licensure of Dietitians by States

- Credentialing of Dietetic Technicians

- Conclusion

INTRODUCTION

Through the decades, the dietetic professional has struggled for identity. This struggle has been within the profession, other professions, and the public in general. Early attempts at a "legal" definition went essentially unnoticed. Practitioners were called dietologists, dietists, dietotherapists, and dietitians. The term *nutritionist* did not surface until the early 1920s.[2] Although The American Dietetic Association (ADA) was not organized until 1917, the term *dietitian* was defined by the Lake Placid Conference on Home Economics in 1899 by a group of dietetic professionals.[3] Their definition was "persons who specialize in the knowledge of food and can meet the demands of the medical profession for diet therapy," which adequately described the professionals for many decades.

Evidence of the relationship between food and the treatment of diseases goes back to 2500 BC determined by stone tablets found with what was perhaps the first diet prescription.[4] Numerous other records of experiments and use of food in medical treatment can be found until the present time. One Italian medical school divided medicine into three areas: diseases treated manually, by medicine, or by diet.[5] Medical treatment with diet is well documented in the early practice of medicine and surgery but not with the scientific basis necessary to declare it a profession. This science of "nutrition" did not really begin to emerge until late in the nineteenth and early twentieth centuries with the identification of nutrient-deficiency diseases and the discovery of vitamins.

This developing science of food and nutrition formed the basis for the organization of a group of practicing professionals. One of the earliest concerns of this group, organized in 1917, was the overwhelming amount of food faddism and fallacies between the general public and other professionals. It was difficult, if not impossible, for the public to determine fact from fiction between the many medical and health claims for specific foods and procedures.

This early concern for protection of the public by disseminating the knowledge of dietitians has continued until the present time. Not only did it lead to the national organization of dietitians that could promote the professionals as having expertise in "dietotherapy, teaching, social welfare, and administration," but it served as the impetus to begin thinking about credentialing of practitioners.

A second concern came forward at the second annual meeting of the ADA in 1919 and that was the "need to distinguish between dietitians with a college degree and special training in some scientific work and the ones with lesser training."[6]

This was perhaps the first formal reference to credentialing. In 1926 annual meeting notes, dietitians were considering formal certification—something beyond membership in the national association. In her 1927 presidential address, Florence Smith urged that the association should establish the standards for dietitians and that state or national registration could be the solution. She indicated that dietitians in California were already considering licensure.[7] It would be fitting that 60 years later, California would become the first state to pass legislation protecting the title of dietitians. National registration would surface again in 1929 in the presidential address of Anna Boller, in which she referenced the protection of the public from food quacks and faddists as motivation for credentialing at the national level.[8]

In 1929, the membership determined that standards for dietitians should be nationally uniform to protect the public against food quackery, food faddism, and fraud. A study of national registration was initiated. The following definition of a dietitian was adopted as result of these discussions and study: "Any person who is qualified for membership in The American Dietetic Association is by virtue of uniform basic training and required experience, entitled to be designated as a dietitian." Discussions about registration and credentialing continued in 1930, and although the association refused to take a stand, they did recommend that all members sign their names in medical charts and for other professional activities as "member of The American Dietetic Association."[6]

Not until the early 1950s did the association appoint a committee to formally study state licensing of dietitians. Interestingly enough, the issue of *specialties* or specialization in dietetics surfaced at this same time, with the suggestion that membership should be expanded to include others who were well qualified in the many *specialities* embraced by the designation of dietetics.[9] At the time, persons qualified in institutional administration were wanting to substitute business-related courses for some of the required courses. Oddly enough, this issue became an issue of membership requirements rather than considering credentialing of various specialties under the broad framework of membership in the association. Certainly, the association was in a growth mode attempting to meet the need for more dietitians. This discussion continued even through 1940, when educational standards recognized *specialized education for specialized areas of practice*. The speciality areas were designated: public health nutrition, administration, and hospital and food clinics. These would stand until the mid-1950s when no speciality designations were made in the educational standards. It is interesting to speculate if credentialing (licensure by the states and certifying of specialists [i.e., food service, public health, clinical, etc.]) might have increased the visibility of the profession and contributed to larger numbers seeking membership. Not until much later were educational and membership requirements varied, and with more flexibility to allow variation among practitioners with similar basic preparation.

In 1958, Plan III was approved (after considerable committee study and debate), and once again educational designations emerged representing specialty areas of practice. Plan III advocated a basic core curriculum for all dietetic students with one area of *emphasis* (business, food management, or education) and one area of *concentration* (general, administrative, or nutrition). The traditional dietetic internships were also changing with the emergence of "medical dietetics" for those wanting only to practice in clinical or medical settings. This plan would stand until the mid-1970s.

About this same time, the debate of a generalist (a dietitian who could perform in all areas of practice [e.g., a single dietitian in a small hospital] or the concept that a dietitian could move from one practice area to another) versus the specialist (a dietitian wanting to restrict his or her practice in one area [i.e., clinical or food service]) surfaced and consumed a lot of time in the House of Delegates. This debate was fueled by the shortage of dietitians overall and the need for them to be more mobile. The generalist role was advanced by the following themes: all dietitians are the same, dietitians can move from one area of practice (food service into public health) to another without additional training, and greater external recognition of the term *dietitian*. By contrast, the specialist role was driven by the following themes: the explosion of knowledge and technology requiring each dietitian to know "more and more about less and less"; the need to differentiate among dietitians with varying skills and knowledge, advanced education, and experience gained on the job; the emergence of part-time employment opportunities; and new, innovative practice areas (school food service, consultants to nursing homes, enteral and parenteral nutrition techniques, and nutrition support).

DEVELOPMENT OF CERTIFICATION/REGISTRATION

The 1960s was a time of multiple important issues being addressed simultaneously, all of which would ultimately affect credentialing. Those relevant to certification were the association tax status, reimbursement for services, recognition of specialists, and state licensure. Most members continued to practice in clinical or hospital dietetics, which led to the need to be more involved in legislative affairs because health and medical care were becoming dominated by governmental regulations. The tax status of the association was 501(c)(3), which was appropriate for an educational and scientific organization. This precluded any participation in lobbying or legislative efforts by members. This tax status was changed in 1966 to 501(c)(6) to allow for more active participation in political and governmental activities.

During this same period, a committee was established by the executive board to study licensure, registration, and certification. The exact charge to the committee was to "review the definitions of licensure, registration, and certification; the pros and cons of each; and implications these would have to the total Association membership."[10] The committee deliberated, consulted with state associations and legal counsel, and reported to the house of delegates in 1966 with a final report.[11] The report proposed that the association proceed with "voluntary registration" for members. The rationale behind the report was that this would be the best way to achieve the desired objectives of the profession (i.e., education for excellence), not only in the *primary* development of dietitians but also for the continuing competency of all dietetic practitioners. This committee report delivered the necessary options and described all the options, but "registration" did not fit the description in the 1965 changes to the Social Security Act. That act specified that "licensed professionals or providers" would be considered for third-party reimbursement. Had licensure been chosen in 1966, the history of credentialing in the 1990s would have been very different.

In retrospect, the presentation of the committee's legal consultant to the house of delegates in 1967 tipped the scales in favor of registration over licensure.[12] He did not believe the association was ready for licensure. They had no model licensure act. He concluded that registration should be considered as the first step. The first model licensure act would be presented to the house of delegates in 1973, and by 1978, 10 states were actively pursuing licensure. The movement of state licensure should have continued, but the membership involvement in the implementation of registration preempted immediate progression to licensure.

The association polled the membership concerning registration and the overwhelming response was in favor of the "principle" of professional registration. This set in motion one of the most rapid tracks of implementation that the association had ever accomplished.[13]

In 1967, the executive board presented a proposal to the House of Delegates at the 50th annual meeting in Chicago and subsequently the coordinating cabinet was designated as the ad hoc committee to draw up a timetable for implementation.[14] Thus in February 1968 (just six months later), the "First Tentative Proposal on Registration" was mailed to the membership for input and comments. Record numbers returned the comment sheets that accompanied the mailing. They were summarized and reported in the May 1968 *ADA Courier*.[15]

A "Revised Tentative Proposal" with a reaction sheet was mailed to the members in August 1968 with instructions to return comments to the chairmen of delegates for the house of delegates to deliberate in the fall. Discussions at that meeting were developed into the "Final Revised Proposal for Professional Registration," which was mailed to members to prepare them for a vote on an amendment to the constitution to implement the proposal.[16] This vote was taken early in 1969 when the amendment was approved with implementation effective June 1, 1969.

Implementation

An interim committee was appointed to assist with implementation with two members elected each year until all appointed members were replaced. In 1972, all committee members had been elected. This was the most effective process of member involvement at the grassroots level that the association had accomplished to that date. A detailed account of the implementation and a review of the first five years of professional registration was published in the *Journal of The American Dietetic Association* in 1974.[13]

The professional registration system adopted by the association differed significantly from other health professional certification systems at that time:

(1) candidates had to pass a national examination and (2) registered dietitians (RD) had to document evidence of continuing education in each five-year period to renew registration. Thus registration was designed as a voluntary process, ensuring competency of dietitians through the qualifications required to take the examination, passing the examination, and formal continuing education. All this was evidence of the concern of the profession for the health, safety, and welfare of the public by encouraging high standards of performance by dietetic practitioners as stated in the amendment to the constitution.[16]

Ninety-three percent of the membership was registered by the end of the 1970s with a majority being registered during the "grandfather" period before establishment of the examination. The first examination was given in 1970 to 56 dietetic interns, all of whom passed. From 1970 to 1973, 83 percent of all taking the examination passed. Test sites were established throughout the United States and some foreign countries to accommodate members in the armed forces.

CDR and Eligibility Requirements

The commission on dietetic registration (CDR) is the agency responsible for maintaining the registration process for the ADA. The 12 members of the commission are elected by members of ADA with the exception of one public member who is appointed. The responsibilities of the commission are to determine the eligibility for registration of both dietitians and dietetic technicians and to develop and administer the registration examinations. The examination for both groups is administered in April and October each year at sites throughout the United States and in other countries with which CDR has reciprocity agreements. The four other countries are Canada, The Netherlands, Philippines, and Ireland.

The eligibility requirements for dietitians to take the registration examination are the following:[17]

1. Education
   • minimum of a baccalaureate degree from an accredited college or university
   • completion of current minimum academic requirements as approved by ADA
2. Supervised practice
   • to be met in an accredited dietetic internship, an accredited coordinated program, or approved preprofessional practice program

Dietetic technicians wishing to take the registration examination must meet the following requirements:[17]

1. Education
   • associate or baccalaureate degree from an accredited college or university

- completion of approved courses in an ADA-approved dietetic technician program or of a didactic program in dietetics minimum academic requirements
2. Supervised practice
    - completion of supervised field experience as stipulated in an ADA-approved dietetic technician program

To remain registered, an RD is required to pay yearly dues and to submit evidence of having attained 75 clock hours of continuing education each five years. A registered dietetic technician (DTR) is required to accrue 50 clock hours each five years.

During the early 1970s the association continued to study other credentialing mechanisms through a national advisory committee on state licensure. As this discussion progressed, the issue of requiring membership for certification was studied by the committee to study the feasibility of developing professional registration independent of the ADA. The committee determined that professional registration independent of membership in the association was both feasible and desirable given the climate of certification activities among the allied health professions, in which membership was not being required as a prerequisite to employment.

In June 1978, the executive board and the committee on operations decided that the association would take no position on the movement toward licensure of dietitians but would leave that function to the states. However, one of the eight goals identified by that group for 1978–1979 was to continue to review and evaluate credentialing procedures and programs for dietitians.[6]

SPECIALTY CERTIFICATION

The greatest new impetus for renewing study of specialization and additional forms of credentialing came from the *Report of the Study Commission on Dietetics* in 1972, which had been partially funded by a grant from the Kellogg Foundation.[18] One recommendation of the commission was to continue to develop systems for the recognition of speciality practice and advanced levels of practice. The report indicated the debate was not one of whether there is speciality practice among registered dietitians but rather how should these specialty dietitians be credentialed or recognized as different from other more general practitioners. The report concluded with the knowledge that most members did not think that further certification (in addition to registration) was necessary but that study of this issue should continue.

In 1975, an ad hoc committee was appointed to study the feasibility of establishing board certification for specialty practice. The committee's final report, presented to the house of delegates in 1979, was defeated. Two important factors contributed to the defeat: (1) the report recommended establishing specialty boards (with testing authority) autonomous of the association, patterning them after medical specialty boards, and (2) the formal recognition of "special interest" groups as dietetic practice groups (DPG) within the Council on Practice (COP). The membership was just becoming comfortable with the "autonomy" of the professional registration committee and was hesitant to begin another group with authority outside of the association.

The COP ironically lobbied against and tipped the scales in favor of defeat of the report. The membership of the DPGs and COP saw themselves as protectors of and the assurance of quality practice. For the most part, they were naive about the political processes of the association because most were truly interested in enhancing their area of practice through networking with others working in the same area. They viewed the specialty boards as producing groups of certified specialists who would dilute the ranks of the DPGs. At the time, they were thinking that practitioners should develop these certifications, but they were not mature enough in their structure to see how they could have affected and possibly controlled the boards. Interestingly enough, the COP and DPGs would be the groups in the 1980s to push again for specialty certification and bring forth a successful program.

Another significant event of the mid-1970s to affect credentialing was the appointment of a professional standards review committee in 1973. This group developed the first document to attempt to promote standards of practice within employment areas of dietetic practice. Results were distributed to members in 1975, followed in 1976 by regional workshops to enable grassroots practitioners to begin to evaluate their practice and allow for "peer review," as was already occurring in most other areas of health care. Two publications, *The Professional Standards Review Procedure Manual,* which introduced dietitians to the patient record audit, and *Guidelines for Evaluating Dietetic Practice,* which was to help dietitians in self-evaluation, also proved helpful for peer review.

A third publication in 1977 was *The Patient Care Audit—A Quality Assurance Procedure Manual for Dietitians,* which continued the association's pursuit of quality practice and the responsibility of the individual practitioner. All these publications and the deliberations of the committees were continuing the discussion of credentialing of individuals.

The association and the COP continued to be concerned about ensuring competency of practitioners who could provide high-quality practice. This resulted in the publication of *Standards of Practice: A Practitioner's Guide to Implementation* in 1986. As a result, states began to train individuals who could serve as resources for dietitians who wished to evaluate their own practice.

Role Delineation Studies

In 1979, the association had begun a series of studies to delineate the actual and appropriate roles and responsibilities of "entry-level" dietitians.[19] The first would examine clinical dietitians followed closely by studies of food service management and community dietetics.[20,21] These reports were followed by two articles that further enlightened members about current and future roles of dietitians.[22,23]

During this period, the CDR worked closely with the Council on Education (COE) and the COP to ensure that education requirements would be derived from practice in various areas and that the registration examination would continue to determine those individuals able to practice at entry level. The role delineation studies would continue to be updated.

Even though the 1972 study commission report had indicated that "there will be increased differentiation of roles and functions of dietitians" and "dietitians will become more specialized," the association would not approve the process of certification of specialists until after the publication in 1984 of the second major study of the profession—*A New Look at the Profession of Dietetics*.[24] Even so, the proliferation of self-acknowledged dietetic specialists continued. In 1985, the house of delegates committee on specialization defined specialization and recommended recognition of advanced levels of practice in three areas: clinical nutrition, community nutrition, and food service systems administration. A president's page of the *Journal of The American Dietetics Association* was written giving details of the specialty certification process and included a survey form for members to return with their comments.[25]

The 1986 House of Delegates approved the concept of specialization and designated the COP as the appropriate organizational unit to pursue functional subspecialty certification with eventual credentialing by the CDR. A major presentation was developed by COP, CDR, and a consultant from the American College Testing Program. The report indicated that the role delineations to identify an advanced level of practice in specific clinical subspecialties would be added to the 1988–89 update of the role delineations.

After decades of committees, debate, and study, the profession of dietetics was coming of age. The first credential since RD in 1969 was about to materialize! In addition to study by the association, other independent studies and reports were adding to the documentation of the need for a new credential.[26] O'Sullivan-Maillet and Gilbride reported that approximately 75 percent of respondents to a survey projected the need for two to nine clinical specialties within the next 10 years.[27] In addition, 25 percent of the graduate programs contacted indicated that they already had or were preparing for educational programs for dietitian specialists. Similarly, Sandrick reported that respondents to her survey indicated that the association should certify specialists in dietetics and that certification should include a written examination.[28]

The definition of "specialty" is a reality! The ADA defined specialty as an advanced level of practice that responds to a defined area of need and requires demonstrated competence exceeding that for entry level. Specialty areas must have a substantial and verifiable knowledge base, an identified dimension of advanced practice, and a reasonable pool of practitioners.

Many dietitians may limit their practice to one particular area. They may or may not be practicing at an advanced level. They may continue to apply entry-level knowledge and skills and have not expanded their knowledge and experience to the point of being a specialist. The COP knew that a formal program of credentialing was the best way to differentiate between dietitians practicing a specialty at an advanced level and a dietitian limiting his or her practice to a single practice area but not functioning as a highly skilled specialist.

By 1990, many dietitians had sought specialty designation from other organizations, primarily the American Society for Parenteral and Enteral Nutrition as certified nutrition support dietitian and the American Association of Diabetes Educators for certified diabetes educator (this credential not being restricted to dietitians—nurses and physicians could also qualify). Some dietitians practicing on nutrition support teams were especially anxious to become certified, as other members of their team (nurses, pharmacists, and physicians) were already board-certified specialists. Their perception was that the ADA had not responded to their needs in a timely manner, although many of them were still valuing the association to provide certification.

The association determined that specialty certification would begin within the broad areas of clinical dietetics because the greater numbers of dietitians were practicing in that area in the late 1980s.

DPGs were asked to submit applications for specialty certification. Each applicant was asked to detail the necessary knowledge base, outline a dimension of practice (including the uniqueness of the practice to distinguish it from other areas), and document the numbers of individuals currently practicing the specialty that would determine a reasonable pool of practitioners. Three areas were selected: pediatric nutrition, renal nutrition, and metabolic nutrition care (which included nutrition support but was broader in concept).

It was determined that credentialing requirements would include educational preparation (basic and specialized), on-the-job training/experience, verification and evaluation of practice, and an examination. To develop examinations and other evaluative measures of practice, the roles, functions, and knowledge and skill levels must be determined. The combined efforts of the COP, CDR, and the Council on Research (COR) set out to determine the wide-ranging tasks (task analysis) that characterize the dietitian's work in nine categories of activities that had been used in the entry-level role delineations, which could be used as a baseline for understanding advanced and specialty competency.

After task analysis, the skills and knowledge necessary to perform those tasks would have to be determined and verified. The last part of this dynamic process was to link education with performance and practice. The COE joined with COP, CDR, and COR to accomplish this last part of the process of credentialing.

The resultant role delineations were described in detail in the *Journal of The American Dietetic Association.*[29,30] The study of advanced-level practice was unique because the knowledge and skills were similar to those of entry-level dietitians. Therefore, differences, if they existed, had to be in other areas—possibly in their approach to practice or in psychosocial areas. No other professional group had attempted to study these differences; hence, there was no model study to follow. The 1989 role delineation for RDs and entry-level technicians had indicated the possibility that the advanced practitioner had greater responsibility in management, finance, and supervision.[31]

Certification and Designation of Board Certified Specialists

The study undertaken to credential specialists determined that there were differences among the areas of renal, pediatric, and metabolic nutrition. It also verified the knowledge and skills unique to each specialty and those that were consistent across the three areas. Other minimum criteria for certification were established:

- *education and experience:* an RD with six years of practice post-RD and currently practicing in the specialty area
- *examination:* passing a written examination developed and administered by CDR
- *fees:* payment of application, testing, and certification fees

The research also generated an empirical model for advanced-level practice with the following minimum characteristics:

- *education and experience:* an RD; a master's degree; eight years of practice experience; current employment in dietetic practice
- *professional achievement:* awards or honors; or authorship of journal articles, books, or book chapters; or major conference presentations
- *approach to practice:* complements technical knowledge and skills with in-depth holistic understanding plus intervention; uses feelings and a process

focus that is adaptable and creative; and values self-knowledge and innovation

- *role positions:* occupies multiple role positions with diverse and complex duties
- *role contacts:* develops network of diverse practice contacts within and beyond local or immediate job area
- *fees:* payment of application and certification fees.[32]

The resulting credentials were board-certified specialist in pediatric, renal, or metabolic nutrition (CS) for dietitians practicing in specialty areas and fellow of the ADA (FADA) for those practicing at advanced levels.

The CDR began credentialing specialists, with the first examination being given in 1993, and credentialed the charter fellows in 1994. Credentialing of entry-level dietitians as RDs is ongoing. Early in 1997, the following number of credentials had been processed: fellows, 288; certified specialists in pediatrics, 163; renal,156; metabolic nutrition, 25.

The certification of entry-level dietitians as RDs continues to involve the largest number of practitioners as it designates those who are deemed competent to practice and not be harmful to the public through their practice. This program is now in its third decade and has contributed significantly to the identity of dietitians throughout the world. Because of the necessity to maintain and renew registration through continuing education requirements, some measure of competency of practitioners is ensured. The CDR continues to improve the system, most recently through significant efforts to assist individual practitioners with self-assessment and a "plan" for continuing education over time. This certification remains at the forefront of credentialing systems and continues to be the envy of other professional organizations.

LICENSURE OF DIETITIANS BY STATES

Licensure efforts in the states continued to grow, particularly since 1982 when California became the first state to enact legislation to restrict the use of the title *dietitian* and to define what activities could be undertaken by dietitians. Later that same year, Louisiana passed a law allowing only persons professionally qualified to represent themselves as dietitians or RDs. In 1983, Texas passed a bill that provided for voluntary licensure of dietitians but did not include protection of a scope of practice. That year, the association ad hoc committee on licensure developed a document, *Licensure/Entitlement for Dietitians*, which detailed definitions and terminology and titles and included a model scope of practice, sample bills for licensure, and an extensive appendix of forms and reference materials.

Alabama became the first state to achieve legal protection of both titles, *dietitian* and *nutritionist,* in 1984. By that time, eight states had some form of legal credentialing, and 60 percent of the state associations reported activity in the pursuit of licensure. Eleven states had achieved licensure by 1985, just three years from the achievement of licensure in California. Other states would follow the trend with a variety of title protection and scopes of practice during the next 15 years. Some would amend or add changes to their laws that enhanced dietitians' opportunities for third-party reimbursement and for inclusion in health care insurance programs. A few states would experience litigation in the pursuit of protecting the health of the public from persons not licensed to practice or from those in violation of the laws. Still other states would make repeated attempts to get licensure laws passed before achieving success.

By the mid-1990s, 36 states had licensure and/or certification programs in place. In the managed care debate of the 1990s in which *multiskilling* and *cross-training* are frequent buzz words, these protected scopes of practice will enhance dietitians' positions in these areas. Many already have skills and knowledge that can be used in other areas of health care practice.

CREDENTIALING OF DIETETIC TECHNICIANS

Although the early dietitians valued the role of less well-trained individuals who could extend the role of the dietitian by carrying out delegated responsibilities and agreed in the 1920s to call them "nutrition aides," it would take the increased demand for dietitians during World War II to enhance the role of these aides. References to "assistant dietitian" and "dietitian's assistant" are found throughout the history of the association.[6]

As RDs began to refine their roles and because dietitians were not available in all areas, the use of "dietetic assistants" and "technicians" became more important. The delegation of authority for supervision led to the formation of the Hospital, Institution and Educational Food Service Society (HIEFSS) in 1960. This group in conjunction with the ADA, set standards and provided educational programs for dietetic assistants and technicians. In 1975, the ADA expanded membership to dietetic technicians. The dietetic assistants would form their own group known as the National Association of Dietary Managers.

The 1970s would see educational programs emerge for technicians in both the clinical dietetics and food service management areas. Some dietitians and educators also saw the need for these educational programs (most were two years in length, leading to an associate degree) to prepare technicians to go on for four-year programs and become dietitians if they wanted career advancement.

The 1972 study commission would emphasize the need for dietitians to increase delegation of some of their responsibilities and roles to other less highly trained individuals.[18]

The process to credential dietetic technicians began in 1981. The formal program began in 1986 with a grandfather clause allowing registration of those technicians who had graduated from approved educational programs. Thereafter, they had to successfully complete a national examination administered by CDR to use the letters DTR after their name, indicative of fulfillment of the credentialing process.

Continuing evaluation of this credential and examination is evidenced by CDR's *Role Delineations for Registered Dietitians and Entry-Level Technicians,* completed in 1989.[31] Credentialing of dietetic technicians continues to grow. Early in 1997 (10 years of the program) the number of technicians registered was 5,090. One factor deterring the increase of numbers in this group is the lack of educational programs for technicians. Not without impact is the view of many dietitians who have not been willing to accept the roles of this group in anything but clerical activities. Certification gives credibility to this group for their education and experiential preparation and for the specific roles of technicians as set out through the role delineations of CDR.[32] Supply and demand will increase the numbers of educational programs in the future to meet the needs for practitioners. In addition, because most technicians and dietitians work in the health care arena, the changes in acute and ambulatory care and the increased emphasis on "prevention" will undoubtedly mean changes in the roles of both.

CONCLUSION

Dietitians continue to want recognition and differentiation among their peers that is visible and can be communicated to other professional practitioners. Many thought registration would be that vehicle. Now, the credentialing program has been designed to do just that and to dispel the paradigm that "all dietitians are alike." The certification of fellows and specialists is here and ready to fill that niche. Although the numbers are small that have taken advantage of this new system, it is reasonable to think that these numbers will grow with effective marketing within the association among peers and with other groups and innovative changes already occurring in dietetic practice. The benefits of credentialing to individual practitioners will never be greater than the value the profession as a whole places on the program. RD has become valued to the point that most individuals consider it synonymous with "dietitian." Employers (most of whom are dietitians) view it as a mandatory credential to practice.

As licensure efforts continue to grow across the United States, the RD has increased in value, not decreased as some feared. Almost all states that have licensure (24) are using RD and the CDR examination (23), and of those that have certification of dietitians (12), nine are using the RD and/or the examination in their programs. One state, Maine, also licenses dietetic technicians. Both RD and licensed professional will continue to be used in state and national legislation.

The credentials of "fellow" and "certified specialist" will continue to grow in importance and may escalate as RDs begin to move toward "independent practice" status in private practice, in consultative roles in business, research, and food production, and in the arena of prevention and health and move away from total dependence on acute care and medical nutrition therapy. Objective credentials such as these enhance the ability of individual practitioners to market themselves without the support of an institution. In addition, they provide other benefits to all dietetic practitioners by identifying role models, peer experts, and specialists, which will enhance networking and growth of the profession. Career enhancement through career ladders can also be accomplished.

Dietitians no longer have to leave the profession to enjoy the job-related recognition and advancement they have desired. Each individual can use this framework in establishing goals for practice, on-the-job training, experiential learning beyond entry level, and career development. In the future, as we change jobs more frequently than we have in the past, these credentials will serve as "passports" or "entrees" into new and diverse job ventures. Educational programs, both traditional graduate programs and nontraditional programs, will use the criteria for these credentials in developing new and varied programs as demanded by future practitioners.

Credentials have been used extensively in international markets and jobs to describe individuals and job qualifications. For dietitians and technicians, this is a plus as we move toward a global practice and world.

Consumers will always demand credentials of some kind. As consumers recognize that the credentials of the ADA provide assurance that the practitioners are competent and can provide services that they want, the demand for these credentials will rise. More significantly, these credentials will enhance the RD's efforts to describe the diversity and to obtain a competitive advantage in the practice of dietetics in the United States and internationally.

DEFINITIONS

Certification Process by which a nongovernmental agency or association grants recognition to an individual who has met certain predetermined qualifications specified by that agency or association (e.g., registration for dietitians and dietetic technicians administered by the commission on dietetic registration).

Credentialing Formal recognition of professional or technical competence as by certification or licensure.

Entry Level Term descriptive of competence attained through fulfillment of the knowledge and performance required for dietitians or technicians as delineated in the standards of education (also, the first position held by a practitioner).

Licensure Process by which an agency of government grants permission to an individual to engage in a given occupation on finding that the applicant has attained the minimal degree of competency necessary to ensure that the public health, safety, and welfare are reasonably well protected.

Practitioner One who practices in a profession or occupation.

Reciprocity Giving of privileges in return for similar privileges, as eligibility requirements.

Registration (See Credentialing)

Scope of Practice Extent of or dimensions of activities performed in an area of practice.

REFERENCES

1. Needham J. *Clerks and Craftsmen in China and the West. Lectures and Addresses on the History of Science and Technology.* Cambridge, MA: University Press; 1970.

2. Barber MI. *History of The American Dietetic Association (1917–1959).* Philadelphia: JB Lippincott Co; 1959.

3. Corbett FR. The training of dietitians for hospitals. *J Home Econ.* 1909;1:62.

4. Jastrow M. *The Civilization of Babylonia and Assyria.* Philadelphia: JB Lippincott Co; 1915.

5. ADA. *A New Look at the Profession of Dietetics: Report of the 1984 Study Commission on Dietetics.* Chicago: The American Dietetic Association; 1985.

6. Cassell J. *Carry the Flame: The History of The American Dietetic Association.* Chicago: The American Dietetic Association; 1990.

7. Smith FH. Presidential address. *J Am Diet Assoc.* 1927;3:145–204.

8. Boller AE. Presidential address. *J Am Diet Assoc.* 1929;5:175.

9. Perry E. Report of the executive board. *J Am Diet Assoc.* 1950;26:949–957.

10. ADA. *Annual Reports and Proceedings, 1960–61.* Chicago: The American Dietetic Association; 1962.

11. ADA. *Annual Reports and Proceedings, 1965–66.* Chicago: The American Dietetic Association; 1967.

12. Grad FP. *Consideration of Legal Definitions of the Dietitian.* Chicago: The American Dietetic Association; 1975. Unpublished report.

13. Bogle ML. Registration: the sine quo non of a competent dietitian. *J Am Diet Assoc.* 1974;64:616–620.

14. ADA. *Annual Reports and Proceedings, 1966–67.* Chicago: The American Dietetic Association; 1968.

15. Report of Committee on Professional Registration. *ADA Courier.* 1968;8.

16. ADA. *Constitution of The American Dietetic Association, as Amended.* Chicago: The American Dietetic Association; 1971.

17. ADA. *Directory of Dietetics Programs, 1997–1998.* Chicago: The American Dietetic Association; 1997.

18. ADA Study Commission on Dietetics. *The Profession of Dietetics*. Chicago: The American Dietetic Association; 1972.

19. Baird SC, Armstrong RVL. *Role Delineations for Entry-Level Clinical Dietitians*. Chicago: The American Dietetic Association; 1981.

20. Baird SC, Burrelli JS. *Role Delineations and Verification for Entry-Level Positions in Foodservice Systems Management*. Chicago: The American Dietetic Association; 1983.

21. Baird SC, Burrelli JS. *Role Delineations and Verification for Entry-Level Positions in Community Dietetics*. Chicago: The American Dietetic Association; 1983.

22. Baird SC, Armstrong RVL. The American Dietetic Association role delineations for the field of clinical dietetics: 1. Philosophical overview and historical background. *J Am Diet Assoc*. 1981;78:370–374.

23. Baird SC, Armstrong RVL. The American Dietetic Association role delineations for the field of clinical dietetics: 2. Methodology and summary of results. *J Am Diet Assoc*. 1981;78:374–382.

24. ADA Study Commission on Dietetics. *A New Look at the Profession of Dietetics*. Chicago: The American Dietetic Association; 1986.

25. Owen AL, Dougherty D, Bogle ML. President's page: specialization in dietetics—the time has come. *J Am Diet Assoc*. 1986;86:1072–1076.

26. COP Ad Hoc Committee. *Specialization Report: ADA House of Delegates Annual Meeting Action Item*. Chicago: The American Dietetic Association; 1990.

27. O'Sullivan-Maillet J, Gilbride JA. *Services of Clinical Dietetic Specialists*. New York: New York University; 1989. PhD dissertation.

28. Sandrick JG. Dietetic specialization: opinions of directors of departments of dietetics. *J Am Diet Assoc*. 1989;89:1458–1464.

29. Bradley RT, Young WY, Ebbs P, Martin J. Characteristics of advanced-level dietetics practice: a model and empirical results. *J Am Diet Assoc*. 1993;93:196–202.

30. Bradley RT, Young WY, Ebbs P, Martin J. Specialty practice in dietetics: empirical models and results. *J Am Diet Assoc*. 1993;93:203–210.

31. Kane MI, Estes CA, Cotton DA, Eltoft CS. *Role Delineations for Registered Dietitians and Entry-Level Dietetic Technicians*. Chicago: The American Dietetic Association; 1990.

32. Bogle ML, Balogun L, Cassell J, Catakis A, et al. Achieving excellence in dietetic practice: certification of specialists and advanced-level practitioners. *J Am Diet Assoc*. 1993;93:149–150.

CHAPTER 6

Dietetic Manpower Team

Robin B. Fellers

". . . a team has members who work collectively in a way that magnifies the group's impact, above and beyond that generated only from individual efforts. This is the effect of synergy. The team's collective effort is more than the sum of its individual efforts."[1 (p.6)]

Outline—Chapter 6

- Introduction

- The Dietetic Team: What Does This Mean?

- Development of the Dietetic Team

- Roles and Responsibilities of Dietetic Teams

- Role Delineation Studies

- Practice Audit

- Conclusion

INTRODUCTION

The 1972 Study Commission on Dietetics pointed out that dietitians make a unique contribution to the health and well-being of society through their knowledge of food, nutrition, and health.[2] Dietitians serve the public's interests by interpreting scientific knowledge about food and nutrition so that optimal nourishment in individuals and populations will result. Good nutrition is a major factor in preventing disease and maintaining a healthy population. Dietitians are unique in the health professions because of their expert knowledge in matters concerning food, nutrition, and health.

This chapter focuses on the work that dietitians do as they provide food and nutrition services to individuals and groups, in health and disease. In most work settings, dietitians work as part of a team. Even in a counseling session when a dietitian is working one-on-one, the outcome is more likely to be effective when the dietitian thinks of the client and referring physician as valued members of a team effort to restore or maintain the client's health.

For most of the profession's history, health care facilities have been the major sites of employment for dietitians. Most of the examples cited in this chapter relate to work done in health care facilities' work settings. This source of employment probably will lose dominance as more health care services, including dietitians' services, are outsourced from acute care hospitals. Future dietetic team members, although still working *in* health care facilities, very well may be *employed by* independently owned dietetic contract services.

THE DIETETIC TEAM: WHAT DOES THIS MEAN?

A registered dietitian (RD) who is employed as a pediatric nutritionist in a community-based clinic specializing in evaluating clients with developmental disabilities described her work this way:

> With health care reform, my main focus for my nutrition care plans is how to keep our clients out of the hospital. My services are also recommended by physical therapists, social workers, occupational therapists, speech pathologists, as well as nurses and physicians in order for their therapies to be more effective. Emphasis on *team* and the role of the nutritionist, and practical experience on an interdisciplinary team should be part of every dietitian's training. (Diane M. Miller, MPH, RD, written communication, August 15, 1996)

Miller's remarks underscore a very important fact about dietitians' work in today's health care settings: very few dietitians work alone. In practical terms, this means that most dietitians in most practice settings associate with other health professionals in a cooperative effort to achieve a goal. Major characteristics of effective teams in health care settings are

- A desired outcome that is shared by all members

- A presence of diverse skills and experience within the team adequate to meet the desired outcome
- A plan for achieving a coordinated effort

Most dietitians are members of one or more teams. Some teams are *interdepartmental*. Others are *intradepartmental*. Some teams are very small, like the team of three—dietitian, client, physician—cited at the beginning of the chapter. Other teams can be quite large, such as a patient care planning team in a rehabilitation facility that could include not only the physician, patient, and dietitian but also nurses and a host of other health professionals.

Interdepartmental teams tend to be well defined and formalized. An example of this type is the patient care team shown in Figure 6-1. Such a team exists to assist the patient/client to attain optimal health. That is the reason for placing the patient/ client at the team center. Sometimes (think of a child), the success of treatment depends as much on a family member or other caregiver as it does on the patient/ client. In these cases, family members must be included in patient care plans. Patients/clients and families are included because without their understanding, consent, and cooperation, no treatment can be effective.

If the patient care team shown in Figure 6-1 existed for diabetes education, team members typically would include a physician, nurse, dietitian, and exercise physiologist. These professionals represent the health disciplines that make the greatest contribution to effective treatment of diabetes mellitus. However, some patients with diabetes mellitus might need services of other health professionals to optimize the treatment benefits. For example, some need assistance with housing, grocery shopping, or transportation for medical appointments. A social worker has the knowledge and skills to identify resources that meet these needs. A pharmacist may be included to provide information about the ways that different medications interact with insulin. Patients with diabetes mellitus can develop gangrene and lose toes, feet, and legs to amputation, so a podiatrist becomes an important part of the diabetes care team.

Intradepartmental teams exist within the department of dietetics. They are composed of dietitians and other employees of the same department. In some hospitals, the dietitians responsible for clinical nutrition services work in their own department, but in others, clinical dietitians are employed in the department of food and nutrition services. This discussion assumes the latter.

Intradepartmental teams are established to accomplish the goal of providing excellent food and nutrition services to patients. The team approach is necessary because the integrated efforts of the dietitian, dietetic technician, diet clerk, dietary manager, chef, cooks, tray aides, and all food service employees are necessary for accomplishing departmental goals. Each employee contributes to the tasks involved in delivering quality food and nutrition services to the right patient at the right time.

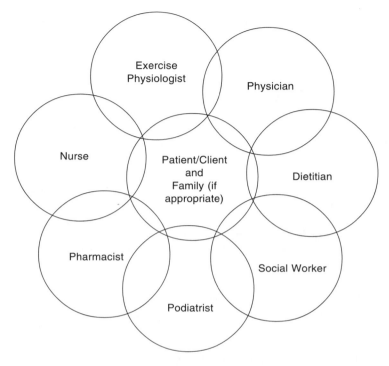

Note: Overlapping circles indicate shared goals, shared information, cooperation, and collaboration.

Figure 6–1 Interdepartmental Patient Care Team for Patients with Diabetes Mellitus

Figure 6-2 shows these relationships in diagrammatic form. Again, the patient/client is the focus of the team's efforts. Dietitians are shown in two of their major roles: administration and clinical nutrition. The other dietetic team members are

- dietetic technicians who assist dietitians with clinical nutrition and management responsibilities
- diet clerks who assist clinical nutrition dietitians by coordinating patient information
- dietary managers who assist dietitians and dietetic technicians with supervision of food production, service, and distribution
- cooks to prepare food, servers to serve meals, and other food service employees

The nature of dietetics is such that very few dietitians can do the work demanded of them without assistance or input of other individuals. Dietitians do their most effective work in teams.

Teamwork in dietetics can be viewed in at least two different ways. One way is to view the team as though it were a sports team with each person trained (or coached) to participate in the game. Further training emphasizes specific skills of a defined position so that the individual team members together contribute to the team's success when it faces a challenger. In the health care setting, diseases and injuries are the health care team's challengers, and a patient care team comprised of the appropriate health professionals assembles to meet the challenge of returning patients to optimal health. This patient care team is similar to the diabetes care team described above. Each member has a defined role and responsibility for returning the patient to health: The dietitian contributes nutrition care, the nurse teaches the patient to administer insulin, and other team members contribute their specific knowledge and skills.

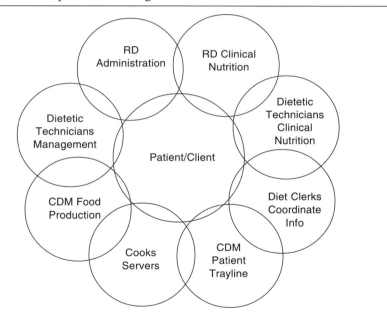

Note: Team members with food service responsibilities are on the left side of the diagram and those with nutrition service responsibility are on the right side. All team members may interact and collaborate. Dietetic professionals on this team are the registered dietitians (RD), dietetic technicians, and certified dietary managers (CDM). Overlapping circles indicate shared goals, shared information, cooperation, and collaboration.

Figure 6–2 Intradepartmental Patient Care Team for Food and Nutrition Services

Yet another way to view team work is to examine the various functions that the individual dietitian is expected to perform. Some of the time, the dietitian on the diabetes education team will be called on to assess the nutritional status of a patient and make recommendations to the physician about nutrition care; at other times, the same dietitian uses management skills to solve a problem arising from tray service to the patient; and sometimes, this dietitian assumes a teaching role to help a group of patients with diabetes learn new dietary habits.

There is historical precedent for the team concept in dietetics. From the earliest days of the profession, dietitians have done their work as members of a team. In a 1925 article published in the first issue of the *Journal of The American Dietetic Association*, MacEachern identified at least three major responsibilities for hospital dietitians.[3] First was the dietitian's responsibility to work with physicians to provide special diets and nutrition education as part of the patient's treatment. (In 1925, this was termed *dietotherapy*.) Second, the dietitian was responsible to the hospital administrator to manage the business of providing nutrition services to patients and staff. (MacEachern noted that the dietitian "has a great deal of power and influence in controlling the food budget of the hospital.") Third, the dietitian was expected to interact effectively with the nursing service. In an era when schools of nursing were hospital based, dietitians were responsible for teaching student nurses about nutrition in health and disease.

From the earliest days of the profession, dietitians were expected to function well in these three roles:

1. as a clinical nutritionist, working with physicians and other allied health professionals, providing nutrition care for patients
2. as a manager, working with hospital administrators, purchasing officers, accountants, and other department heads, managing resources necessary to provide food and nutrition services to patients, staff, and visitors
3. as a teacher, working with students, health care employees, patients/clients, community groups, and the general public

These expectations, documented as early as 1925, go hand-in-hand with a dietitian's primary competencies: to be an expert in the interrelationship of food, nutrition, and health; to be a competent manager of resources needed to provide food and nutrition services; and to be an effective teacher.

Effective team participants are individuals who possess certain interpersonal characteristics. Essential for all health care workers is a willingness to work with people. In fact, a desire to help people achieve a healthier lifestyle is the reason frequently cited by college students who select nutrition/dietetics as their major course of study. Teamwork means more than simply enjoying personal interactions, however. Successful teams are composed of individuals who value and respect each others' contributions, who trust each other, and who can look beyond their personal goals to work cooperatively toward the team's goals. Sharing is an essential quality for a successful team. Team members share responsibility, achievement, success, and sometimes, failure. A well-functioning team is indeed greater than the sum of its parts.

DEVELOPMENT OF THE DIETETIC TEAM

Dietetic team members are shown in Figure 6–2. People who wish to qualify as dietitians, dietetic technicians, or dietary managers all must undergo some form of postsecondary education. Table 6–1 summarizes the required education and training for dietetic professionals and compares their typical roles and responsibilities.

Dietitians or, more accurately, registered dietitians are college educated and receive preprofessional training to be eligible to take the national registration examination for dietitians. At best, this process requires approximately five years. Therefore, whenever a shortage of dietitians exists, it takes a long time to meet the demand.

Hospitals are complex organizations with numerous departments that require the services of many different types of employees. More than 60 years ago, hospital administrators reported that patients expected prompt and accurate diagnoses, coupled with scientifically based treatments that would contribute to rapid recovery.[3] These expectations are just as legitimate and important today.

Advances in medical knowledge and technology along with changing economic and social conditions have continually influenced the work of dietitians even though dietitians were never available in sufficient numbers to meet the demand for their services. This long-standing deficiency in meeting the demand for qualified dietitians existed throughout the profession's developing years. It was particularly acute during the 1950s when the Hill-Burton Act provided federal assistance to build new hospitals and expand existing facilities. These had to be staffed with qualified dietetic practitioners. The dilemma was that there simply were not enough dietitians to fill the available positions, and it took at least five years to recruit, educate, and train new ones.

Resourceful problem solving is a time-honored characteristic that has enabled the profession of dietetics to survive for almost a century. Dietitians of the 1950s found solutions to staffing problems within their own departments. They identified existing employees with on-the-job experience, proven aptitude, and potential for developing skills necessary to perform many of the routine daily tasks previously assigned to professional dietitians. Dietitians developed training programs housed first within their institutions, then taken up by universities, statewide agencies, and eventually, The American Dietetic Association (ADA). The ADA Correspondence Course for Food Service Supervisors was developed and implemented nationwide by 1960. Graduates of these programs were trained to be support personnel for professional dietitians, and became known as food service supervisors. This title persisted until 1974 when a committee to develop a glossary on terminology for the association and profession[4] recommended a change to dietetic assistant. The committee said this distinguished a food service supervisor with ADA-sponsored training from one who had grown into the job through work experience. The *dietetic assistant* title was changed yet again in 1984 to dietary manager. Today, dietary managers have their own professional organization and credential: certified dietary manager (CDM). Throughout these changes, dietitians have continued to regard dietary managers as valued members of the dietetic team. Refer to Table 6–1 for a summary of education, training, roles, and responsibilities for dietary managers.

A persistent need for a more technically oriented team member coupled with growth and development of two-year community colleges made it possible for dietitians to solve manpower shortages in another way. Dietetic technician programs were established at two-year community colleges to train technical support personnel. The education and training requirements, along with other information about roles and responsibilities of dietetic technicians, are shown in Table 6–1.

These three dietetic professionals: RDs, dietetic technicians—registered (DTR), and CDMs possess credentials that were originally developed by the ADA in response to health care system needs. Between them, RDs, DTRs, and CDMs form a dietetic team for staffing food and nutrition services in hospitals, nursing homes, life care centers, community nutrition clinics, school nutrition programs, colleges and universities, and other such facilities around the nation.

ROLES AND RESPONSIBILITIES OF DIETETIC TEAMS

The development of dietetic teams was outlined in the first part of this chapter. The remaining section is a discussion of roles and responsibilities of the dietetic team members. Health care in the 1990s is increasingly complex, diversified, and changing. Most health care facilities and many community nutrition programs use the dietetic team concept. And as was pointed out in the Introduction, most dietitians work as part of a team. In the increasingly complex world of health care, how do dietetic professionals know that their education, training, and credentialing will enable them to provide safe, effective food and nutrition services to the public? One way to answer this question is through role delineation studies.

ROLE DELINEATION STUDIES

A role delineation study is research undertaken to answer the question: How do we know who does what in the workplace? The major reason for conducting such studies is to develop empirical data to prove that licensure and credentialing examinations reflect knowledge and skills necessary for safe, competent professional practice. A role delineation study is a survey. Usually, it is a questionnaire mailed to people who practice in a particular profession or perform a specific type of work. Respondents answer questionnaires designed to describe what they do now or anticipate doing in the future as they fulfill their job responsibilities.

The first comprehensive role delineation studies in dietetics were completed by the ADA in the 1980s. From these came three publications that described the work of dietitians in three areas of practice: community dietetics, food service systems management, and clinical dietetics. These reports specified what dietitians in each area of practice should be doing, based on information gathered from panels of experienced practitioners representing various areas of dietetic practice and various work settings.

Dietetic technicians were well represented in dietetic practice by the time a second role delineation study was undertaken in 1988–89.[5] In fact, registration for dietetic technicians was implemented in 1987. Answers were sought for several questions. One question was related to the work of dietitians and dietetic technicians to determine what they were doing in various practice settings. Another area of inquiry was to find out what differences existed between the roles of dietitians and dietetic technicians. Yet another was to determine the effect of years of experience on the roles and responsibilities of dietitians and dietetic technicians. The results of this study demonstrated that differences between the work of dietitians and dietetic technicians occurred in level of responsibility rather than the work assigned to each professional. In other words, both dietitians and dietetic technicians had the knowledge and skills to undertake all the basic tasks in dietetics—nutrition, food service management, education. The difference or delineation occurred because dietitians were found to perform these tasks at a higher level than dietetic technicians. This meant that in clinical nutrition settings, dietetic technicians were likely to be assigned to patients requiring routine, uncomplicated nutrition care, but dietitians were likely to have responsibility for patients with complex conditions and critical care needs. In a food service management setting, dietetic technicians were likely to be performing routine management and supervision tasks, whereas dietitians were more involved in policy setting and advising.

The ADA's 1988 role delineation study included 129 activities that a dietetic professional would be expected to perform. An example of an activity was: "Calculate nutrient intakes." Other activities are listed in Table 6–2. Respondents to the questionnaire answered three questions about each activity:

- The nature of the person's involvement in each activity. Respondents were asked to indicate whether they were involved in the activity, and if so, whether the involvement was as an advisor, policy setter, supervisor, or performer (meaning that the respondent was responsible for doing the task).

Table 6–1 Comparison of Characteristics of Professional Members of the Dietetic Manpower

	Dietary Managers	Dietetic Technicians	Dietitians
Education/Training	Postsecondary education program approved by Dietary Managers Association (DMA) (site-based or independent study*) for those employed in food service positions: 120 clock hours classroom instruction 150 clock hours supervised field experience	2-year community college programs, approved by ADA (site-based or independent study) for full- or part-time students who may or may not be employed in food service positions: Associate degree (ADA-approved) including 450 clock hours of supervised field experience or Graduates of BS degree/ADA-approved didactic program in dietetics who add the supervised field experience component from an ADA-approved dietetic technician program	4-year baccalaureate degree from an ADA-approved *didactic program in dietetics* consisting of: Baccalaureate degree (ADA-approved) and ADA-accredited supervised preprofessional experience (at least 900 clock hours), usually administered through a different institution or 4-year baccalaureate degree from an ADA-accredited *coordinated program in dietetics* consisting of: Baccalaureate degree including 900 hours supervised reprofessional experience administered through the degree-granting institution

continues

Table 6–1 continued

	Dietary Managers	Dietetic Technicians	Dietitians
Degree Attained	None; although some dietary managers could have earned degrees previously from 2- or 4-year colleges. One route to eligibility to take the certified dietary manager (CDM) examination is to have a BS degree in nutrition	Associate degree (graduates of a 2-year ADA-approved dietetic technician program) Baccalaureate degree (graduates of a 4-year ADA-approved didactic program in dietetics)	Baccalaureate degree Master's degree (in some universities the coordinated programs and the supervised preprofessional experience programs are at the graduate degree level)
Credential	CDM National examination administered by the Certifying Board of Dietary Managers	DTR National examination administered by the Commission on Dietetic Registration (CDR)	RD National examination administered by the CDR
Professional Organization	DMA One Pierce Place, Suite 1220W Itasca, IL 60143-1277	The ADA 216 West Jackson Boulevard Chicago, IL 60606-6995	The ADA 216 West Jackson Boulevard Chicago, IL 60606-6995
Primary Employment Opportunities	Long-term care facilities Life care centers Hospitals Schools Correctional facilities	Hospitals Long-term care facilities Community nutrition programs	Hospitals Long-term care facilities Community nutrition programs Corporations (e.g., pharmaceutical, food manufacturers, food distributors, contract management) Self-employment

continues

Table 6–1 continued

Type of Work		
Manages/supervises food service operations	Supervises/provides patient/client nutrition services Supervises/manages food service operations Provides nutrition education	Manages/provides patient/client nutrition services Manages food service operations Develops/provides nutrition education programs Manages dietetic consulting services

*These programs are also called *correspondence* or *distance learning.*

Table 6–2 Professional Activities of Entry-Level Registered Dietitians (ELRD), Experienced Registered Dietitians (BELRD), and Dietetic Technicians (DTR) (as reported by 50 percent or more of respondents to the 1989 role delineation study)

Numbers in each column represent percentage of respondents who reported performing these activities.

Food and Nutrition-Related Activities	ELRD (%)	BELRD (%)	DTR (%)
Clinical nutrition-related activities			
Identify nutrition-related needs	90	82	77
Teach/counsel clients/families	88	79	66
Document client care	86	76	73
Calculate nutrient intake	85	76	70
Evaluate food-related behavior of clients	85	75	64
Confer with physicians about client care	85	75	<50
Compare biochemical data with expected values	84	71	50
Calculate nutrient requirements	83	70	52
Adapt oral diets to individual needs	82	72	75
Assess learning needs of clients	82	71	<50
Review medical record for nutrition data	81	72	72
Take preliminary diet histories	80	69	74
Take comprehensive diet histories	79	69	61
Plan oral diets with multiple modifications	79	69	64
Refer clients to other sources of help	79	69	<50
Monitor physiological status of clients	76	65	<50
Evaluate intake of specific nutrients	76	68	55
Prescribe supplements for oral diets	75	64	53
Evaluate influence of psychological status on eating	75	67	<50
Participate in the health care team	72	63	54
Monitor quality of care	69	69	51
Diagnose nutrition problems	67	60	<50
Prescribe oral diets	63	53	<50
Prescribe enteral products	57	<50	<50
Assist clients with menu selections	56	<50	64
Perform anthropometric measurements	54	<50	<50
Monitor changes in body composition	53	<50	<50
Compare physical development with charts	52	<50	<50
Community nutrition-related activities			
Provide nutrition education to groups	79	75	<50
Prepare educational materials for groups	75	70	<50
Management-related activities			
Develop menus for clients—special needs	65	68	57
Assess client satisfaction with menus	63	64	82
Monitor quality of service	55	64	68

continues

Table 6–2 continued

Food and Nutrition-Related Activities	ELRD (%)	BELRD (%)	DTR (%)
Conduct staff training and development	51	64	<50
Develop menus for clients—normal needs	55	63	59
Monitor food quality	52	57	67
Select products to be purchased	<50	56	<50
Maintain safety and sanitation in food	<50	55	65
Counsel staff	<50	54	<50
Develop job descriptions	<50	53	<50
Monitor staff compliance with regulations	<50	52	<50
Check trays for accuracy	<50	<50	67

Source: M.T. Kane et al., Role Delineation for Dietetic Practitioners: Empirical Results. Copyright The American Dietetic Association. Adapted by permission from *Journal of The American Dietetic Association*, Vol. 90, pp. 1124–1133, © 1990.

- Frequency of the performance of each activity. Respondents were asked to indicate whether they were involved in the task less than once a month, monthly, weekly, daily, or more than once a day.
- Importance or criticality of the activity. Respondents rated the consequences of their involvement in each activity, especially with respect to risks associated with poor performance of the task.

Role delineation results reported for RDs were divided into two groups. Data were reported for entry-level RDs (ELRD) with zero to three years of experience, and beyond-entry-level RDs (BELRDs) with more than three years of experience. Nearly half the ELRDs reported that they worked in acute care hospitals, assigned to inpatient services. Other major employment settings were outpatient clinics and community nutrition programs. Not many ELRDs reported having financial responsibility. In fact, only 12 percent were responsible for preparing budgets. Therefore, most ELRDs can expect their first jobs to include assignment to providing clinical nutrition services.

Specific activity categories in which ELRDs were involved are listed below. The percentages given refer to the number of respondents reporting involvement in each type of activity. A respondent could report involvement in more than one activity. So for the first category in the list, more than two-thirds of the ELRDs said they were involved in providing nutrition care to individuals. Only one-third said they were involved in managing food and other material resources; and so on, down to approximately one-tenth who reported involvement in research, a group that probably included ELRDs completing their master's degrees as well as ELRDs assigned to in-house cost-benefit and quality assurance studies.

- Providing nutrition care to individuals—68 percent
- Managing food and other material resources—33 percent
- Providing nutrition programs for groups—32 percent
- Teaching dietitians, other professionals, and/or students—32 percent
- Managing human resources—25 percent
- Marketing services and products—21 percent
- Managing financial resources—18 percent
- Managing facilities (intradepartmental physical facilities)—16 percent
- Conducting research—11 percent

The specific nutrition care activities that are most likely to be assigned to an ELRD are listed in Exhibit 6–1.

As the ELRD gains experience, roles and responsibilities change. The number of experienced dietitians (BELRD) who reported providing nutrition care to individuals declined slightly, to 59 percent. All task categories related to management increased, demonstrating that as RDs gain experience, they also become more involved with management activities. Only three categories, dietitians in community nutrition, education, and research, showed very little change in involvement over time. The specific activities that more experienced dietitians were most likely to be doing are listed in the BELRD column in Table 6–2.

In the community nutrition area of practice, dietitians, regardless of experience, were much more likely than dietetic technicians to be involved with community nutrition programs, health promotion, and media work.

These data clearly show that as dietitians gain experience, many accepted management responsibilities. The following changes occurred:

- Their position titles reflected increased responsibility (e.g., Director of Clinical Nutrition Services, Director of Food and Nutrition Services).
- Their administrative assignments involved supervision of other dietitians, dietetic technicians, and departmental employees.
- They were given responsibility for setting policies.
- They had budget preparation responsibility.

Activities most frequently reported by dietetic technicians are found in Exhibit 6–1. In descending order of frequency, dietetic technicians reported activities in these categories:

- Providing nutrition care to individuals—47 percent
- Managing food and other material resources—42 percent

Exhibit 6–1 Specific Nutrition Care Activities Most Likely To Be Performed by Entry-Level Registered Dietitians and Entry-Level Dietetic Technicians

Entry-Level Registered Dietitians Nutrition-Related Activities

Screen and assess clients
    Identify nutrition-related needs.
    Assess learning needs.
    Review medical record for nutrition data.
    Take diet histories—preliminary and comprehensive.
    Evaluate intake of specific nutrients.
    Compare biochemical data with expected values.
    Evaluate food-related behavior of clients, including psychological influences.
    Calculate nutrient requirements.
    Calculate nutrient intake.

Provide nutrition services to clients
    Document client care.
    Assist clients with menu selections.
    Adapt oral diets to individual needs.
    Plan oral diets with multiple modifications.
    Prescribe supplements for oral diets.
    Monitor physiological status of patients.
    Teach/counsel clients/families.
    Prepare and provide education programs to groups.

Use team approach to client care
    Participate in the health care team.
    Confer with physicians concerning client care.
    Refer clients to other sources of help.

Entry-level dietetic technicians   Nutrition-related activities.

Screen and assess clients
    Identify nutrition-related needs.
    Review medical record for nutrition data.
    Take preliminary diet histories.
    Calculate nutrient intakes.

Provide nutrition services to clients
    Document client care.
    Adapt oral diets to individual needs.
    Assess client satisfaction with menus.

Source: M.T. Kane et al., Role Delineation for Dietetic Practitioners: Empirical Results. Copyright The American Dietetic Association. Adapted by permission from *Journal of The American Dietetic Association*, Vol. 90, pp. 1124–1133, © 1990.

- Managing human resources—23 percent
- Managing facilities (intradepartmental physical facilities)—19 percent
- Managing financial resources—14 percent
- Providing nutrition programs for population groups—11 percent
- Teaching dietitians and other professionals/students—9 percent
- Marketing services and products—8 percent
- Conducting research—3 percent

Dietetic technicians are most likely to work in positions in which they provide nutrition services to hospital and nursing home patients. Compared with ELRDs, dietetic technicians are more likely to have management responsibilities. This reflects the fact that dietetic technicians are frequently employed in hospital and nursing home food service management positions. These and other work settings are listed in Table 6–3.

Overall, the 1989 role delineation study pointed out very important differences between the work done by ELRDs and BELRDs and between dietetic technicians and dietitians. Results from the study provided insights into the types of activities performed by dietetic team members and work settings. Dietitians and dietetic

Table 6–3 Comparison of Work Settings between Entry-Level Registered Dietitians (ELRD), Experienced Registered Dietitians (BELRD), and Registered Dietetic Technicians (DTR)

Work Settings	ELRD (%)	BELRD (%)	DTR (%)
Clinical dietetics—hospitals	48	33	38
Clinical dietetics—long-term care	18	16	29
Community nutrition	21	17	11
Outpatient nutrition counseling	28	23	3
Hospital food service	16	20	33
Long-term care food service	13	16	33
College faculty	6	9	<1
Consulting—private practice	6	8	2
Consulting—health care facilities	5	12	<1
Consulting—other	4	5	1
Other food service operations	6	11	10
Food companies	1	2	1
Pharmaceutical companies	<1	<1	<1
Other	10	10	7

Note: Some respondents reported more than one work setting.

Source: M.T. Kane et al., Role Delineation for Dietetic Practitioners: Empirical Results. Copyright The American Dietetic Association. Adapted by permission from *Journal of The American Dietetic Association*, Vol. 90, pp. 1124–1133, © 1990.

technicians performed similar activities but at different levels that seemed to reflect the different levels of education and training required for dietitians and dietetic technicians.

PRACTICE AUDIT

The commission on dietetic registration updated the 1989 role delineation study with a practice audit in 1995.[6] Similar in many respects to the 1989 study, a slightly different focus in the 1995 study precludes direct comparisons between the two. Generally, results from the 1995 audit confirmed those from the earlier role delineation study.

Acute care hospitals, long-term care facilities, and community nutrition programs remain the most common work settings for dietitians and dietetic technicians. However, as hospitals eliminate duplicated services and inpatient services focus more on caring for the very sick, more dietitians reported employment in outpatient facilities than in 1989.

The category of clinical services was the most frequently reported function for dietitians (67 percent) and dietetic technicians (72 percent). The practice audit specified only 22 activity areas (compared with 129 tasks listed in the 1989 role delineation study). Results of the activities in clinical services for ELRDs and entry-level dietetic technicians (ELDT) showed the following: For all functions, the ELRDs reported a higher level of responsibility than the ELDTs.

- Nutrition screening and assessment: 89 percent of ELRDs and 87 percent of ELDTs
- Provision of nutrition care to individuals: 88 percent of ELRDs and 87 percent of ELDTs
- Nutrition care plans for individuals: 88 percent of ELRDs and 81 percent of ELDTs
- Nutrition education and counseling of individuals: 87 percent of ELRDs and 69 percent of ELDTs

More dietetic technicians (48 percent) than dietitians (20 percent) reported performing food service management functions. However, more dietitians (25 percent) than dietetic technicians (13 percent) performed public health/community nutrition functions. This pattern also was apparent in the wellness/disease prevention function: 22 percent of the dietitians and 8 percent of dietetic technicians.

The 1995 practice audit confirmed that as dietitians and dietetic technicians gain experience, they were more likely to assume responsibility for managing financial resources and for performing other management tasks.

Dietitians and dietetic technicians performed similar work, but the major difference between the two dietetic team members occurred in the level of responsibility. For all 22 areas of activity examined in the practice audit, dietitians reported higher levels of responsibility than dietetic technicians. This difference was clearest in comparing responsibilities for enteral and parenteral nutrition, nutrition education to public groups, and research activities.

No role delineation or practice audit studies comparing dietitians, dietetic technicians, and dietary managers have been published. It is therefore not possible to make empirical comparisons of the role of dietary managers in dietetic practice or as members of dietetic teams.

CONCLUSION

The practice of dietetics has three components:

- nutrition and food services in health and disease
- management of food and other resources
- education of patients/clients, the public, students, and other health professionals

The very first dietitians were expected to perform all these tasks. During an era of hospital and health care expansion in the 1950s, dietitians met the demand for their services by training promising employees to perform routine dietetic responsibilities. These employees, the first nondietitian members of the dietetic team, were formally designated food service supervisors. More recent titles were dietetic assistant, dietary manager, and currently, CDM.

Dietetic technicians are graduates of two-year associate degree programs. Through the commission on dietetic registration, dietetic technicians may take a national credentialing examination and, if successful, use the credential DTR. They are capable of performing many of the same tasks as an RD but at a different level of responsibility.

Dietitians, dietetic technicians, and dietary managers are the professionally qualified members of the intradepartmental dietetic team. All dietetic professionals should also function at various levels as part of interdepartmental teams involved in patient care. Indeed, dietitians and dietetic technicians do their most effective work as members of a team.

Although many dietetic professionals work in acute care hospitals and are assigned to clinical nutrition responsibilities, there are also employment opportunities for dietetic professionals in long-term facilities, community nutrition programs, and other work settings.

Role delineation studies have clarified roles and responsibilities of dietitians and dietetic technicians in various work settings and at various stages of experience. The primary responsibility for entry-level practitioners is provision of clinical nutrition services (nutrition assessment, planning, and care) to individuals in various types of health care facilities. All ELDTs are more likely than ELRDs to work in food service settings, but as all practitioners gain experience, they accept positions with increasing levels of responsibility in which management skills and knowledge are essential for success. Dietitians and dietetic technicians, however, are distinct in their roles, responsibilities, and contributions to the dietetic manpower team.

DEFINITIONS

Associate Degree Degree granted by a two-year postsecondary educational institution, usually a community college.

Clinical Nutrition Nutrition services provided to patients in health care settings, usually including assessment of nutritional status, development of treatment plans, and some form of dietary modification; term often used with respect to nutrition therapy for disease states.

Empirical Data Information developed from observation or experience of actual events.

Health Care Facility Hospitals, nursing homes, outpatient clinics, rehabilitation centers, public health clinics, and similar organizations in which health services are available.

Interdepartmental Between different departments.

Intradepartmental Within the same department.

Outsourced Service formerly provided by an organization's employees that is contracted to an independent supplier.

REFERENCES

1. Manion J, Lorimer W, Leander WJ. *Team-Based Health Care Organizations: Blueprint for Success.* Gaithersburg, MD: Aspen Publishers, Inc.; 1996.
2. ADA. *The Profession of Dietetics: Report of the Study Commission on Dietetics.* Chicago: The American Dietetic Association; 1972.

3. MacEachern MT. The hospital dietary department—a forecast. *J Am Diet Assoc.* 1925;1:3–8.

4. Arkwright MS, Collins ME, Sharp JL, Yakel RM. Titles, definitions and responsibilities for the profession of dietetics—1974. *J Am Diet Assoc.* 1974;64:661–665.

5. Kane MT, Estes CA, Colton DA, Eltoft CS. Role delineation for dietetic practitioners: empirical results. *J Am Diet Assoc.* 1990;90:1124–1133.

6. Kane MT, Cohen AS, Smith ER, Lewis C, et al. 1995 commission on dietetic registration dietetics practice audit. *J Am Diet Assoc.* 1996;96:1292–1301.

CHAPTER 7

The American Dietetic Association

Margaret L. Bogle and Kathy Stone

"In the history of the dietetics profession, there have never been more diverse or more interesting opportunities for dietitians and dietetic technicians. New levels of competence will continue to open doors in food and nutrition arenas."[1]

Outline—Chapter 7

- Introduction

- Strategic Framework of the Association
  - Member initiative
  - Public initiative
  - Policy initiative

- Membership Categories
  - Benefits of membership

- Governance of the Association
  - Board of Directors
  - House of Delegates
  - Council on Practice (Former)
  - Dietetic practice groups
  - Restructuring
  - Commission on Accreditation/Approval of Dietetic Education
  - Commission on Dietetic Registration
  - Election of Officers

- Affiliated Units of The American Dietetic Association

INTRODUCTION

The American Dietetic Association (ADA), formed by a small group of dietitians in 1917 stands as the professional organization of more than 60,000 food and nutrition experts. In the 80 years since its founding, the association has been the major forum for the networking of dietitians, presentation of research related to food and nutrition, and the political activities necessary to govern this large organization.[2,3] (See Chapter 1 for historical perspective.)

Although the original constitution and bylaws of the association have been amended frequently, the focus of the association has remained constant from the beginning: *maintaining a concern for the continuing interests of dietitians and dietetic professionals in their education, practice opportunities, and research for the future.* Ensuring that these professionals are able to protect the nutritional health and well-being of the public was formalized with the registration process in 1969 but was evident in the earliest deliberations of the association and continues today, through the commission on dietetic registration (CDR) and its focus on lifelong education of the dietitian presented in the document "Professional Development 2001: Guide to Proposed Recertification System."[4]

The association has always sought external study and validation of their efforts on behalf of the profession and individual practitioners. This was evidenced best by the commissioning of two study groups, in 1972 and again in 1984.[5,6]

The first commission was instructed (1) to review and evaluate the resources and potential of the profession, (2) to identify areas for growth and enhancement, and (3) to determine and recommend improved methods and techniques for providing dietetic services. By using a futuristic approach, the commission was directed to assess the role of the association and to critically review the organizational structure with reference to the association's being able to meet the needs of the members. Recommendations were studied and implemented by the association in areas of education, practice, certification of practitioners, and organizational structure.

The 1984 commission report indicates that it was charged as a follow-up study to determine what portions of the 1972 recommendations had been implemented, what findings or problems identified in the first report still existed, and an assessment of current status of education and practice. Further, the second commission was asked to explore future directions of the association and the profession in an ever-changing society.

The terms *The American Dietetic Association* and *profession of dietetics* have become almost synonymous, as evidenced by the published reports. This clearly shows the long-standing concerns of the two groups as similar: protection of the public in areas of nutritional health and disease prevention and the welfare of the practitioner (or individual member). The organization of the association and the leadership of elected members have worked through the years to keep these concerns in focus.

The current mission statement of the ADA sums up this important concept: *The American Dietetic Association is the advocate of the dietetics profession, serving the public through the promotion of optimal nutrition, health, and well-being.* It is this mission that sets the agenda of the association and its programs.

The vision of the association is: *Members of The American Dietetic Association will shape the food choices and improve the nutritional status of the public.* This vision delineates the responsibility of each member for professional practice and sets the stage for the philosophy statement of ADA: *Members of The American Dietetic Association serve the profession best by serving the public first.*

These statements along with the agreed on values—excellence, leadership, integrity, respect, communication, collaboration, fiscal responsibility, and action—form the basis for this most successful organization of dietetic professionals.

STRATEGIC FRAMEWORK OF THE ASSOCIATION

The 1996–99 strategic framework is entitled "Creating the Future" and established the proactive position of the association. This plan is directed toward providing members with professional strategies and skills to move forward into the twenty-first century as the recognized experts in food and nutrition. Three initiatives are identified: members, public, and policy.

Member Initiative

The member initiative will concentrate on adapting skills and expertise to new career opportunities made possible by technologies, the information revolution, and changes in health care and services.

Public Initiative

The public initiative will continue the efforts of the association to position the association and its members as the authoritative voice on scientifically sound food and nutrition information. Recognition of the registered dietitian (RD) as the person who provides appropriate food and nutrition information for medical nutrition therapy continues to be a goal. It is especially relevant today at a time when food and nutrition fads and fallacies continue to proliferate at a rapid pace.

One ongoing program that supports the public initiative, "The Ambassador Media Spokesperson" program, was started in 1982 with the cooperation and financial support of an industry partner. The ADA selects individual members to be ambassadors in various media markets across the United States. They are given extensive training in print, radio, and television media for them to be spokespersons for ADA. They are quoted in many newspapers, participate in radio presentations as well as appear on local and national television programs. All activities further the image of the dietitian as the expert in food and nutrition.

Policy Initiative

The policy initiative is designed to promote the continuation of the association and its work with policy makers at state and national levels. This includes legislative efforts, support of existing food and nutrition-related policies, and the drafting of new legislation (especially in the area of reimbursement for medical nutrition therapy) important to all dietetic practitioners.

MEMBERSHIP CATEGORIES

Membership in the ADA currently exists for the following categories: active, associate, retired, returning student, and honorary (Appendix F).

The largest category is active member, which, in general, includes persons who have bachelor's or advanced degrees and meet academic requirements specified by ADA; or are RDs; or those who have completed a supervised practice program accredited/approved by the commission on accreditation/approval of dietetic education (CAADE). In addition, dietetic technicians who are registered (DTR) by CDR; or have completed an associate program accredited/approved by CAADE; or meet the academic requirements specified by ADA with a CAADE-approved dietetic technician program experience are eligible. Any person who has completed a term as president of the association or one who has previously paid dues to obtain "life" membership is also an "active member."

The associate member category is an option for those persons with a bachelor's degree meeting ADA academic requirements but not eligible for active membership. Undergraduate or associate degree students enrolled in a CAADE-accredited/approved program; or graduate students meeting the minimum academic requirements in a CAADE-approved/accredited program may also apply for associate membership. Others qualifying for the associate category are students in supervised practice programs accredited/approved by CAADE or those students who are enrolled in regionally accredited, postsecondary education programs that are *not* approved/accredited by CAADE. A student should consult the current bylaws of ADA for additional information on this and all categories of membership.[7]

The third category, retired members, is available to any member of ADA who is no longer employed in dietetic practice or education and is at least 62 years of age and to those members retired on total (permanent) disability.

The returning student member is open to any active member returning to school on a full-time basis and working toward a degree in a dietetic-related course of study. The category of honorary member is reserved for persons who have made notable contributions to the field of nutrition and dietetics. They must receive an invitation to become an honorary member from the ADA board of directors (BOD).

The dues, rights, and privileges of each of the membership categories appear in the bylaws of ADA.[7] The dues may change from year to year by two-thirds vote of the members of the house of delegates (HOD). The student should review the current bylaws of the association for additional details. The dues are different for each category, with a portion of the national dues offsetting the cost of the *Journal of The American Dietetic Association* and the *ADA Courier* and a rebate returned to the state affiliate association for each member from that state. In addition, the 28 national dietetic practice groups (DPG) charge for membership in their groups and provide newsletters and other educational materials for members in the specific practice areas.[7]

Benefits of Membership

Membership in the association benefits the individual and collective members in many ways. For example:

- quality standards for entry-level education
- 28 practice groups for networking in specific areas of practice
- positions on food and nutrition issues
- the annual meeting and exhibition (showcasing the latest in technology and products from more than 300 leading food and nutrition organizations)
- credentialing programs for technician, entry-level, specialty, and advanced-level practice
- monthly issues of the *Journal of The American Dietetic Association* (providing peer-reviewed articles on current food and nutrition research and practice)

- the *Courier*, which features association news
- peer-reviewed educational materials for use in the practice of dietetics
- collaboration with international groups promoting global nutrition activities

Benefits from the ADA Foundation and the National Center for Nutrition and Dietetics (NCND) are discussed later in this chapter.

GOVERNANCE OF THE ASSOCIATION

The organizational structure of the association has changed over time; however, in general the governance has been through "volunteers" who are elected from the members-at-large to office serving as the BOD, an HOD representing the membership of state affiliates, and an executive director/chief operations officer to oversee and manage a paid staff at the "headquarters" office in Chicago.

In recent years, under the leadership of Beverly Bajus, chief operating officer, the paid staff have become "partners" with the various volunteer groups, forming "teams" to accomplish the variety of tasks necessary to keep the organization functional and implement the strategic plan.

Board of Directors

At the present time, the BOD is composed of the president, president-elect, the secretary/treasurer, the speaker of the HOD, the speaker-elect, the president of the ADA Foundation, the chief operating officer, and five directors elected at large and two public members elected by the BOD. The BOD meets regularly throughout the year to conduct the business of the association. The chairs of CDR and CAADE serve on the BOD ex officio without vote.

The BOD is responsible for the association's mission and vision, broad policy making, and governance. In addition, the board manages the property and fiscal affairs (budget); directs the implementation of approved actions and programs; and monitors outcomes of the association's activities and programs. Numerous other specific functions are listed in the bylaws.[7] Much of the business of the board is accomplished through the following committees: executive, budget and fiscal affairs, legislative and public policy, diversity, and scholarship.

House of Delegates

The HOD is presided over by the speaker. Membership in the house from each of the 50 states, Puerto Rico, and the American Overseas Dietetic Association is based on numbers of members in the state, with each state affiliate having at least one representative, or delegate, as they are called. States with more than 250 members will have more than one delegate. In addition, the council on professional issues sends five delegates, one each for research and education and three from practice areas as follows: food and nutrition management, clinical nutrition, and consultation and business practices. Three dietetic technicians, elected at large, also serve as delegates. The HOD is divided into seven regions, with a coordinator elected from each region by the members in that region. These area coordinators, the speaker, and speaker-elect provide the leadership for the HOD. The HOD meets at least yearly at the annual meeting of the association and frequently convenes a midyear meeting when activity warrants an additional meeting.

The council on professional issues is charged with representing all areas of practice and DPGs. The council consists of 15 delegates; 8 representing practice; 3 representing education; 3 representing research; and 1 dietetic technician-at-large. The council meets at the time of the house meeting plus one additional meeting per year. Functions of the council include

- fostering leadership and management skills among dietetic professionals
- developing, approving, and evaluating standards of education in collaboration with CAADE
- providing direction for advancement of research activities
- evaluating and maintaining standards of practice
- managing the formation, merger, or dissolution of DPGs

Council on Practice (Former)

The bylaws of ADA adopted in 1977 established the Council on Practice (COP). As an outgrowth of the special interest groups, COP was charged with the issues of dietetic practice. This resulted in the development of standards of practice (for practitioners) and practice criteria sets for guiding practice in specific diseases and conditions. The COP was organized initially into five divisions of practice: clinical dietetics and research, management practice, community dietetics, and education and dietetic consultation. Ultimately, the education and research areas were combined, leaving clinical nutrition as a separate division, and consultation and business practice became a division. This reflected the changes that were occurring in practice at the time. At the same time that the divisions were forming, the special interest groups that were in existence were renamed DPGs. In 1978, 13 groups applied for formal recognition as DPGs, which required at least 50 member signatures on a petition for recognition.[8]

The COP had several standing committees that produced significant documents relative to the practice of dietetics. In addition to facilitating the activities of the DPGs, the COP was identifying continuing education needs and opportunities, establishing and monitoring quality assurance guidelines, and identifying methods for the recognition of the dietetic practitioner. The COP was also instrumental in establishing recognition of specialty practice through certification of specialists in renal, pediatric, and metabolic nutrition and advanced-level practice through the fellow program of the ADA (FADA).[9,10] (See Chapter 5 for additional information on the certification process of specialists and fellows.)

The quality management (QM) committee was established in 1979, first as the quality assurance committee and later renamed. This committee participated in several diverse quality management–related projects for the DPGs and ADA. This committee was initiated by and resided within the COP until its formal incorporation into the HOD as a committee of the house in 1996. The first QM committee included six members representing management, clinical, consulting, community, education, and dietetic technician practice areas. Also represented on the committee were members from the council on education, the legislative advisory committee, and the ADA liaison to the Joint Commission on Accreditation of Hospital Organizations (the Joint Commission).

The QM committee has had direct influence in the shaping of several Joint Commission standards for hospital food service and patient nutrition care and assisted in the analysis of standards for revision of several accreditation manuals, including those for mental health, ambulatory care, and long-term care. The committee also conducted training workshops for QM representatives of DPGs and state dietetic associations. This committee assumed the task of documenting the quality and value of dietetic services for the association. The importance of this task has evolved into major proportions with the dramatic changes in health care in the United States.

Standards of Dietetic Practice

To evaluate the quality of dietetic services, it is necessary for each practitioner to adhere to nationally recognized standards of practice. The standards of practice for ADA were developed by the QA committee to assist the individual practitioner in systematically planning, implementing, evaluating, and adapting performance regardless of area of practice.[11] The standards were published in 1986 to assist practitioners in providing quality care and were broad statements that continue to be used. The DPGs used these standards of practice to develop criteria sets by which their specific areas of practice could be evaluated. The six Standards of Practice are:[11]

1. Establishing performance criteria, comparing actual performance with expected performance, documenting results, and taking appropriate action.

2. Developing, implementing, and evaluating an individual plan for practice based on assessment of consumer needs, current knowledge, and clinical experience.
3. Utilizing unique knowledge of nutrition, collaborating with other professionals, personnel, and/or consumers in integrating, interrepting, and communicating nutrition care principles.
4. Engaging in life-long self development to improve knowledge and skills.
5. Generating, interpreting, and using research to enhance dietetic practice.
6. Identifying, monitoring, analyzing, and justifying the use of resources.

Dietetic Practice Guidelines

Practice guidelines define how dietetic care and services are delivered. They are a set of statements or specifications that help practitioners or patients/clients choose appropriate dietetic services. They may relate to any area of practice.[12] These guidelines outline preferred protocols or practice patterns and often address prevention and/or treatment of specific diseases or conditions. Practice guidelines are validated through extensive field testing by a pool of practitioners using their day-to-day practice.

The DPGs published numerous sets of practice guidelines for various practice settings. For example, the renal dietitians DPG has published nine sets of guidelines for the care of renal patients. The goal of these guidelines is to help dietitians provide acceptable minimum and uniform nutrition care and to assess the efficacy of nutrition care provided to patients with end-stage renal disease.

Clinical Indicators

Clinical indicators are measurement tools used to monitor and evaluate key aspects of patient care. The indicators include processes, treatments, and high-frequency aspects of patient care. Clinical indicators describe events, complications, or outcomes. Nutrition intervention of patients who are not receiving food or are on clear liquid diets beyond a certain number of days without nutrition support is an example of a clinical indicator.

Dietetic Practice Groups

In 1970, the HOD discussed the concept of members forming special interest groups. By 1971, there were 10 groups of ADA members networking within their special interest groups or areas of practice. In 1975, the special interest groups were visible within the association sharing the values, broad interests, and mission of ADA while focusing on the needs of their respective members. Many members belonged to more than one special interest group, depending on their individual needs for networking.

Currently, there are 28 DPGs.[13] Exhibit 7–1 shows the diversity of the practice areas included.

Each of these groups network to serve members working in or having an interest in a particular area of nutrition practice. Members join DPGs by checking the appropriate category on the ADA membership renewal form and paying a fee for each DPG selected. Many members continue membership in more than one DPG.

Formation of new DPGs occurs after interest groups become large enough to seek official status. A petition is submitted with no less than 500 signatures indicating interest to form a DPG and specifying individuals willing to serve as officers for the first year plus a budget. A minimum number of members (300) is

Exhibit 7–1 Dietetic Practice Groups

- Public Health Nutrition (PHNPG)
- Gerontological Nutritionists (GN)
- Dietetics in Developmental and Psychiatric Disorders (DDPD)
- Vegetarian Nutrition (VN)
- Hunger and Malnutrition (HM)
- Environmental Nutrition (EN)
- Oncology Nutrition (ON)
- Renal Dietitians (RPG)
- Pediatric Nutrition (PNPG)
- Diabetes Care and Education (DCE)
- Dietitians in Nutrition Support (DNS)
- Dietetics in Physical Medicine and Rehabilitation (DPM&R)
- Dietitians in General Clinical Practice (DGCP)
- Perinatal Nutrition (PN)
- HIV/AIDS
- Nutrition Entrepreneurs (NE)
- Consultant Dietitians in Health Care Facilities (CD-HCF)
- Dietitians in Business and Communications (DBC)
- Sports, Cardiovascular, and Wellness Nutritionists (SCAN)
- Management in Health Care Systems (MHS)
- School Nutrition Services (SNS)
- Clinical Nutrition Management (CNM)
- Dietetic Technicians in Practice (DTP)
- Food and Culinary Professionals (FCP)
- Dietetic Educators of Practitioners (DEP)
- Nutrition Educators of Health Professionals (NEHP)
- Nutrition Education for the Public (NEP)
- Research

required to maintain official status. Aside from maintaining a minimum number of members, the DPGs have other uniform requirements. These include publication of a newsletter at least quarterly for their members, maintaining governing documents, showing evidence of tangible benefits to their members, conducting an annual meeting of the members, and maintaining a balanced budget. Other optional services provided by some DPGs include catalog production of member-produced products for marketing to other dietitians and the public, annual seminars or workshops, tools for member use to educate clients, mentoring activities, tape-lending libraries, and numerous articles and publications discussing topics of interest in a specific area of practice.

DPGs are also involved in many alliances with organizations with whom ADA or the DPGs have a formal contract. Activities are coordinated through ADA's alliance program and include joint projects, attendance at meetings, and sharing of information and expertise.

Membership in DPGs, because of the opportunity to network within a smaller group of professionals with similar interests, provides tremendous member satisfaction and contributes to the high membership renewal rate that ADA enjoys. The fact that DPGs are a national network affords an opportunity to discuss ideas with members who may have different experiences because of geographic location and allows members to spot trends earlier based on these networking situations. DPGs provide significant opportunities for leadership responsibilities both within the DPG and the greater association.

Restructuring

In 1992, the BOD began discussing the concept of restructuring the association. The concept was based on streamlining decision making and improving efficiency and coordination of the ADA units. Ultimately, the HOD passed a revision to the bylaws in 1995 that positioned the COP in the HOD and made the QM committee a committee of the house. Instead of three separate councils: council on research, council on education, and council on practice; a council on professional issues was created with representation in the HOD. Thus, the COP, as such, was replaced, although its activities continued.

The implementation became effective March 1996. The speaker and speaker-elect of the house are representatives of practice, research, and education to the BOD. The former divisions of the COP are now represented in the HOD by nationally elected delegates for education, research, and practice.

Commission on Accreditation/Approval of Dietetic Education

The review and maintenance of educational standards and the monitoring of educational programs is accomplished through CAADE, chaired by a member elected at large. This commission conducts its business with the use of three review panels whose chairs are elected at large: the panel to approve didactic programs in dietetics, the panel on accreditation of dietetic internships, and the panel on accreditation of coordinated programs. Other panels may be utilized as needed. Volunteer members with experience in the various areas are selected to serve on these panels after extensive training. The commission acts autonomously from the association in rendering the approval of various programs. Procedures are in place for appeal of any decision of the commission.

Commission on Dietetic Registration

The CDR is another autonomous body and is responsible for ensuring the safety of the public through the credentialing of RD, DTRs, specialists (certified specialists [CS]), and FADAs. The CDR is composed of seven RDs and one DTR elected at large by the membership of ADA. In addition, one public member is appointed. Additional members are appointed to panels of the CDR to conduct their business (i.e., test panels, specialty and fellow panels, etc.). (See Chapter 5 for additional information on CDR activities.)

Election of Officers

The yearly ballot for election of officers and leaders is prepared by the nominating committee, which is elected by members of each area. Members serve for two years.

AFFILIATED UNITS OF THE AMERICAN DIETETIC ASSOCIATION

State and District Associations

Each of the 50 states and Puerto Rico are affiliates of ADA and are organized with state and district associations. Membership in ADA determines the membership in state affiliates as states charge no membership fees. A member of ADA is automatically a member of a state affiliate.

The state organizations for the most part parallel the national organization. Each state elects their delegates to represent them in the HOD. The number of district organizations is determined by the states as well as how they fit into the state organization. The district groups provide educational and informational programs for the grassroots members. Most states have one or two meetings per year that provide continuing education opportunities for the members. Delegates from the state affiliates take state and/or member issues to the HOD for all members to have input into the functioning of the ADA.

National Center for Nutrition and Dietetics

The association operates the NCND, which positions the dietetic professional as the food and nutrition expert. In addition, the center serves the public by providing objective nutrition information to consumers by promoting such programs as national nutrition month each year in March and consumer nutrition hot line. A recently instituted service provides consumers with an opportunity to speak with RDs through a 900 telephone number.

Another relatively new program is the nationwide nutrition network, which is available to RD member subscribers. This program provides opportunities for consumers, physicians, and businesses seeking nutrition services to be referred to RDs in their areas. More than 6,000 referrals were made to RDs in 1996.

The NCND provides a valuable service by providing The Good Nutrition Reading List, which presents resources available from libraries, ADA, and bookstores. Topics covered include food allergies and sensitivities, sports nutrition, diabetic meal planning, and many others. Other nutrition education materials for use by dietetic professionals are available by calling the NCND and ADA customer service 800-877-1600, extension 5800. Some materials are free and others are available at a nominal price plus shipping and handling charges.

The American Dietetic Association Foundation

Some of the programs of the NCND are sponsored by or underwritten financially by the ADA Foundation, which was responsible for beginning the formation of the center. The ADA Foundation was established in 1966 as a means of providing monies for scholarships for prospective dietetic students and for members to continue their graduate education through fellowships. In the ensuing years, the foundation has experienced tremendous financial growth through its alignment with corporate sponsors and through ADA member campaigns. This additional financial growth has allowed the foundation to give increasing numbers of scholarships and to provide funding for significant research projects needed by the association or the profession.

The foundation exists to further the mission of the association, especially in providing information to the public and consumers through the NCND. The current building, which houses the association, the foundation, and the NCND, was originally negotiated by the foundation and made possible by an extensive fund-raising effort.

Washington Office

Since 1986, the association has staffed an office in Washington, D.C., to further the legislative efforts of the profession. This allows the association to be in touch with legislative issues, relative to the profession, as they occur. Although these legislative and lobbying efforts required a tax status change for the association, the benefits are beginning to accrue to individual members directly and to consumers and the public indirectly. With the help of a large consultant firm in Washington, bills have been introduced in Congress that would allow for third-party reimbursement to registered dietitians for medical nutrition therapy. This collaborative effort has given much more visibility to the RD and the association through interaction with numerous federal agencies as well as Congress.

ADA SERVICES

This chapter attempts to give the student an appreciation of the ADA and its related programs. To keep current on new initiatives and programs of the association, the student is encouraged to read the publications of the association and those of DPGs (i.e., *Journal of The American Dietetic Association, ADA Courier)*, association bylaws, and various newsletters of the DPGs. In addition, the association has several books, pamphlets, and other nutrition materials for sale by contacting publications at 1-800-877-1600. These materials are also available at the annual meeting in the book mart.

CONCLUSION

The American Dietetic Association is the professional organization for dietitians. Its programs and initiatives spotlight the member, the public, and its role in policy making on behalf of members and the public. The ADA is governed by elected and appointed volunteer members of boards, commissions, and committees, all of whom perform specific functions according to the Bylaws of ADA.

Important as the functions are that ADA provides for members, the Association is recognized as the authoritative voice in reaching the public with guidance regarding food and nutrition issues. The third area, that of actively promoting policy that enhances the health and well being of all individuals, is accomplished through well organized activities both by members and by the Washington Legislative office.

The philosophy statement of ADA succinctly expresses how members relate to the profession for a larger purpose: "members of the ADA serve the profession best by serving the public first."

DEFINITIONS

Board of Directors The elected officers who perform specific functions in governing the association.

Bylaws Authoritative rules and regulations governing an association or group.

Chief Operating Officer Person employed by the association to direct the headquarters operations and implement the fiscal affairs of the association. May also serve as an official spokesperson for the association on direction of the board of directors.

Governance Activities involved in conducting the affairs of an organization.

House of Delegates Body of representatives elected by the states who establish the standards, membership requirements, and other professional issues for the association.

Strategic Framework Operational plans and strategies that shape the overall activities and function of an organization.

REFERENCES

1. Polly Fitz, President of The American Dietetic Association. 1997–1998.
2. Barber M. *History of The American Dietetic Association (1917–1959)*. Philadelphia: JB Lippincott Co; 1959.
3. Cassell J. *Carry the Flame: The History of The American Dietetic Association*. Chicago: The American Dietetic Association; 1990.
4. CDR professional development 2001: guide to proposed recertification system. *ADA Courier*. 1997;36(1).
5. ADA. *The Profession of Dietetics: Report of the Study Commission on Dietetics*. Chicago: The American Dietetic Association; 1972.
6. ADA. *A New Look at the Profession of Dietetics: Report of the 1984 Study Commission on Dietetics*. Chicago: The American Dietetic Association; 1985.
7. ADA. *Bylaws of The American Dietetic Association, as amended October 20, 1996*. Chicago: The American Dietetic Association; 1996.
8. ADA. *Council on Practice Policy and Procedure Manual*. Chicago: The American Dietetic Association; 1996.
9. Wellman N, Bogle M. President's page: beyond the RD. *J Am Diet Assoc*. 1990;90:1117–1121.
10. Owen A, Dougherty D, Bogle M. President's page: specialization in dietetics—the time has come. *J Am Diet Assoc*. 1986;86:1072–1076.
11. ADA. Quality Assurance Committee. *Standards of Practice: A Practitioner's Guide to Implementation*. Chicago: The American Dietetic Association; 1986.
12. Council on Practice Quality Assurance Committee: Learning the language of quality care. *J Am Diet Assoc*. 1993;93:531–532.
13. Council on Professional Issues. DPG's mark 20th anniversary. *ADA Courier*. 1997;35(4): 3–4.

PART III

Areas of Practice

The Dietitian
in Clinical Practice

Carolyn Moore

"The dietetic practitioner interacts with complex beings who eat food rather than nutrients. The psychosocial aspects of diet modification may therefore determine ultimate clinical usefulness and ethical practice."[1]

Outline—Chapter 8

- Introduction

- Employment Settings of Clinical Dietitians

- Organization of Clinical Nutrition Services
  - Managed health care

- Responsibilities in Clinical Dietetics
  - Nutrition services
  - Medical nutrition therapy
  - Major functions and time involvement

- Clinical Nutrition Service Team
  - Clinical nutrition managers/chief clinical dietitians
  - Clinical dietitians
  - Dietetic technicians
  - Dietetic assistants
  - Clinical dietitian practitioners

- Advancement Opportunities in Clinical Dietetics

- Legal and Ethical Issues

- Future of Clinical Dietetics

- Conclusion

INTRODUCTION

The discipline of clinical dietetics originated in 1899 when *dietitian* was defined by the American Home Economic Association as "individuals with a knowledge of food who provide diet therapy for the medical profession." Until 1917, dietitians were affiliated with this association but, after 1917, they belonged to the newly formed The American Dietetic Association (ADA).[2]

The earliest dietitians worked primarily in hospitals or were associated with food assistance programs. During the 1930s and 1940s, dietitians became involved either in food production and/food service or in the planning and provision of diets designed to meet special medical needs. The title *therapeutic dietitian* was used to describe the person who provided food for medical reasons, such as to prevent a nutrient deficiency or to help with the treatment of disease.[3] Examples of early diet therapy included the Sippy diet, which used milk and cream to treat ulcers, and the Kempner rice diet, which was used to treat hypertension, each named for the physicians who had designed them.

As the dietitian's role in the hospital became one of providing specialized care and modifying diets to treat various medical conditions, the title *clinical dietitian* began to replace *therapeutic dietitian*.[2]

In early 1970s, reports of widespread malnutrition among hospitalized patients helped to increase the visibility of the role of clinical dietitian.[4,5] Rather than providing diet therapy as ordered by physicians, clinical dietitians began to take a more active role in screening and monitoring the provision of nutrition support. Development of individual nutrition care plans became important functions of clinical dietitians. As the role of diet in the etiology of chronic diseases became better defined, clinical dietitians began to spend a greater percentage of their time participating in the prevention of diseases such as heart disease, cancer, and diabetes.

EMPLOYMENT SETTINGS OF CLINICAL DIETITIANS

In 1995, the number of registered dietitians reporting being employed in dietetics was 84 percent of the membership.[6] The fact that such a large number of registered dietitians (RDs) were working in the field of dietetics reflects the diversity of job opportunities. Health care was the major employment setting for dietitians, accounting for 6 out of 10 jobs held by RDs.[6] Table 8–1 summarizes the employment settings of dietitians in 1995. The four major health care facilities using the clinical skills of dietitians were inpatient/acute care hospitals (39.0 percent), extended day care centers (9.7 percent), clinics and ambulatory care centers (8.3 percent), and health care facilities (6.8 percent). When recent employment data were compared with previous reports, remarkable stability among employment settings is shown.[7]

ORGANIZATION OF CLINICAL NUTRITION SERVICES

Clinical nutrition services may be organized in a variety of ways, depending on the setting. Clinical nutrition services in most hospitals are managed by a clinical nutrition manager, director of clinical nutrition, or chief clinical dietitian (Figure 8–1a). Typically, the chief clinical dietitian reports to an individual with primary responsibility for food service and financial management of the entire food and nutrition department. In some instances, clinical dietetics may be organized as a separate department that reports to an executive or administrator with other patient care responsibilities such as nursing or pharmacy (Figure 8–1b). There are advantages and disadvantages to both types of organization. Combining clinical nutrition with food services can facilitate communication about patient food

Table 8–1 Primary Employment Setting of Registered Dietitians in 1995

Employment Setting (Primary Position)	Percentage
Hospital (inpatient/acute care)	39.0
Clinic or ambulatory-care center	8.3
Extended care facility	9.7
Health maintenance organization, physician, or other health care provider	2.1
Community/public health program	10.9
School food service (kindergarten through 12th grade and college/university)	3.1
College or university faculty	5.2
Private practice, primarily individual client counseling	3.3
Consultation, primarily to health care facilities	6.8
Consultation, primarily to other organizations	2.0
Other for-profit organizations	4.2
Other nonprofit organizations	4.2
Total	100.0

Source: J.A. Bryk and K.T. Soto, Report on the 1995 Membership Database of The American Dietetic Association. Copyright The American Dietetic Association. Adapted with permission from *Journal of The American Dietetic Association*, Vol. 97, pp. 197–203, © 1997.

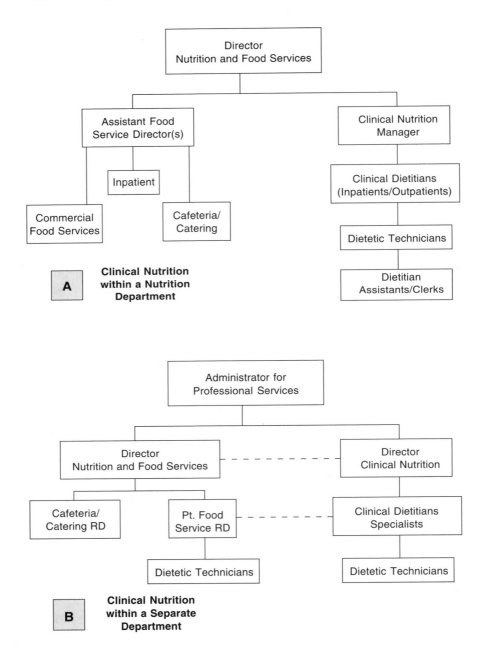

Figure 8–1A and B Examples of Nutrition and Food Service Organizational Charts. Example A is courtesy of The Methodist Hospital, Houston, Texas. Example B is courtesy of Nutrition Center, Arkansas Children's Hospital, Little Rock, Arkansas.

choices and menus. By contrast, having clinical nutrition as a separate department may increase visibility as an important patient care service unit distinct from food service.

Managed Health Care

Many hospitals and health care institutions are now operated under managed care organizations, and managed health care is rapidly becoming the primary means of delivery of health care in the United States. The cost and access to health care are major reasons for this trend. Health maintenance organizations (HMO) are the main type of managed care plans dietitians are likely to be associated with, although there are others such as integrated delivery systems or groups of delivery systems.[8] The basic concepts of managed care are that all medical care will be provided in exchange for a set fee, a primary physician is designated, and prevention of disease is stressed as a means of controlling costs before conditions require expensive treatment.[9]

Medical Nutrition Therapy (MNT) is being increasingly recognized as effective in treating disease and preventing disease complications, resulting in health benefits and cost savings for the public.[10] Several studies have documented the economic benefits of MNT, and dietitians are urged to document the outcomes of clinical nutrition services to demonstrate its role in cost-effectiveness.[11] The process followed in MNT is described in more detail later in this chapter, and the terminology is used throughout the chapter.

RESPONSIBILITIES IN CLINICAL DIETETICS

Nutrition Services

In 1995, The Joint Commission on Accreditation of Healthcare Organizations (the Joint Commission) developed standards for nutritional care and assessment of patients.[12] The major components of nutritional care services that are usually provided for hospitalized patients are summarized in Figure 8–2. These nutritional services are described.

Nutritional Screening

Nutritional screening is a process that is initiated to identify patients or clients with nutritional problems characteristic of, or that may lead to, malnutrition. Screening helps to establish the patient's need for MNT and helps to focus intervention on those individuals most likely to benefit from the nutritional support.[13,14] The parameters used to determine a patient's nutritional status are

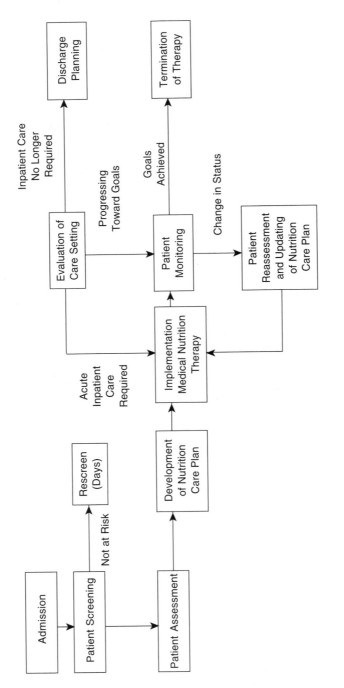

Figure 8–2 Provision of Medical Nutrition Therapy for Hospitalized Patients. *Source:* Reprinted from the American Society for Parental and Enteral Nutrition (A.S.P.E.N.), Guidelines for the Use of Parenteral and Enteral Nutrition in Adult and Pediatric Patients, JPEN; 17(4):1SA–52SA. A.S.P.E.N. does not endorse this material in any form other than its entirety. For information on ordering a complete set of guidelines, contact A.S.P.E.N., 8630 Fenton Street, Suite 412, Silver Spring, MD 20910; 301-587-6315.

clinical, biochemical, anthropometric (weight, height, percentage body fat, and/or lean body mass), and nutritional history data. The nutritional screen is used to determine when a detailed nutritional assessment is indicated.

Nutritional Assessment and Nutritional Care Plan

A nutritional assessment is a comprehensive process for evaluating nutritional status by using medical, dietary, and medication histories; anthropometric measurements; and laboratory data. The assessment should include a review of the subjective and objective assessment of the patient's current nutritional status and nutritional requirements. A nutrition care plan is developed that includes the immediate and long-term goals of therapy.[14] The recommended nutrition therapy should be based on the most appropriate modality. For instance, if the patient can eat, use food; if the gut works, use it; last resort, use intravenous nutrient therapy. Periodic reassessment is determined by the patient's disease or condition, medical stability, tolerance of and complexity of nutrition therapy, and achievement of goals.

Monitoring of Patients

Periodic review of the patient is necessary to determine beneficial and adverse effects and clinical changes that could influence continuing therapy. Frequency of monitoring is determined based on the patient's medical condition and complexity of nutrition therapy. Routine monitoring typically includes evaluation of physical condition, fluid status, nutrient deficiencies and excesses, weight and laboratory data, and tolerances to nutritional therapy.[14]

Nutrient Analysis

An evaluation of nutrient intake over time may be performed. Although frequently called "calorie counts," all nutrients need to be evaluated including protein, fat, carbohydrate, vitamin, and mineral intake. Intake of nutrients from food consumed and/or nutritional support (supplements, tube feedings, or parenteral nutrition) is calculated. Many computerized programs are available for nutrient analysis. This information is used to determine if specialized nutritional support such as enteral (supplementation or tube feedings) or parenteral (central or peripheral) nutrition is needed, or if nutrient recommendations are being met.

Medical Nutrition Therapy

MNT is becoming synonymous with clinical nutrition practice in the sense that the services provided are essentially the same. The term arose with the national attention on health care reform and growth of managed care. It became increasingly important to show that nutrition services are beneficial and essential in providing cost-effective care.

MNT is vital to the medical management of acute and chronic diseases, reducing costs by speeding recovery and reducing complications. Fewer hospitalizations, shorter hospital stays, and less need for other treatments are the results. In preventing disease development, MNT reduces risk of disease, maintains health, and improves quality of life.[11]

The process used in MNT is the following:[10] MNT involves the assessment of the nutritional status of patients with a condition, illness, or injury that puts them at risk. This includes review and analysis of medical and diet history, laboratory values, and anthropometric measurements. Based on the assessment, nutrition modalities most appropriate to manage the condition or treat the illness or injury are chosen and include the following:

- diet modification and counseling leading to the development of a personal diet plan to achieve nutritional goals and desired health outcomes
- specialized nutrition therapies including supplementation with medical foods for those unable to obtain adequate nutrients through food intake only; enteral nutrition delivered via tube feeding into the gastrointestinal tract for those unable to ingest or digest food, and parenteral nutrition delivered via intravenous infusion for those unable to absorb nutrients

The RD in clinical dietetics, along with the other members of the dietetic team, is the qualified professional best delivering MNT. Unfortunately, the concept of MNT has not been fully incorporated into all managed care plans. This is the reason the ADA is pursuing enactment of legislation that would establish MNT in Medicare regulations, thus giving it greater visibility and wider incorporation into managed care plans. The legislative efforts are discussed in Chapter 17.

Major Functions and Time Involvement

A profile of the amount of time spent by clinical dietitians in the functions they perform was reported by Shanklin et al.[15] Dietitians spent 51 percent of their time performing client-related activities, 10 percent in managerial functions, 1 percent in professional activities, 5 percent in nonprofessional activities, and 20 percent in transit time.

In the area of client-related activities, the major functions performed were documentation of nutritional care (16 percent), preliminary nutritional screening (11 percent), health team conferences (10 percent), and nutritional care evaluation and reassessment (10 percent). Patient diagnosis and the complexity of the dietary modifications influence the time required by dietitians to perform these functions.

In general, dietitians spend more time providing clinical services to patients with diagnoses involving the endocrine (e.g., diabetes) or renal (kidney) system.

The type of diet order also influences the amount of time a dietitian spends in patient care. Calorie-controlled diabetic diets, modified mineral content as for cardiac conditions, and individualized diets for specific patient needs are very time-consuming. The calculation and design of complex dietary modifications is especially time-consuming for dietitians caring for pediatric patients. Pediatric patients may require more frequent monitoring. Patient's growth and energy requirements must also be factored into the diet plan, and for some, modifications may need to be made daily.

CLINICAL NUTRITION SERVICE TEAM

Clinical nutrition services may be provided by a number of team members in health care facilities. Inpatient nutritional care in hospitals is usually the responsibility of several positions:

- clinical nutrition managers/chief clinical dietitians
- clinical dietitians
- dietetic technicians
- dietetic assistants

Outpatient clinics and ambulatory care centers may use all four positions but are more likely to employ only clinical dietitians. Extended day care facilities and HMOs or physician offices may have clinical dietitians on staff; however, more often these facilities will use a consulting dietitian to provide MNT for patients and clients. The consulting dietitian may be in private practice or part of a group practice.

Clinical Nutrition Managers/Chief Clinical Dietitians

Clinical nutrition managers are primarily responsible for directing the activities of clinical dietitians, dietetic technicians, and dietetic assistants. Major tasks performed include hiring of clinical nutrition employees, evaluating employee job performance, providing inservices and on-the-job training, reviewing productivity reports, writing job descriptions, scheduling employees, developing policies and procedures, designing performance standards, and developing and implementing goals and objectives of the department.[16] The clinical nutrition manager is also responsible for communicating with the staff of other departments and administration. Ultimately, the clinical nutrition manager ensures that performance is actually accomplished to achieve the goals and objectives of the department.

Clinical Dietitians

The primary responsibility of clinical dietitians is to provide nutritional care for patients. Clinical dietitians in hospitals are involved in the nutritional screening of patients to determine the presence of or risk of developing malnutrition, performing nutritional assessments, and developing nutrition care plans. Clinical nutrition services may be provided to general patient care units or may be based on a medical specialization (e.g., critical care, diabetes education). Clinical dietitians are important members of the total health care team because they consult and collaborate with physicians, pharmacists, nurses, social workers, chaplains, and others when providing nutritional care.

Clinical dietitians are the source of authoritative knowledge in the areas of MNT and patient education. They routinely communicate with other disciplines regarding developments in MNT and patient education through inservices team rounds and multidisciplinary patient care conferences.

Successful clinical dietitians in acute health care facilities must also be able to apply managerial concepts to provide effective nutritional care. Management tasks often performed by clinical dietitians include inservice training, on-the-job training, employee interviews and evaluations, writing job descriptions, planning cycle menus, and evaluating the quality of patient food.[16]

Clinical dietitians working in settings other than acute health care facilities tend to be involved in a wider range of tasks. Their responsibilities often include more managerial and administrative tasks that are similar to the duties of a clinical nutrition manager. In addition, they may provide more preventive nutrition therapy through modification of lifestyle.

Clinical dietitians may be members of one or more dietetic practice groups. Besides Dietitians in General Clinical Practice, some elect to join the Gerontological Nutritionist group, Dietetics in Development and Psychiatric Disorders, Oncology Nutrition, Renal Dietitians, Pediatric Nutrition, Diabetes Care and Support, Dietitians in Nutrition Support, Perinatal Nutrition, HIV/AIDS, and others. The diversity of specialty and subspecialty areas of practice reflects the broad range of interests and opportunities open to the clinical dietitian.

Dietetic Technicians

The primary responsibility of dietetic technicians, in a clinical setting, is to assist the clinical dietitian. Typically, the major functions performed by dietetic technicians are gathering data for nutritional screening and assigning a level of risk for malnutrition according to predetermined criteria. They may help with nutritional assessments by gathering laboratory and anthropometric data, collecting and analyzing nutrient intake information, obtaining nutritional histories, and reviewing medical histories. Dietetic technicians may administer nourishment and dietary supplements for patients and monitor patient tolerance. They may also provide information in helping patients select menus and give simple diet instructions. Dietetic technicians maintain a high level of knowledge of nutritional care. Management responsibilities of dietetic technicians may include supervision of dietetic assistants.

Dietetic Assistants

Dietetic assistants assist the clinical dietitian and/or dietetic technician in some of the more routine aspects of nutritional care. They are often responsible for processing diet orders, checking menus against standards, setting up standard nourishments, and tallying special food requests. Dietetic assistants may also help distribute and pick up patient menus and pass and collect trays. They may be involved in evaluating patient food satisfaction and help gather food records to be used to evaluate nutrient intake.

Clinical Dietitian Practitioners

Evelyn Bakken, RD (personal written communication, June 8, 1997), is a clinical dietitian at the Valley Care Medical Center, Livermore, California. She is chair of the dietitians in general clinical practice dietetic practice group (DGCP), having been active in the group in several different capacities. Her interests are broad, as can be seen from the list of other practice groups she also belongs to: diabetes care and education, pediatric, renal, clinical nutrition managers, and vegetarian. She is also active in both the California Dietetic Association and the Diablo Valley District Dietetic Association.

With a background in both clinical nutrition and food service management, she is a strong advocate of her profession and says:

> I believe in the growing importance of the dietitian in general clinical practice. This group of over 2,000 members is in the forefront of opportunities for patient care due to recent reductions in specialty areas of practice in response to the managed care changes. In over 40 years in the profession, I have seen the growth and development of nutrition as it relates to patient care and as it is being recognized in medical nutrition

therapy. Being a member of the DGCP has given me valuable tools and references not available elsewhere. Prior leaders of this group have set high standards and are outstanding examples of the dietetic profession. I think that while being mindful of the past, we must act today and be concerned about the future expansion of our dietetic profession.

Another enthusiastic dietitian, Lisa Fieber, MS, RD, LD of Fairfield, Illinois (personal written communication, June 10, 1997), says that baptism by fire may be the best way to describe how she got into clinical dietetics. Shortly after completing her MS degree and passing the registration examination, she had an opportunity to take a position as director of dietetics in a small hospital with a 60-bed nursing home attached. As the sole dietitian, she dealt with all aspects of clinical nutrition from baby formulas to total parenteral nutrition and functioned as a general practitioner.

She later diversified and currently operates a consulting business that specializes in long-term care and the developmentally disabled. She also teaches at the local community college, conducts medical literature research for physicians and consumers, counsels patients in her private practice, and teaches consumers to cook and eat healthier. Her offices are located in a home complete with a cooking school kitchen. She also serves as past chair and webmaster on the executive board of the DGCP.

Ms. Fieber says of her practice: "The greatest advantage of my clinical experience is that I have learned to give that extra personal touch. Whether in or out of the office, I want my patients to understand that I care about them and their health. When they come to my home office, not only can I discuss their dietary problems with them, I can take them into the kitchen to assess their culinary skills, teach them healthier cooking/eating habits, and develop menus/recipes specific to their medical condition."

ADVANCEMENT OPPORTUNITIES IN CLINICAL DIETETICS

Since the early 1970s, career ladders have been used in technical fields ranging from engineering to nursing. They have been developed for several reasons:

- to provide better care
- to increase motivation of staff
- to increase recognition of staff and the profession
- to retain staff
- to enhance quality and competency of staff

Clinical nutrition departments are implementing career ladders for dietitians to offer promotional alternatives to clinical dietitians other than traditional management positions such as the clinical nutrition manager. Any career incentive program must be consistent with the overall goals of the organization and department.

Bogle[17] describes a career ladder for clinical dietitians in effect in a specialty (pediatrics) health care facility. Not only does it serve as an advancement avenue for individual dietitians, it also serves to differentiate dietitians within an institution. Before the implementation of the career ladder, all dietitians in the institutions were in the same grade for personnel purposes. Even though most of the staff were certified specialists in pediatric nutrition, the career ladder allows for advancement as the dietitians attain more education (graduate degrees), provide consultative services, assume more responsibility, and become autonomous practitioners. The ladder has six levels, including one for dietetic technicians and a pediatric nutrition resident-in-training. Each level has specific criteria to be accomplished before moving to or applying for another level. These criteria are also used in evaluating job performance. In addition, this ladder program offers a choice for the dietitian who does not choose to work full time or who cannot (for family or other reasons) assume greater responsibility and autonomy.

In the past, many health care facilities have used career advancement programs comprised of entry-level dietitians and specialists. Advancement was usually based on an opening occurring in a specialty area. However, career ladders that incorporate three- to five-level programs offer a wider range of opportunities for growth and development of staff. A range of salaries, increased clinical and management responsibilities, and increased recognition of expertise contributes to better staff retention.[18]

Recently, the ADA has taken a lead in recognizing advanced education and experience as well as certifying advanced-level practitioners and specialists. A role delineation study for advanced-level and specialty practice was used to determine characteristics of entry-level professional and advanced-level professional practice.[19-21] A fellow of the ADA now recognizes advanced experience and education. Board certification in metabolic support, pediatric nutrition, and renal education are recognized areas of specialization by the ADA.[22]

Similarly, the American Diabetes Association certifies individuals, including clinical dietitians in diabetes education (Certified Diabetes Educator, CDE). The American Society of Parenteral and Enteral Nutrition also certifies clinical dietitians in the area of nutritional support (certified nutrition support dietitian). Both professional organizations have education, certification examinations, and continuing education requirements similar to the ADA that must be satisfied to maintain specialist certifications.

Typical responsibilities of three different levels of clinical dietitians (staff, senior, and specialist) in a large acute care hospital are shown in Table 8–2 with a summary of the knowledge, skill, and experience requirements of each in Table 8–3.

LEGAL AND ETHICAL ISSUES

The code of ethics of the ADA (Appendix A) is the guide to professional practice by the clinical dietitian.

The ADA has published a position statement regarding feeding terminally ill patients[23] and permanently unconscious patients.[24] In both situations, clinical

Table 8–2 Clinical Dietitian Responsibilities

Function	Staff	Senior	Specialist
Nutritional screening	X	X	X
Nutritional assessments/care plans:			
General patients	X	X	X
Critical care/complex patients		X	X
Diet instructions	X	X	X
Diet calculations, eating plans, menu checking,			
evaluation of meal service	X	X	X
Evaluates nutrient intake and provides follow-up care	X	X	X
Direct activities of dietetic technicians and dietetic			
assistants	X	X	X
Provides clinical inservices to dietitians, dietetic			
technicians, and dietitian assistants	X	X	X
Participate in performance evaluation of dietetic			
technician and dietetic assistants	X	X	X
Medical team rounds and multidisciplinary team meetings	X	X	X
Evaluation of clinical monitors for quality management	X	X	X
On-call duties (weekend/week night)	X	X	X
Clinical nutrition committee membership	X	X	X
Clinical responsibility in focus area—patient education			
or assessment		X	X
Maintain reference in area of clinical focus		X	X
Revises standards of care and clinical procedures		X	X
Conducts peer review of clinical dietitian chart notes		X	X
Trains new staff and interns		X	X
Clinical responsibility in area of specialization			X
Provides updates in specialization area			X
Participates in research and presents findings			X
Scheduling dietitian coverage in absence of supervisor			X
Chairs clinical committees		cochairs	chairs

Courtesy of The Methodist Hospital, Houston, Texas.

Table 8–3 Knowledge, Skill, and Experience Requirements for Clinical Dietitians

Function	Staff	Senior	Specialist
Registered dietitian (the ADA)	Yes	Yes	Yes
Licensure	Yes	Yes	Yes
Clinical experience (years)	Entry	3	5
Advanced knowledge and certification	No	No	Yes
Outside continuing education hours	No	Yes	Yes

Courtesy of The Methodist Hospital, Houston, Texas.

dietitians are charged with taking an active role in developing criteria for feeding terminally ill and permanently unconscious patients in collaboration with other members of the health care team.

When developing the nutritional care plan for terminally ill patients, three major criteria should be considered.[23] These are (1) the medical condition as documented by the physician, (2) the patient's informed preference for the level of nutritional support at various stages of dying, and (3) the current ethical and legal practices that influence the formulation of policies.

In 1996, the Joint Commission on Accreditation of Healthcare Organizations (the Joint Commission) set standards stating that "the patient's right to treatment or service is respected and supported" and "patients are involved in all aspects of their care."[25] The intent of the Joint Commission was to ensure that patients and/or family are involved in giving informed consent, making care decisions, formulating advance directives regarding withholding of life-sustaining treatment, and determining the type and extent of care at the end of life. If at any time a patient's right of self-determination is at odds with a clinical dietitian's own moral and/or religious beliefs, the need to reassign the patient's care to another dietitian may be necessary.

Within health care facilities, an ethics committee is usually responsible for developing and implementing guidelines for patient care. The hospital ethics committee is often involved with educating physicians, health care personnel, and the public. Clinical dietitians should serve as a member or a consultant to the committee to help with the development of policies and procedures related to MNT and hydration issues. They may also make decisions in specific cases involving complex ethical or moral issues related to nutrition.

FUTURE OF CLINICAL DIETETICS

Changes in health care are occurring rapidly. In the next 20 years, health care services now provided at community hospitals are expected to be provided at alternative sites. It has been projected that future health care systems will be dispersed over wide geographic areas. Ambulatory care centers are expected to replace, in large part, the typical hospital.[26] These changes are and continue to affect the practice of clinical dietitians.

In managed care organizations, the emphasis is on keeping individuals enrolled in their programs healthy and therefore lead to reduced hospital admissions with greater continuity of care in communities. As the practice of managed care grows, more clinical dietitians are expected to be used in ambulatory care centers rather than in acute care settings. At the same time, many hospitals are expected to convert existing beds into other uses such as rehabilitation centers, skilled nursing facilities, and outpatient clinics. MNT and consultation of clinical dietitians will continue to be needed at these facilities.

In the future, employment of dietitians by hospitals is also expected to grow slowly as more hospital food service operations are contracted to private companies who will provide their own dietitians. By contrast, employment opportunities in rehabilitation centers, nursing homes, and residential care centers are expected to grow as the population continues to age.[27]

By the year 2005, the settings with the greatest projected employment demand for clinical dietitians will include physician offices (54 percent), offices of other health care professionals (63 percent), nursing and home health care facilities (91 percent), and residential care (129 percent).[27] Aging of the population and changes in reimbursement will be major factors influencing change in demand for services of clinical dietitians. Industries with the smallest projected percentage increase in need for dietitians include acute care hospitals (7 percent), education (16 percent), and government (0.5 percent).[27]

The future roles of clinical dietitians can be expanded by developing new skills and competencies.[28] Increased employment opportunities are expected to become available as clinical dietitians expand their role into areas of providing more community-based care and preventive care. Efforts that increase access to health care will also increase employment opportunities for clinical dietitians. By emphasizing primary care and prevention through promotion of a healthy lifestyle, clinical dietitians can expand their role and remain an important health care provider in the future.

CONCLUSION

The clinical dietitian plays a major role in helping persons during illness through nutrition interventions and MNT. Equally important is helping individuals prevent the onset of chronic disease by the application of optimal nutrition practices throughout life. A current challenge for the professional practitioner in clinical dietetics is the inclusion of MNT in managed care plans through documentation of cost-effectiveness data and demonstration of quality practice.

Even though employment may move outside the hospital or clinic, the services provided by the clinical dietitian will remain vital to the health and well-being of people in illness and injury.

DEFINITIONS

Ambulatory Care Center Health care facility in which ambulatory patients are treated.

Clinical Dietetics Area of practice in dietetics dealing with treatment of persons during illness or injury by using nutrition assessment, planning, and implementation of nutrition care plans and monitoring the patients' status.

Clinical Nutrition Services Activities provided in the practice of clinical dietetics.

Diet Therapy Treatment by diet; this term now replaced by clinical nutrition therapy or medical nutrition therapy.

Extended Care Facility Institution that "extends" health care beyond the hospital setting as when further long-term care is needed.

Managed Care Organization Groups providing comprehensive health care services in which access, cost, and quality are controlled by direct intervention before or during service.

Medical Nutrition Therapy (MNT) Application of nutrition in the management of illness or injury.

Outpatient Clinic Treatment area of a hospital or health care facility in which patients are treated on an outpatient (as opposed to inpatient) basis.

REFERENCES

1. Coulston AM, Rock CL. A summary of the current state of knowledge in clinical nutrition and dietetic practice: suggestions for future research in dietetic practice and implications for health care. In: *The Research Agenda for Dietetics.* Conference proceedings. Chicago: The American Dietetic Association; 1993:1–24.

2. Cooper LF. The dietitian and her profession. *J Am Diet Assoc.* 1938;14:751–758.

3. Huyck I, Rowe MM. *Managing Clinical Nutrition Services.* Rockville, MD: Aspen Publishers; 1990.

4. Butterworth E. The skeleton in the hospital closet. *Nutr Today.* 1974;9:4.

5. Bistrian B, et al. Protein status of general surgical patients. *JAMA.* 1974;230:858–860.

6. Bryk JA, Soto KT. Report on the 1995 membership database of The American Dietetic Association. *J Am Diet Assoc.* 1997;97:197–203.

7. Bryk JA, Soto KT. Report on the 1993 membership database of The American Dietetic Association. *J Am Diet Assoc.* 1994;94:1433–1439.

8. Laramee SH. Nutrition services in managed care: new paradigms for dietitians. *J Am Diet Assoc.* 1996;96:335–336.

9. Fielder KM. Managed health care: understanding the role of the nutrition professional. *J Am Diet Assoc.* 1993;93:1111–1112.

10. ADA. Position of The American Dietetic Association: cost-effectiveness of medical nutrition therapy. *J Am Diet Assoc.* 1995;95:88–91.

11. ADA. Position of The American Dietetic Association: nutrition services in managed care. *J Am Diet Assoc.* 1996;96:391–395.

12. The Joint Commission. *The Joint Commission on Accreditation of Healthcare Organizations Comprehensive Accreditation Manual for Hospitals 1995*. Oakbrook Terrace, IL: Joint Commission on Accreditation of Healthcare Organizations; 1995.

13. Nagel MR. Nutritional screening: identifying patients at risk for malnutrition. *Nutr Clin Prac.* 1993;8:171–175.

14. Standards for nutritional support: hospitalized patients. American Society of Parenteral and Enteral Nutrition. *Nutr Clin Prac.* 1995;10:208–218.

15. Shanklin CW, Hernandez HN, Gould RM, Gorman MA. Results of a statewide time study in Texas. *J Am Diet Assoc.* 1988;88:38–43.

16. Digh EW, Dowdy RP. A survey of management tasks completed by clinical dietitians in the practice setting. *J Am Diet Assoc.* 1994;94:1381–1384.

17. Bogle ML. Career development in clinical nutrition: implementing a career ladder. *Building Block Life.* 1992;15:1–3, 11.

18. Smith AE. Improving career outlook in clinical dietetics. *Clin Nutr Manage.* 1993;12:1–2.

19. ADA. *Role Delineation for Registered Dietitians and Entry-Level Dietetic Technicians.* Chicago: The American Dietetic Association; 1990.

20. *Role Delineation for Advanced-Level and Specialty Practice in Dietetics: Results of an Empirical Study 1992.* Vol. 1. Monterey, CA: MacMillan/McGraw Hill; 1992.

21. Bradley RT, Young WY, Ebbs P, Martin J. Characteristics of advanced-level dietetics practice: a model and empirical results. *J Am Diet Assoc.* 1993;93:196–202.

22. Bogle ML, Balogun L, Cassell J, Catakis A, et al. Achieving excellence in dietetic practice: certification of specialists and advanced-level practitioners. *J Am Diet Assoc.* 1993;93:149–150.

23. ADA. Position of The American Dietetic Association: issues in feeding the terminally ill adult. *J Am Diet Assoc.* 1992;92:996–1005.

24. ADA. Position of The American Dietetic Association: legal and ethical issues in feeding permanently unconscious patients. *J Am Diet Assoc.* 1995;95:231–234.

25. Robinson GE. Applying the 1996 JCAHO nutrition care standards in a long-term care setting. *J Am Diet Assoc.* 1996;96:400–403.

26. Brylinsky C. Shifting clinical dietetics to new markets. *Clin Nutr Manager Newslett.* 1995;15:4–5.

27. Kornblum TH. Professional demand for dietitians and nutritionists in the year 2005. *J Am Diet Assoc.* 1994;94:21–22.

28. Parks SC, Fitz PA, Maillet JO, Babjak P, et al. Challenging the future of dietetics education and credentialing—dialogue, discovery, and directions: a summary of the 1994 Future Search Conference. *J Am Diet Assoc.* 1995;95:598–606.

CHAPTER 9

Management in Food and Nutrition Systems

Lea L. Ebro

"Knowledge of food and management skills is essential to most areas of practice in dietetics. Many Dietetic Practice Groups, including those in clinical nutrition, community nutrition and business practice, routinely translate nutrition science into food choices for specific audiences."[1]

Outline—Chapter 9

- Introduction

- Areas of Employment
  - Food service in acute care
  - Food service in long-term care
  - Food service in noninstitutional settings
  - School nutrition programs
  - Clinical nutrition management
  - Commercial food services
  - Further areas of opportunity

- Roles and Responsibilities

- Characteristics of Successful Food and Nutrition Managers

- Career Ladder Opportunity

- Ethical Bases of Practice

- The Future

- Conclusion

INTRODUCTION

Food and food service is prominent in the history of the profession of dietetics. One of the main purposes of the first organizing meeting of The American Dietetic Association (ADA) was to discuss ways of meeting food shortages during World War I, and many of the first members of the association served overseas, feeding hospitalized soldiers and persons living under wartime conditions. Cooking schools also helped lay the groundwork for the dietetic profession, as did the scientists who produced the first tables of food values. Early day soup kitchens in Boston and school lunch programs were among the forerunners of institutions that fed the public.[2]

Food service in hospitals was the primary early focus of dietitians. During the 1890s, food service in hospitals was managed by the chef, the housekeeper, or the nursing department. In the early 1900s, however, many dietitians were in charge of dietary departments and had the responsibility for all food services plus teaching nurses and providing diet therapy for patients with metabolic disease. Hospital dietitians dealt with budgets, department organization, personnel management, and quality food service as well as special diets for patients. Nutrition was recognized as an aspect of medicine, and food prescriptions were handled as apothecary compounds, thus creating a demand for special diet kitchens. The hospital dietitian had the same status as the superintendent of nurses and was recognized as the nutrition expert.[3]

Dietitians with food service management responsibilities became members of the "food administration" section in ADA, and their area of practice was referred to as "administrative dietetics." Gradually, this terminology changed, and now the terms *food service systems management* or *management in food and nutrition systems* are more widely used. The term *institution administration* is also used but to a lesser extent.

Management is required in all areas of dietetics. Spears defines the manager as one who is responsible for people and other organizational resources and possesses management skills including technical, human, and conceptual.[4] In this chapter, we focus on the dietitian in food service management, although some discussion of the clinical manager is also included.

AREAS OF EMPLOYMENT

Most dietitians begin their careers in clinical practice. About half of those beyond entry level (i.e., after 10 years of practice), however, are employed in food and nutrition management as indicated in the 1993 and 1995 membership databases.[5,6] (See Figure 9–1.)

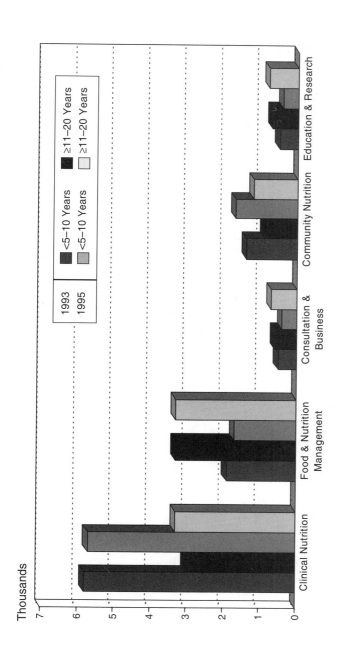

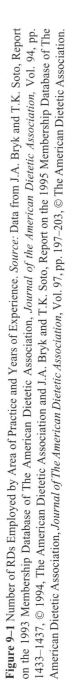

Figure 9–1 Number of RDs Employed by Area of Practice and Years of Experience. *Source:* Data from J.A. Bryk and T.K. Soto, Report on the 1993 Membership Database of The American Dietetic Association, *Journal of the American Dietetic Association*, Vol. 94, pp. 1433–1437, © 1994, The American Dietetic Association and J.A. Bryk and T.K. Soto, Report on the 1995 Membership Database of The American Dietetic Association, *Journal of The American Dietetic Association*, Vol. 97, pp. 197–203, © The American Dietetic Association.

Dietitians in food service management typically affiliate with four ADA Dietetic Practice Groups (DPG): Management in Food and Nutrition Systems, Dietitians in Business and Communication, School Nutrition Services, and Food and Culinary Professionals. In addition, managers in clinical areas may belong to the Clinical Nutrition Management Group. Management dietitians may also be identified through a wide range of titles. For instance, Taylor identified position titles of coordinator, specialist, and executive dietitian.[7] Among more traditional titles, Liu found position titles of directors/associate directors of food and nutrition services, directors of clinical nutrition, directors of multiunit services, and food/nutrition consultants.[8] Molt, in her doctoral dissertation, described titles such as director, chief, or chief administrator among dietitians working in hospital food service, school food service, and college and university residence halls.[9]

The 1990 Role Delineation for Registered Dietitians (RD) and Entry-Level Dietetic Technicians[10] categorized practice areas by work settings. The categories used were food service in acute care, food service in long-term care, and food service in the noninstitutional population. To encompass the broader management area, clinical nutrition management, commercial food services, and school nutrition programs have been added to this list. A brief discussion of each of these areas follows.

Food Service in Acute Care

Food service in acute care is described as food service in hospitals or similar health care institutions in which patients receive short-term medical treatment. The length of stay may range from one day up to an average of five days. There are several characteristics of this type of food service: (1) fast turnover of patients with day-to-day fluctuations in the number of meals prepared; (2) special diets requiring different types of food preparation (in some institutions, as many as 30 to 50 percent of all patients will require special or modified diets); (3) selective menus for patients used in many hospitals, increasing the number of food items prepared; (4) multiple serving systems, such as individual tray service for patients, cafeteria service for hospital personnel and the public, catering for hospital staff, and vending services for personnel and the public at night; and (5) various types of food service for patients. In some, food is prepared in bulk, then preportioned and held until the time of meal service, when it is reheated and served. In others, food is prepared centrally just before meal service and either portioned individually or sent in bulk to the patient area. In whatever type of system is used, the dietitian may have overall responsibility for food production and service or may share management with others such as chefs and managers. Whatever the scope of his or her responsibility, however, the dietitian must be knowledgable in food production techniques, food purchasing, safety and sanitation, strategic planning, human relations, and financial and managerial skills.

Food Service in Long-Term Care

The provision of food for clients in nursing homes and extended care facilities and in correctional institutions is included in this category.[11] The dietitian may be hired as a consultant in these facilities at less than full time.

Food service in these types of institutions will differ from that in acute care in that clients are long term, and the majority will be served in group settings rather than individually and by central food production at meal time. Fewer special diets are usual, as most of the long-term clients will be following a normal, healthy eating pattern. The food service, especially in smaller nursing homes and extended care facilities, may be managed by a dietetic technician or by a certified dietary manager under the direction of a dietitian consultant. In correctional institutions, day-to-day management is often provided by nonprofessionals, again, under the direction of a consultant dietitian when available. All aspects of food service management are equally as important in long-term care as in the hospital setting, with the added necessity of ensuring nutritional adequacy and acceptability over longer periods of time. There are federal and state regulations relating to the provision of food services to clients in almost all long-term facilities that must be followed for the institution to receive funding and provide quality care. The qualifications for the food service manager are also stated in the regulations.

Food Service in Noninstitutional Settings

This type of food service includes colleges and universities, school lunch and breakfast programs, business and commercial enterprises, and hotels and restaurants. It is estimated that 99 percent of all organizations provide some type of food service for clients and/or employees.[12]

These types of food services vary in several ways. They may be for profit or nonprofit (generally, those serving the public will be for-profit while those in schools or for company employees in businesses nonprofit); clients choose to patronize the food service offered (in contrast to the earlier institutional groups); and the types of food service may vary widely. A college or university, for instance, may offer cafeteria, dining room, restaurant, catering, and/or vending services. School and employee food service is often by cafeteria service, along with vending and dining room service in some. The dietitian's responsibility is in providing food that is safe and acceptable to the customers, that meets financial expectations, and that promotes good nutrition.

Mary Molt, RD, LD, PhD, has been a dietitian in the housing and dining services at Kansas State University for more than 20 years. She has progressed from an assistant in one dining hall to assistant director of all food services and member of a management team with responsibilities for residence life, maintenance, housekeeping, and family housing as well as dining halls. The dining service operates a central food store, three dining centers serving 3,100 students in nine residence halls, and a cooperative living house. She manages eight professional staff, 100 employees, and a budget of more than $6 million. In addition, she teaches and provides supervised practice experience for students in the dietetics and hotel restaurant management programs at the university.

Molt has been a very active member of the ADA Practice Group Management in Food & Nutrition Systems and also reviews examination questions for the Council on Dietetic Registration. She is a national leader in the National Association of College and University Food Services and is well known to dietitians and students in food service management as the author of *Food for Fifty*.[13]

Molt credits the teachers and mentors she has had for insisting on high standards that she now follows in her practice. She has, in turn, become a role model in setting professional standards and developing leadership qualities in students and dietitians. When asked about her career advice for dietetic students, she provides almost a guide to practice: The future for management practice in dietetics lies in the ability to be competitive, do a job better than anyone else, and market one's uniqueness and successes. She believes dietitians must embrace change and make it work for them and that their talents and skills require continual updating. "Management dietitians of the future must be self-reliant and politically astute as there is always the need to sell the value of ones services when competing for resources."

Role model, mentor, teacher, food service manager, and top-notch dietitian are all terms that describe Mary Molt.

School Nutrition Programs

School nutrition programs, offering either lunch or breakfast, or both, are available to more than 90 percent of all students and about 25 million are fed daily.[14] Because the programs are administered by and partially funded by the federal government, they must meet specific guidelines for nutritional quality of meals and for student eligibility (free meals are provided based on family economic circumstances). The emphasis is on long-term health benefits for children through the establishment of good eating habits, and nutrition education is stressed as a part of the program.

Dietitians in school nutrition programs need both managerial and nutrition education skills. Many in this career area affiliate with the School Nutrition Services DPG and may also be members of the American School Foodservice Association.

In 1990, the National Food Service Management Institute (NFSMI) was founded for the purpose of improving the quality and operations of child nutrition programs.[15] Activities through the institute provide direct assistance to school food service personnel through research, education and training materials, workshops and technical assistance, and establishment of a clearinghouse for sharing of materials.

An example of the research conducted by the NFSMI was to determine the job functions and tasks of school nutrition managers. The job functions rated most important were program accountability, sanitation and safety, customer service, equipment use and care, and food production. The manager in a school food service program has responsibilities in at least seven other areas: nutrition and menu planning, food procurement, food acceptability, financial management, marketing, personnel management, and professional development.[16]

Clinical Nutrition Management

Clinical nutrition management refers to the activities of practitioners in hospitals and health care institutions who perform primarily management functions. This can include the responsibility for one or more units and for other professionals in clinical areas. Although the employment setting is not in food services, many of the management functions performed are the same. Specifically, the management of human resources and of financial and material resources will be the primary job functions. The clinical dietitian who progresses to a management position from an entry-level position will usually have previous experience and will not be involved in day-to-day activities directly related to patient care.

Commercial Food Services

Shanklin and Dowling describe commercial food service as retail and hospitality food service establishments that prepare food for immediate consumption on or off premises.[17] The types of establishments employing dietitians include independent restaurants, casual/family dining restaurants, and fine dining restaurants. In the same study, supermarket chains, limited service (fast-food) chains, and hotel chains were identified as having high potential for dietetic services. Five specific areas of need in these institutions were said to be nutrition education, healthful menu planning, recipe and menu analysis, marketing, and quality control.

Lechowich and Soto[18] reported a study of opportunities in commercial food services from the industry standpoint and found that although the opportunities exist, relatively few dietitians are employed in these areas. Skills in areas such as public relations, communications, marketing, and purchasing are usually expected; therefore, additional training and experience are often needed by the dietitian to be fully qualified for these roles.

Marcella Gelman, RD, MS, is a dietitian working for the Vons Companies, Inc., a 316-store supermarket chain in southern California and Nevada. Her career with the company began after a BS degree at the University of Georgia with a double major in dietetics and institution administration and the MS degree at Oklahoma State University in food service systems administration. She was first hired as the quality assurance consumer coordinator to handle product complaints and was promoted a year later to supervisor of consumer affairs. At present, she is the manager for safety and environmental affairs.

The company has been through reorganizations, and Gelman's responsibilities have also changed over the years. She fully expects they will continue to change in the future. Management skills such as managing resources and individuals are very key skills that are valuable in this and in any industry according to Gelman.

Further Areas of Opportunity

Other opportunities for dietitians in food and nutrition management include positions in food corporations (research, consumer affairs, communications), disaster planning centers, military bases, homeless shelters and food distribution centers, worldwide religious ministries and government food programs, and academic units with food/nutrition/hospitality programs.

ROLES AND RESPONSIBILITIES

Three major studies, conducted by ADA since 1989, have described the roles and responsibilities of dietitians in the various areas of practice in which they are employed. The first study was the Role Delineation Study[10] followed by the 1995 Commission on Dietetic Registration Practice Audit[19] and the Educational Competencies Steering Committee Study on Competencies.[20] Both dietitians and dietetic technicians were included in these three studies.

In the role delineation study, the average percentage of time spent in various activities is shown in Table 9–1. The shaded number indicates the highest percentage.

In the same study, it was reported that experienced dietitians were involved in advising, policy setting, and supervising to a greater extent than the inexperienced dietitians and that entry-level dietitians were more involved in "doing." The

Table 9–1 Average Percentage of Time by Categories of Food Service Activities

Category	Entry-Level RD			Beyond-Entry-Level RD			Entry-Level Dietetic Technician		
	Food Service Acute	Food Service Long Term	Food Service Noninstitutional	Food Service Acute	Food Service Long Term	Food Service Noninstitutional	Food Service Acute	Food Service Long Term	Food Service Noninstitutional
Managing food service, material resources	24.3	29.0	29.8	25.6	27.0	31.1	27.9	33.9	58.3
Providing nutrition care to individuals	25.0	26.0	2.3	14.0	29.7	1.4	43.3	34.1	0.5
Providing nutrition programs for population groups	3.3	2.4	5.0	2.2	2.3	5.5	1.3	0.9	2.5
Managing financial resources	8.1	6.1	10.5	13.9	10.0	15.9	3.0	6.9	9.1
Marketing services and products	2.4	0.8	4.1	3.5	1.0	7.0	0.1	0.8	1.5
Teaching dietitians and other professionals/students	3.7	2.1	3.3	3.4	2.6	3.0	1.3	0.5	0.1
Conducting research	0.3	0.0	0.2	0.3	0.1	0.2	0.0	0.1	0.1
Managing human resources	26.8	19.9	34.6	26.0	14.6	21.2	9.7	8.0	11.3
Managing facilities	5.8	6.0	10.3	9.1	8.8	12.0	3.5	8.7	14.0
Other	0.3	7.7	0.0	2.1	3.8	2.8	10.0	6.1	2.8

Source: Reprinted with permission from *Role Delineation for Registered Dietitians and Entry-Level Dietetic Technicans,* © 1990, The American Dietetic Association.

experienced dietitians were also involved in a broader range of activities including teaching, research, and marketing.[21]

In the 1995 practice audit conducted by the Commission on Dietetic Registration[19] dietitians in food service management were not singled out for study; instead, areas of activity were reported for all those surveyed. The main findings from this study were

- Both dietitians and dietetic technicians work in a variety of settings but are concentrated in acute care, long-term care, and community settings.
- Both dietitians and dietetic technicians perform a variety of functions, with the most common being clinical services, food services, nutrition information, and public health functions.
- The areas of activity in which dietitians and dietetic technicians are involved depend mainly on their work settings and the functions they perform.
- Levels of responsibility tend to increase with years of experience.

Reinforcing the earlier statement that food and management skills are essential for those in all areas of practice, in this study it was shown that food production, distribution, and service (32 percent of all practitioners); menu planning (45 percent); safety and sanitation (40 percent); and marketing (57 percent) activities were performed. Among dietetic technicians, more than 50 percent of all respondents performed the first three activities just described.

In the third study,[20] a steering committee was appointed to determine competencies expected for practice in dietetics at the entry level. The committee developed a set of core competencies for all entry-level dietitians and further competencies for areas of emphasis in practice. The competencies identified for the entry-level dietitian in food service systems management were the following:

1. Manage development and/or modification of recipes and formulas.
2. Manage menu development for target populations.
3. Manage production of food that meets nutrition guidelines, cost parameters, and consumer acceptance.
4. Manage procurement, distribution, and service within delivery systems.
5. Manage the integration of financial, human, physical, and material resources.
6. Manage safety and sanitation issues related to food and nutrition.
7. Supervise customer satisfaction systems for dietetic services and/or practice.
8. Supervise marketing functions.
9. Supervise human resource functions.
10. Perform operations analysis.

CHARACTERISTICS OF SUCCESSFUL FOOD AND NUTRITION MANAGERS

Dietitians in food and nutrition management need to exhibit leadership qualities similar to those in all areas of business, health care institutions, schools, etc. They must manage personnel and financial resources, produce quality products and service, and communicate effectively both within the organization and to the larger community. The development of "transformational leaders," defined as those who possess personal characteristics that allow them to influence the work situation, was studied by Arensberg et al.[22] Among clinical nutrition managers, they determined that the area of communications scored the lowest among 50 items on a leadership behavior questionnaire. The transformational leader helps people and organizations to function at a high level, to master change, and to move ahead in planning for the future. Obviously, the dietitian with more experience is likely to be the most effective in transformational leadership.

Witte and Messersmith[23] also studied clinical nutrition managers and found that training needs identified by the managers were computer-assisted management (82 percent), budget development (75 percent), marketing (73 percent), and budget management (68 percent). These are management rather than clinical skills.

A list of leadership competencies needed by health care food service directors is shown in Exhibit 9–1.[24] These competencies are described as typical of "visionary" leaders who are effective in their positions and in the organization. Molt[9] found that experiences helpful in developing leadership skills among management dietitians were activities in present positions, working with others, working in professional organizations, volunteer service, and analyses of the organization.[7]

CAREER LADDER OPPORTUNITIES

Entry-level dietitians with management responsibilities are employed primarily in food service or clinical nutrition service operations. The predominant responsibilities at the entry level involve technical skills that ensure that food is procured, managed, prepared, and delivered to patients and other clients and that appropriate nutrition services are provided. With experience and perhaps graduate study, conceptual skills are used to identify problem areas requiring attention, to select appropriate techniques, to analyze alternative strategies, and to select solutions consistent with organization goals.

From entry-level positions, dietitians may advance to the assistant or associate director level and eventually to director or chief administrator of a department.

Exhibit 9–1 Leadership Competencies Needed by Health Care Food Service Directors

---

Successful health care food service directors will:

- Exhibit astute collaborative management techniques to unify diverse points of view through consensus building, to cultivate mutually advantageous relationships in and out of the institution, and to achieve cooperation through teamwork.
- Demonstrate effective communication techniques to achieve a common understanding of personnel and departmental policies, and effective interpersonal skills through two-way communication with personnel inside and outside the department.
- Achieve an organizational structure, mission statement, policies, and procedures that effect necessary changes while managing risk taking for the department.
- Possess common-sense intelligence based on sound technological knowledge of food service, practice experience, and consideration of external business and administrative needs.
- Bear effective personnel management techniques based on sound character, compassion, insight, and personal integrity.
- Exhibit personal behaviors and attitudes consistent with professional and institutional goals.
- Demonstrate continuing pursuit of professional knowledge and growth.
- Possess effective supervisory/managerial techniques to derive optimal employee performance and appropriate documentation.
- Achieve ways to enhance performance and growth of employees.
- Possess an understanding of the politics of the institution and an ability to interface effectively with superiors.
- Exhibit effective use of resources (e.g., fiscal, personnel, materials) to facilitate planning and current operations.
- Possess analytic and decision-making techniques to achieve maximum quality for customers/clients.
- Personify behaviors and techniques that foster professional growth and leadership in department personnel.
- Demonstrate the ability to formulate a creative vision for the department that integrates mutually satisfying department and institutional goals.

Source: M. Watabe-Dawson. Visionary Leaders Are Key to Success in Food Service. Copyright The American Dietetic Association. Reprinted by permission from *Journal of The American Dietetic Association*, Vol. 95. p. 13, © 1995.

These dietitians generally have several years of experience and an advanced degree.[25,26] Often, management dietitians pursue advanced degrees in business administration, personnel management, finance, industrial engineering, or law to meet the challenges of career advancement. In major medical centers with large staffs, there are career ladders for staff dietitians in food services and in clinical nutrition management. Directors of food and nutrition services may progress to directing multiunit operations in the medical center or become higher level administrators responsible for human resources. They may manage multidepartmental units or a complex of smaller hospitals, specialty clinics, or long-term care retirement centers that are a part of a medical center or a business and industry.

Dietitians directing food and nutrition services must have a diversified multipurpose, broad-based education and experiences from which to draw for expanded roles. They must be familiar with computer technology, business organization, marketing, labor relations, industrial engineering, writing and media relations, public relations, financial management, data evaluation, policy formation, and personnel management. Other skills essential to the success in expanded roles are problem solving, decision making, negotiation, behavior modification, and dealing with adaptive challenges.[27,28]

ETHICAL BASES OF PRACTICE

Dietitians in managerial positions must provide leadership through demonstration of ethical conduct and by instituting systems that facilitate ethical practices among all personnel. Policies pertaining to, for example, institutional purchasing, resource allocation, financial management, human resource issues, patient care issues, and professional integrity will develop and foster ethical procedures in practice. The Code of Ethics of the ADA is the guide for dietitians in establishing these systems.[29] (See Appendix A.)

The framework in which such policies are developed is the hallmark of an effective value structure, which includes the following:[30]

1. The guiding values and commitments make sense and are clearly communicated.
2. Organization leaders are personally committed, credible, and willing to take action on the values they espouse.
3. The espoused values are integrated into the normal channels of management decision making and are reflected in the organization's critical activities.
4. The organization's systems and structures support and reinforce its values.
5. Managers throughout the organization have the decision-making skill, knowledge, and competencies needed to make ethically sound decisions on a day-to-day basis.

Ethical practice has been described in resource allocation decision, which is similar to the systems approach for problem solving.[31] For working through ethical problem areas, this seven-step process includes (1) describing the facts of the situation, (2) identifying the problems that are present or anticipated, (3) describing the values at stake, (4) identifying the resources available to address the problem, (5) identifying the options for a decision, (6) proposing a solution, and (7) evaluating the outcomes.

Human relationships and human resource management in the workplace are critical functions of the resource management dietitian. Several guiding principles toward this end have been deliberated by Brodeur[32] as follows:

- Treat people as an end, not as a means.
- Pay personnel justly.
- Do not lie to or manipulate other individuals.
- Institute mechanisms for participatory decision making.
- Ensure that personnel policies are just and do not discriminate.
- Treat all with dignity and respect.
- Ensure fair disciplinary policies.
- Do not allow physical or sexual harassment in the workplace.

THE FUTURE

The future practitioner in food and nutrition management will need to be prepared for expanded roles and new opportunities. Derelian[27] describes the expanded roles as falling into three categories: (1) taking on new responsibilities within dietetic practice, (2) taking on new responsibilities not generally associated with dietetics, (3) and creating new roles for the profession.

Halling and Hess, in 1995, outlined several observations relating to the separation of food and food service from clinical nutrition and voiced concern that a vital part of the profession could be lost.[1] Since then, a new DPG that focuses on foods has been formed (the food and culinary professionals) and an emphasis area in food service systems management has been identified for the education of dietitians.[20] These activities provide heightened visibility for this important area of practice in a time when there is a high level of consumer interest in good eating and what constitutes "healthy" food, and they are thus very positive steps.

There are further opportunities for dietitians in the commercial food service industry in marketing, menu planning/analysis/policy, provision of food and nutrition information, and promotion and sales.[18] It is also suggested that by partnering with hospitality and culinary programs, alliances may be built that position dietitians as providers of services in the commercial food industry.

It is predicted that school food and nutrition programs will undergo major restructuring by the year 2000 and that the result will be changes in present approaches to operating and managing programs.[33] Despite several anticipated forces leading to the changes, school food and nutrition programs will continue to provide a valuable service to the nutrition and health of school-age children. Professionals trained to use new technologies, deal with competitive and environmental concerns as well as the government, and who continue to provide quality food service and nutrition education will be needed.

Managerial roles in college and university food services are similar to those in hospital food services, however, managerial positions are less likely to be filled by registered dietitians.[34] This may be an area of practice in which the services of a dietitian need to be "sold" because of the need for nutrition education as well as the provision of appealing food choices for this vulnerable age group.

CONCLUSION

The food service industry is one of the largest industries in the country. The efficiency and effectiveness of these food services are important to the health of the American public and to the economic well-being of the country. The opportunities for dietitians in food service management are many and, to the extent their competency and competitiveness in assuming these positions is manifested, the future is unlimited.

DEFINITIONS

Food Production Preparation of food involving purchasing, storage, and processing or preparing food for service.

Food Services Production and service of food; also refers to the unit or group responsible for providing feeding of groups, usually in an institutional setting.

Food Service Systems Activities that together form the inputs, transformation, and outputs making up an entire food operation.

Human Resources Personnel in an organization or institution.

Leadership Process of setting goals and priorities and maintaining standards among associates and subordinates.

Management Administration of the activities and functions within an organizational unit.

Operations Analysis and Planning Development and enforcement policies, procedures, and reports.

Quality Assurance Certification of the continuous, optimal, effective, and efficient outcomes of a service or program.

Resource Allocation Equitable distribution of financial, physical, and human capital.

Role Delineation Study of activities and specified responsibilities for which a practitioner is responsible.

Systems Approach Use of a process consisting of a sequence of procedures involving transformations and feedback.

Transformation Action or activity used in changing input into output in a system.
Work Processes Sequence of actions and interactions between customers and suppliers that results in a product or service.

REFERENCES

1. Halling JF, Hess MA. Vision vs. reality: ADA members as food/food management experts. *J Am Diet Assoc*. 1995;95:169–170.
2. Cassell JA. *Carry the Flame: The History of The American Dietetic Association*. Chicago: The American Dietetic Association; 1990.
3. Barker A, Foltz M, Arensberg MBF, Schiller MR. *Leadership in Dietetics: Achieving a Vision for the Future*. Chicago: The American Dietetic Association; 1994.
4. Spears MC. *Foodservice Organizations: A Managerial and Systems Approach*. 3rd ed. Englewood Cliffs, NJ: Prentice Hall; 1995.
5. Bryk JA, Soto TK. Report on the 1993 membership database of The American Dietetic Association. *J Am Diet Assoc*. 1994;94:1433–1437.
6. Bryk JA, Soto TK. Report on the 1995 membership database of The American Dietetic Association. *J Am Diet Assoc*. 1997;97:197–203.
7. Taylor M. *Quality of Work Life Assessment of Dietitians in Business and Industry*. Stillwater: Oklahoma State University; 1984. Unpublished MS thesis.
8. Liu YA. *Incentives Perceived by Management Dietitians To Reduce Absenteeism Rate of Foodservice Personnel in Health Care Systems*. Stillwater: Oklahoma State University; 1996. Unpublished PhD dissertation.
9. Molt MK. Dietitians' ratings of helpfulness of experiences to their leadership development. *NACUFS J*. 1995;19:41–50.
10. ADA. *Role Delineation for Registered Dietitians and Entry-Level Dietetic Technicians*. Chicago: The American Dietetic Association; 1990.
11. Focus on: dietitians work in correctional system. *ADA Courier*. 1989;68(29):3.
12. Grossman ME, Magnus M. Order up food services. *Personnel J*. 1989:70–72.
13. Molt, M. *Food for Fifty*. 10th ed. New York: Prentice Hall; 1997.
14. Pilant VB. Current issues in child nutrition programs. *Top Clin Nutr*. 1994;9:1–8.
15. *Child Nutr. Q*. Publication of the National Food Service Management Institute. University of Mississippi. 1995;1:(1).
16. National Food Service Management Institute. *Job Functions and Tasks of School Nutrition Managers and District Managers/Supervisors*. University, Mississippi: University of Mississippi; 1995.
17. Shanklin CW, Dowling R. Opportunities in commercial foodservice: the member's perspective. *J Am Diet Assoc*. 1995;95:236–238.
18. Lechowich KA, Soto TK. Opportunities in commercial foodservice: the industry perspective. *J Am Diet Assoc*. 1995;95:1163–1166.

19. Kane MT, Cohen AS, Smith ER, Lewis C, et al. 1995 commission on dietetic registration dietetics practice audit. *J Am Diet Assoc.* 1996;96:1292–1301.

20. Gilmore CJ, Maillet JO, Mitchell BE. Determining educational preparation based on job competencies of entry-level dietetics practitioners. *J Am Diet Assoc.* 1997;97:306–316.

21. Kane MT, Estes CA, Colton DA, Eltoft CS. Role delineation for dietetic practitioners: empirical results. *J Am Diet Assoc.* 1990;90:1124–1133.

22. Arensberg MBF, Schiller MR, Vivian VM, Johnson WA, et al. Transformational leadership of clinical nutrition managers. *J Am Diet Assoc.* 1996;96:39–45.

23. Witte SS, Messersmith AM. Clinical nutrition management position: reponsibilities and skill development strategies. *J Am Diet Assoc.* 1995;95:1113–1120.

24. Watabe-Dawson M. Visionary leaders are key to success in foodservice. *J Am Diet Assoc.* 1995;95:13.

25. Dowling R., Lafferty LJ, Norton C. The management component of our profession. *J Am Diet Assoc.* 1990;90:1065–1067.

26. Bogle ML, Balogun L, Cassell J, Catakis A, et al. Achieving excellence in dietetic practice: certification of specialists and advanced-level practitioners. *J Am Diet Assoc.* 1993;93:149–150.

27. Derelian D. President's page: expanded roles mean expanded opportunities. *J Am Diet Assoc.* 1995;95:708.

28. Heifetz RA, Laurie DL. The work of leadership. *Harvard Business Rev.* 1997; 75: 124–134.

29. ADA. *Code of Ethics.* Chicago: American Dietetic Association; 1987.

30. Paine LS. Managing for organizational integrity. *Harvard Business Rev.* 1994;72: 106–117.

31. Meslin EM, Limieux-Charles L, Wortley JJ. An ethics framework for assisting clinical managers in resource allocation decision making. *Hosp Health Serv Adm.* 1997;42: 33–47.

32. Brodeur D. Health care institutional ethics: broader than clinical ethics. In: Monagle JF, Thomasma DC, eds. *Health Care Ethics: Critical Issue.* Gaithersburg, Md: Aspen Publishers; 1994.

33. White G, Sneed J, Martin J. School food service in the year 2000. *School Food Serv J.* 1992; 46:June–July:68–70, 130.

34. Sultemeier PM, Gregoire MB, Spears MC, Downey R. Managerial functions of college and university foodservice managers. *J Am Diet Assoc.* 1989;89:924–928.

CHAPTER 10

Community Nutrition Practice

Helene M. Kent

"It is the position of The American Dietetic Association that nutrition education is essential for the public to achieve and maintain optimal nutritional health. Nutrition education should be an integral component of all health promotion, disease prevention, and health maintenance programs, through incorporation into all appropriate nutrition communication, promotion, and education systems."[1]

Outline—Chapter 10

- Introduction
  - Public health nutrition
- History
- Field of Public Health
  - Prevention
  - Levels of prevention
- Areas of Activity
- Activities of Community Nutritionists
- Career Paths
  - Classes of positions
  - Specialty areas of practice
- Ethical Issues

- Future Issues

- Conclusion

INTRODUCTION

Community nutrition is the branch of nutrition that addresses the entire range of food and nutrition issues related to individuals, families, and special groups with a common bond such as place of residence, language, culture, or health issue. Community nutrition programs include those programs that provide increased access to food resources, food and nutrition education, and health-related care. Public health nutrition is the component of community nutrition that is publicly funded and provided through a public health agency to promote health, prevent disease, and provide primary care. The community dietitian or community nutritionist or public health nutritionist is the dietetic professional who works in the area of community nutrition.

Community nutrition/dietetics professionals are members of community and public health agency staffs who are responsible for nutrition services that emphasize communitywide health promotion and disease prevention and address the needs of individuals in primary and/or ambulatory care. These dietetic professionals establish linkages with other professionals involved with the broad range of human services including child care agencies, services to the elderly, educational institutions, and community-based research. They focus on promoting health and preventing disease in the community by using a population and systems focus and a client or personal health service approach.[2]

Public Health Nutrition

Practice in community nutrition is characterized by a focus on the community and includes those activities that are focused on groups rather than individuals. The largest subunit of community nutrition is the practice of public health nutrition. Whereas the practice area of community nutrition tends to be large and has a small body of defining literature, public health nutrition is well defined and includes a large body of literature discussing its role and defining characteristics. Public health nutritionists tend to work in federal, state, or local agencies.

To understand what a public health nutritionist does requires familiarity with the field of public health. Public health has been defined as "the science and art of preventing disease, prolonging life, and promoting health and efficiency through organized community effort, so organizing these benefits as to enable every citizen to realize his birthright of health and longevity."[3] The public health population–based or epidemiologic approach is distinguished from the clinical or one-on-one care approach.[4] Public health focuses on society as a whole, the community, and the aim of optimal health status. The mission of public health is the fulfillment of society's interest in ensuring the conditions in which individuals can be healthy.[5] The goal of the discipline of public health nutrition is to promote optimal nutrition and health for all members of the population by improving nutritional status and maintaining health.[6]

Kaufman presents a definition of the public health nutritionist as "the member of the public health agency staff who is responsible for planning, organizing, managing, directing, coordinating and evaluating the nutrition component of the health agency's services. The public health nutritionist establishes linkages with related community nutrition programs, nutrition education, food assistance, social or welfare services, care services to the elderly, other human services and community based research."[4]

HISTORY[7–9]

Efforts in the 1800s were primarily toward building the foundation for public health nutrition services; organizing state health departments and voluntary health agencies, initiating early nutrition investigations, and establishing milk stations and school lunch programs in large cities to supplement the food of the poor and to combat high rates of morbidity and mortality of infants and children. Since 1900, public health nutrition has developed as an area of professional practice. At the turn of the century, pioneer researchers in nutrition began to discover and to describe the relationship of food intake and energy expenditure to health. Simultaneously, home economists and social dietitians, the forerunners of today's public health nutrition workers, were helping impoverished immigrant mothers who were unfamiliar with local foods provide nutritious meals for their families. These forerunners were employed by local private health and welfare agencies. They counseled and educated mothers, both individually and in small groups.

During the twentieth century, many changes occurred that influenced the growth and development of public health nutrition services, such as advances in nutrition science and technology, social, political, demographic, and economic changes. Such changes included the high rates of disease and deaths among mothers and children; food shortages during the wars; increasing numbers of children in child care as more mothers went to work; the development of new programs to serve special groups such as the mentally retarded, chronically ill and disabled, recent immigrants, and the aged; the continuing presence of poverty and hunger; the rising prevalence of behavior-related problems (e.g., adolescent pregnancy and substance abuse); and a greater recognition of the benefits of health promotion and disease prevention. Continuing concerns include nutrition policy and planning; development and evaluation of programs; organization, administration, and management of programs; quality of nutrition services; and the transfer and application of research into nutrition practice.

In the 1920s, nutrition researchers began to relate the newly identified vitamins and minerals to specific nutritional deficiency diseases such as rickets, scurvy, pellegra, and anemia, which were then significant public health problems. During the same period, in an effort to reduce maternal and infant mortality, maternal and child health units in several states and large local public health departments began to employ public health nutritionists as consultants and educators.

The term nutritionist came into use in the mid-1920s and was widely accepted by 1930. Hunger and malnutrition were rampant during the Great Depression of the 1930s. Their prevalence, and a growing awareness that nutrition affected individuals and communities, led government leaders to recognize that there was a need to expand public health nutrition services.

Title V of the 1935 Social Security Act gave the first national impetus to the expanded employment of public health nutritionists as consultants in state maternal and child health programs. During the 1940s, the number of nutritionists employed increased, and some state nutrition units added district or regional consultants. These consultants provided training for physicians, nurses, health educators, and teachers.

During the 1950s, policy makers observed the abundance and quality of the American food supply. In this decade, health problems related to dietary excesses such as obesity, diabetes, hypertension, heart disease, and dental caries were identified as emerging public health problems. As public health agencies developed programs in chronic disease control, adult health, and health services for the aging, specialized public health nutritionists were employed to work with these chronic disease programs. The increased mobility of young families at a time when the elderly population was expanding resulted in the proliferation of nursing homes as a new type of health care facility. Institutional nutrition by dietary consultants began as state and local agencies responsible for the licensing of nursing homes and for improving the quality of care in these facilities.

Title V of the Social Security Act was amended in 1963 in response to the growing awareness that the United States still had excessive infant mortality rates and maternal and child health problems. Special project grant funding was made available to initiate maternal and infant care projects and health services projects for children and youth. Funding was also provided for special programs for prevention of mental retardation, rehabilitation of the retarded, and prevention of handicapping conditions through newborn intensive care, university-affiliated child development centers, and expanded services to high-risk mothers and infants.

In the 1960s, the country witnessed widespread awareness of nutrition issues. The agenda was set for expanding the food assistance programs and developing new systems for nutrition surveillance in nutrition service. The Head Start Program was initiated in this decade, and others soon followed.

The 1972 Child Nutrition Act provided funding to launch the Special Supplemental Food Program for Women, Infants, and Children (WIC). During the 1970s, federal legislation created new types of community foods and nutrition resources that required linkages with public health nutrition programs. The US Department of Agriculture's Expanded Food and Nutrition Program, for example, was implemented by the Cooperative Extension System in every US state and territory. The Food Stamp Act was also revised and expanded during this time. The Older Americans Act provided for congregate and home-delivered meals for the elderly through local agencies on aging. In 1977, an amendment to the Child Nutrition Act authorized funding for nutrition education training, which provided expanded nutrition education to school children, parents, and school food service personnel.

Public health concerns during the 1970s began to focus on the quality and safety of the food supply and on the role of diet in preventing chronic degenerative diseases. In 1978, the Senate Select Committee on nutrition and human need published the first dietary goals, the predecessor to the 1980 dietary guidelines for Americans. The 1979 Surgeon General's report, *Healthy People,* especially cited nutrition and diet among the significant factors affecting the health of the population.

The Department of Health and Human Services and the Department of Agriculture published the *Dietary Guidelines for Americans* in 1980 (which have been revised each five-year period thereafter). The Department of Health and Human Services developed *Health Promotion and Disease Prevention: Objectives for the Nation,* to be achieved by 1990. In 1990, the objectives were expanded upon and "Healthy People 2000" objectives were developed with a midcourse review issued in 1995.[10] Objectives for 2010 are also in process. Nutrition was 1 of the 15 areas addressed in this publication. Achieving the nutrition objectives required the provision of information and education to the public to motivate changes in dietary behavior and lifestyles. Nutrition professionals were challenged to develop and expand their roles as educators, consultants, and care coordinators.

By the terms of block grant funding for major public health and nutrition programs instituted in 1982, the responsibility to plan for their population needs was delegated to state and local agencies. This approach challenged nutritionists as they needed to compete for diminishing levels of public funding to maintain services. The 1980s saw advances in nutrition research and practice including new communication and data management technologies, changes in legislation, and an increasing public interest in nutrition and fitness.[8,11]

FIELD OF PUBLIC HEALTH

Kaufman has identified the public health population–based or epidemiologic approach as distinguished from the clinical one-on-one patient care approach.[4] The public health approach is the following:

- Uses interventions that promote health and prevent communicable or chronic diseases by managing or controlling the community environment.
- Promotes a healthy lifestyle as a shared value for all people.
- Directs money and energy to the problems that affect the lives of the largest number of the community's people.
- Targets the unserved or underserved populations by virtue of income, age, ethnicity, heredity, or lifestyle who are particularly vulnerable to disease, hunger, or malnutrition.
- Requires the collaboration of the public, consumers, community leaders, legislators, policy makers, administrators, and health and human service professionals in assessing and responding to community needs and consumer demands.
- Continuously monitors the health of the people in the community to ensure that the public health system achieves its objectives and responds to current needs.

Prevention

The prevention of illness is the purpose of public health as well as in community nutrition practice. Prevention may take place at any point along the spectrum from prevention of disease to the prevention of impairment or disability. Prevention has three essential components: personal health, community-based, and social policies/systems–based. Each component has distinct roles, importance, and focus. Community nutrition practice involves making appropriate and coordinated use of each. Personal health deals with prevention issues at the individual level, such as working with a client to improve the diet for health promotion purposes. Community-based prevention is targeted toward groups such as the Five-a-Day campaign that focuses on increased consumption of fruits and vegetables. Social policies/systems–level prevention focuses on changing policies and law so that the goals of prevention practice are achieved (e.g., laws regarding food safety, tobacco, or alcohol).

Levels of Prevention

For each of the three components of prevention, there are three levels of prevention. *Primary prevention* or health promotion efforts involves prevention of the disease itself. Primary prevention involves health promotion to maintain a state of wellness and focuses on changing or enhancing the environment, community, family, and individual lifestyles and behaviors.

Secondary prevention is the detection, diagnosis, and intervention early in the disease process to minimize detrimental and disabling effects. Secondary prevention focuses on risk appraisal and reduction and includes screening, detection, early diagnoses, treatment, and follow-up before a disease has developed overt symptoms. Interventions or treatments are designed to reduce risk among those who may be more susceptible to a health problem because of their family history, lifestyle, environment, or age.

Tertiary intervention is directed at treating and rehabilitating persons with diagnosed health conditions to prevent or delay their disability, pain, suffering, and premature death. These interventions are provided more commonly by ambulatory health care centers, hospital inpatient and outpatient facilities, and private practitioners and are used most by older persons.[4]

AREAS OF ACTIVITY

Community and public health nutritionists work in a variety of settings that focus on improving the community's health. Positions are characterized by an emphasis on health and wellness and an application of nutrition science to maintain health and cure disease. Community dietitians often work in federal, state, or local public health agency neighborhood or community health centers, industries, ambulatory care clinics, home health agencies and specialized community projects, nonprofit and for-profit private health agencies, institutions, private practices, community-based programs operated by nonprofit programs, or programs associated with industry and hospitals.

Each state has a department of health employing public health nutritionists. Many states also employ dietitians/nutritionists in related departments such as the Indian health service, health and human services or welfare, department of education (school nutrition programs), and in agencies for the aging. The land-grant university in each state administers the cooperative extension programs in which nutritionists, nutrition educators, and expanded food and nutrition education programs are employed.

ACTIVITIES OF COMMUNITY NUTRITIONISTS

According to the ADA, approximately 13 percent of all registered dietitians (RDs) work in community health. More than three-quarters of those employed in public health work for WIC. WIC provides supplemental foods and nutrition education and improves access to health services for low-income pregnant, breastfeeding, and nonbreastfeeding women, infants, and children up to five years of age. Maternal and child health services and other public health programs employ an additional one-fourth of all public health nutritionists. Other public health positions include adult health, institutional management, and work with children with special health care needs.[12]

For individuals to benefit from nutrition research findings, nutritionists working in the community must be able to translate science into practical dietary guidance. In practical terms, this means providing information about foods that are available and affordable in local markets. All nutritionists must be experts in normal and clinical nutrition and be competent in bringing about changes in eating behavior. To be a credible nutrition resource, the RD who works in public health nutrition must understand the fundamentals of nutrition and food science and dietetics, along with their underlying bases in human physiology, chemistry, biochemistry, and behavioral sciences. This includes in-depth knowledge of nutritional needs during stages in the life span as people of all ages will be served in the various programs. Awareness of family-centered care and case management is important as is the ability to function as a clinical or public health team member for diagnostic, evaluative, and follow-up programs providing services for clients in a comprehensive, culturally sensitive, and community-based service system.[4] The nutritionist must develop political and communication skills and be knowledgeable about public policy development and strategic planning.[6,9,11]

Some nutritionists focus primarily on population-based interventions for health promotion/disease prevention. Others who provide more direct nutrition care usually focus their energies on providing nutrition services to medically high-risk persons. There are, however, many nutritionists whose positions are a mix of functions that include community assessment and program development along with client-focused clinical care.

Other duties may include nutrition training for other agency staff as well as providing technical assistance to other professionals; serving as a resource to the public, media, business, and industry; and advocating for needed nutrition policy at the local, state, and/or federal level. Others may include advising the agency administrator, policy makers, and staff on current nutrition research findings that can contribute to the public's health and to the organization's mission, policies, and programs.

CAREER PATHS

The term *public health nutritionist* has usually been reserved for the member of the nutrition team who has a master's degree in public health nutrition. This training includes acquiring skills required to participate in policy analysis and program development. He or she knows the practical aspects of assessing nutritional needs of a community and develops skills in planning, evaluating, and implementing programs to meet these needs. Academic training includes knowledge of biostatistics and skills in collecting, compiling, analyzing, and reporting demographic, health, and food consumption data and understanding the epidemiology of health and disease distribution patterns in the population and studying trends over time.

Classes of Positions

According to Dodds et al., public health nutrition personnel can be placed in three major classes based on the major focus of their responsibilities: management, professional, and technical.[9] Each of these series is subdivided into several positions. The categorization is shown in Table 10–1.

The entry-level dietitian or nutritionist would usually begin at the professional level. Both the managerial and professional classes generally require registration with the commission on dietetic registration as well as licensure (where applicable) as a nutritionist or dietitian. In addition, a master's degree in public health that includes course work in advanced nutrition is recommended for those in management in public health nutrition. For the clinical nutrition class, a master's degree in advanced human and clinical nutrition is recommended.

Specialty Areas of Practice[9]

Adult health promotion/chronic disease prevention and control specialists may work in health care facilities, worksite health promotion, and community health

Table 10–1 Positions of Public Health Nutritionists

Class	Title of Position	Functions
Management	Public health director Assistant public health director	Policy making, planning, management, supervision, fiscal control
Professional	Public health nutrition consultant Public health nutritionist Clinical nutritionist Nutritionist	Planning and evaluation, consultation, care coordination, case management, counseling
Technical	Nutrition technician Nutrition assistant	Education, screening, record keeping, outreach

Source: Adapted with permission from J.M. Dodds and M. Kaufman, *Personnel in Public Health Nutrition for the 1990s. A Comprehensive Guide.* © 1991, The Public Health Foundation.

agencies. Knowledge of nutritional management of specific chronic diseases and behavioral and lifestyle change methodologies is required.

Specialists working with special health care needs related to developmental diseases and chronic disabling conditions need clinical knowledge of child growth and development with an emphasis on the effects of mental retardation, developmental disabilities, and rehabilitation. Knowledge of techniques of feeding under special conditions is also required.

Maternal and child health specialists understand principles of nutrition in pregnancy and lactation and in infancy, childhood, and adolescence. This includes the physical, psychological, and socioeconomic aspects of these early periods of life.

Communication and media specialists must have knowledge of how individuals learn and of nutrition education methodology. They must also know how to use media effectively to design and implement nutrition promotion campaigns by using a variety of communication channels including television, radio, newspapers, magazines, and computers in many settings.

Data management and nutrition surveillance nutritionists require additional training in biostatistics, epidemiology, and computer-based data management. Their responsibilities include the development of user-friendly systems for collecting, analyzing, interpreting, and presenting numerical data to be used in community program planning.

Environmental health and food safety specialists have advanced knowledge and skills in food science, food processing technology, microbiology, epidemiology, and food safety laws and regulation. They must be able to interpret federal, state, and local regulations regarding food safety.

Institutional food service systems management for health care and group care facilities specialists have in-depth knowledge of food service systems management, health care financing, clinical nutrition, and nutritional care planning.

Home health specialists have advanced knowledge of diet therapy for chronic disease and chronic disabling conditions of adults and children.

Research specialists need to know how to prepare grant proposals, manage data, coordinate field-based studies, and design research protocols.

Educators of public health nutrition professionals must have the knowledge and skills to prepare students for practice in public health or community health agencies.

ETHICAL ISSUES

Ethical action refers to decisions about which actions, relationships, and policies ought to be considered right or wrong.[13] Many ethical questions faced by community dietitians/nutritionists are similar to those in other disciplines. For instance, the community RD must be honest when information is communicated about diet and health to judge if there is sufficient knowledge to warrant translation of scientific findings into dietary advice at a point in time. Schiller, in discussing the role of ethics in the practice of diabetes, says that health care practitioners may be guided by ethical principles that include:

- justice (to ensure that all people are treated fairly)
- beneficence (which obligates one to do good)
- the good of society (which must be considered in balance with the good of the individual)[14]

The American Dietetic Association Code of Ethics (Appendix A) is specific for professional actions involving practice and conduct.

FUTURE ISSUES

Community nutrition practice is changing as the overall health care system evolves. Expanding opportunities during a time of decreasing funding require dietitians working in the community to be well prepared academically to compete. At the same time, more nutrition personnel with advanced clinical skills are needed to provide intensive nutritional care in the home and community to medically high-risk pregnant women, disabled and chronically ill infants and children, chronically ill adults, and the elderly.

Public health agencies will assume more population-focused responsibilities, and nutrition professionals will likely shift from a client-focused system with direct care services responsibilities to a population/systems focus with more administrative and planning-related functions.[15] Some in public health will continue to provide personal health services, particularly in areas where providers are limited or where certain high-risk populations are underserved. This shift from a client to a population focus will occur at different rates. In communities where access to clinical, prevention, and therapeutic services is limited, the transition will be slow. Public health and community nutrition professionals will need to be proactive and creative in assuming their responsibilities.[2]

Technical competence relating to the role of nutrition in health and disease throughout the life span will be needed. Additional skills in advocacy and knowledge of how to affect public policy will also be required. Coalition and partnership building, communication skills, behavioral change strategies, and cultural competence are needed to meet commmunity needs. Practitioners with a client focus will need to ensure that services are culturally sensitive and relevant.[15]

Dietitians must cope with future demographic and economic changes, including a growing elderly population, children living with single parents, increased needs for child care, a larger proportion of minorities, and allocation of limited resources. Concerns about the adequacy and safety of the food supply must be continually addressed.[6] Critical health issues include the access to health and nutrition services for everyone, the role of nutrition in health care reform, and community-based programs for the delivery of nutrition services throughout the life span. The role of nutrition risk factors in health promotion/disease prevention is an important issue, and new technologies as well as research will be needed to assess this role fully.

The public is demanding accurate information about nutrition and health and ways to incorporate the information into individual lifestyles. Practitioners who wish to prepare themselves for the health care environment of the future will care for community health, expand access to effective care, provide contemporary clinical care, provide primary care, participate in coordinated care, ensure cost-effective and appropriate care, practice preventive health care, involve patients and families in decision-making processes, promote healthy lifestyles, assess and use appropriate technology, improve the health care system, manage information, understand the role of the physical environment in health care, provide counseling on ethical issues and function ethically, accommodate and expand accountability, participate in a racially and culturally diverse society, and understand the necessity for and participate in continued professional learning.[16] Many of these are already key components in community nutrition practice.

CONCLUSION

Community nutrition involves professionals who interact with the community to promote health and prevent chronic disease. Dietitians/nutritionists working in community nutrition have positions in a variety of areas including public health, community aging programs, cooperative extension, outpatient and public health clinics, state and local government, and agencies dealing with chronic disease conditions. The emphasis in community nutrition is on meeting the nutrient needs of individuals during all ages of life, thus maintaining health and preventing disease.

DEFINITIONS[9]

Case Management Process by which the comprehensive health and social needs of a patient or client are assessed, provided, coordinated, monitored, and evaluated.

Class All positions sufficiently similar as to kind or subject matter of work, level of difficulty and responsibility, and qualifications required to warrant the same title, entrance requirements, and pay schedule.

Client The recipient of services or products.

Client-Based Focus Use of assessment and diagnostic methods to identify individuals at high medical and/or nutrition risk and provide interventions in the form of one-on-one counseling or small group counseling and education as part of clinic or health care.

Community Group of persons whose members share a common bond such as living in the same geographic area or sharing the same culture or language.

Community Assessment Formal process of collecting and evaluating relevant information about the ecology of a particular community and applying the data to determine met and unmet needs of the population.

Community Health Services Health services provided for a specific group of people who have a common bond such as language, geographic area, socioeconomic needs, or similar health problems.

Consultation Act of providing technical information, technical assistance, and making professional recommendations to others.

Counseling Interactive process of exchanging information to give professional advice or recommendations to a client and/or caregiver in developing a mutually acceptable plan of care.

Health Care Team Group of health professionals who work together with the common objective of providing comprehensive and coordinated health care services to individuals and their families.

Health Promotion/Disease Prevention Education and preventive health measures directed toward basically healthy populations to foster wellness and prevent illness.

Nutrition Assessment Evaluation of an individual's nutritional status based on anthropometric, biochemical, clinical, and dietary information.

Nutrition Surveillance Continuous assessment of the nutritional status of a particular population for the purpose of detecting changes in trends or distribution of nutrition-related health problems.

Outreach Function of identifying and contacting potential clients, who are then screened to determine their eligibility for program services.

Population-Based Focus Use of epidemiologic methods to describe health and nutrition needs in the community and serve as the basis for designing interventions to reach the general population of large segments of the population at particular risk.

Program Planning Process by which administrators assess needs and develop a plan to meet those needs.

Screening Obtaining data by measurement, test, or interview to identify problems or to secure information required to establish health or nutritional status and/or need and/or eligibility for services.

REFERENCES

1. ADA. Position of The American Dietetic Association: nutrition education for the public. *J Am Diet Assoc.* 1996;96:1183–1187.

2. Public Health Nutrition Practice Group. *The American Dietetic Association Guidelines for Community Nutrition Supervised Practice Experience.* Chicago: The American Dietetic Association; 1995.

3. Winslow CEA. The untitled field of public health. Mod Med. 1920;2:183.

4. Kaufman M. *Nutrition in Public Health: A Handbook for Developing Programs and Services.* Rockville, MD: Aspen Publishers; 1990.

5. Institute of Medicine. *The Future of Public Health.* Washington, DC: National Academy Press; 1988.

6. *Strategies for Success: Curriculum Guide for Graduate Programs in Public Health Nutrition.* Washington, DC: Association of the Faculties of Graduate Programs in Public Health Nutrition; 1990.

7. Kaufman M, ed. *Personnel in Public Health: Nutrition for the 1980s.* McLean, VA: Association of State and Territorial Health Officials Foundation; 1982.

8. Egan MC. Public health nutrition: a historical perspective. *J Am Diet Assoc.* 1994;94:298–304.

9. Dodds JM, Kaufman M. *Personnel in Public Health Nutrition for the 1990s: A Comprehensive Guide.* Washington, DC: The Public Health Foundation; 1991.

10. *Healthy People 2000: Midcourse Review and 1995 Revision.* Department of Health and Human Services. USPHS: Washington, DC, 1995.

11. Association of Schools of Public Health. *Graduate Education for Public Health.* Washington, DC: Association of Schools of Public Health; 1988.

12. *ASTPHND Biennial Profile of Personnel in Public Health Nutrition.* Recruitment of Public/Community Nutritionist Workshop. Association of State and Territorial Public Health Nutrition Directors; 1994.

13. Monsen ER, Vanderpool HY, Halsted CH, McNutt KW, et al. Ethics: responsible scientific conduct. *Am J Clin Nutr.* 1991;54:6.

14. Schiller MR. Ethics in the practice of dietetics. *Top Clin Nutr.* 1997;12:1–11.

15. Story M, Haughton B, Olmstead-Schafer M. Future training needs in public health nutrition. Results of a national Delphi survey. Unpublished.

16. Shugars DA, O'Neil EH, Bader JD, eds. *Healthy American: Practitioners for 2005, An Agenda for Action for US Health Professions Schools.* Durham, NC: Pew Health Professions Commission; 1991.

Dietitians in Education and Research

M. Rosita Schiller

"Knowledge is the one precious commodity that can be given away without a loss."[1]

Outline—Chapter 11

- Introduction

- Dietitians in Education
  - Elementary and secondary schools
  - Colleges and universities
  - Medical and dental education
  - Nursing and allied health nutrition education
  - Industry-based education
  - Worksite nutrition education

- Dietitians in Research
  - Academic health centers
  - Food companies
  - Industry
  - Government

- Career Maps for Education and Research

- Importance of Education and Research to the Profession

- ADA Education and Research Practice Groups

- Ethical and Legal Bases of Practice
- Case Study of a Dietitian Educator
- Case Study of a Dietitian in Research
- Conclusion

INTRODUCTION

Almost every dietitian serves as an educator some of the time. For example, administrative dietitians conduct inservice programs for food service employees. Public health nutritionists give classes for home care nurses. Clinical dietitians participate in medical nutrition education, and they often conduct group classes for patients with diabetes or coronary heart disease. Consultant dietitians may give food demonstrations for chefs. Dietitians working with Special Supplemental Women, Infants, and Children (WIC) food programs may teach Head Start children how to prevent or reduce the incidence of obesity and adult-onset diabetes.[2] In industry, dietitians are called on to teach sales representatives about specialty nutrition products. Many dietitians are preceptors for dietetics students. Regardless of specialty, many dietitians give classes during national nutrition month. Yet, these dietetics practitioners are unlikely to classify themselves as "educators."

Many dietitians conduct research as a small part of their work. This is especially true for dietitians who specialize in nutrition support, pediatrics, renal dietetics, oncology, acquired immunodeficiency syndrome (AIDS), diabetes, or other clinical subspecialties. Such dietitians often critique research articles or collect research data. They are encouraged to do outcomes research studies to demonstrate the effectiveness of medical nutrition therapy. They may collaborate with physicians who are conducting nutrition-related studies. These dietitians are unlikely to call themselves "researchers."

This chapter focuses on full-time career opportunities in education and research. It offers a bird's eye view of teaching or research positions in schools, colleges and universities, medical centers, government agencies, and industry.

DIETITIANS IN EDUCATION

Elementary and Secondary Schools

Most school-based nutrition education is incorporated into health and science classes in primary, middle, and high schools.[3] A dietitian who teaches at these levels needs to meet state teacher-training and certification requirements. Generally, those who teach grades K–12 have responsibilities that extend well beyond food, nutrition, and health.

Some state departments of education have nutrition education and training sections that often employ registered dietitians (RD) who have advanced degrees in education. Such positions include creating curricula to integrate nutrition with other subjects, developing teaching materials, identifying instructional resources, and training teachers to deliver nutrition education.[4]

Job opportunities for dietitians in child nutrition programs are increasing. Such positions allow dietitians to work closely with both teachers and students to expand nutrition from the lunchroom to the classroom.[5] School-based health centers, a rapidly growing model for the delivery of comprehensive, primary health care to elementary, middle, and senior high school students affords another opportunity for dietitians interested in working with children and adolescents.[6]

Colleges and Universities

There are teaching opportunities for dietitians at culinary institutes, technical schools, and both two- and four-year colleges. Such positions are often associated with programs for chefs, food service supervisors, dietetic technicians, dietary managers, entry-level dietitians, and hospitality managers. The emphasis is on teaching in the classroom, laboratory, or practice setting. Course responsibilities may include food preparation and food science, basic and applied nutrition, meal management, cultural food practices, food service management and equipment, nutrition assessment and therapy, nutrition counseling and education, and community nutrition.

University teaching can be at the baccalaureate, master's, or doctoral level. At the baccalaureate level, professors usually focus on one or another area of dietetics: clinical dietetics, food service management, or community nutrition. In addition, these faculty often teach introductory courses in foods and nutrition. Those who teach at the master's and doctoral levels are usually quite specialized, focusing on a narrowly defined area such as a class of nutrients, energy requirements, diabetes, obesity, AIDS, pregnancy, or nutrition and aging. In addition to classroom teaching, professors may write textbooks and laboratory manuals, develop computer programs, and provide individualized instruction for students.

University faculty roles are quite varied. In addition to their teaching responsibilities, university faculty are required to conduct research and provide service within the institution, community, or profession. They spend a good bit of time in advising student research, serving on committees, consulting with community groups, sharing their expertise with the media and the public, and providing leadership for nutrition-related initiatives.

Higher education can include teaching other groups of students. For example, some institutions offer nutrition courses for nonmajors to fulfill requirements for general education, teacher certification, or health and physical education. Programs in the allied health professions may include nutrition courses. Dietitians can teach courses in nutritional anthropology or epidemiology, often included as part of master's in public health (MPH) programs.

Many colleges and universities offer nutrition education for the student body through university health centers.[7] Dietitians are the most common providers and are usually coordinators for these programs. Besides one-on-one counseling, there can be group presentations in residence halls and point-of-service education in cafeterias. College students can get involved in such activities through peer education programs sponsored by some campuses.[8]

Medical and Dental Education

A few graduate-trained dietitians are engaged in medical and dental nutrition education. Such a role requires assertiveness, creativity, persistence, and tenacity to convince administrators of the unique role that dietitians can play in this regard. Besides an in-depth knowledge of nutrition science and medical nutrition therapy, medical and dental nutrition educators must possess leadership, self-direction, strong communication skills, conceptual thinking skills, time management, and flexibility.[9]

Nutrition education can occur at any level of a medical or dental curriculum. It may consist of nutrition science with clinical applications during the first two years. As students enter the clinical part of their program, diet lunches and seminars are effective.[10] Nutrition rounds and seminars can be incorporated when students are in clerkships. Practicing dietitians can be involved in problem-based learning as an effective way to make nutrition relevant for future medical practice.[11]

Dietitians may also teach in medical residency training programs, especially family practice and pediatrics. Here, the dietitian's role is extremely varied. They often model patient nutritional care services for physicians. They may give conferences and grand rounds, develop medical nutrition education resources, design case studies, and help physicians incorporate nutrition into the history and physical examination. They find ways to make nutrition "insidious and pervasive," such as write columns for local newspapers or conduct nutrition radio spots.[9]

Nursing and Allied Health Nutrition Education

Nutrition services are often provided by nondietitians, depending on the practice setting and contributions of various health professionals. For example, nurses regularly monitor food intake, evaluate laboratory values indicative of nutritional status, and give patients nutritional advice.[12] Dental hygienists and health educators often screen for health/nutritional problems and provide education and intervention. All health professionals should understand the role nutrition plays in wellness and disease prevention, and they need training on appropriate interventions. It is generally agreed that nutrition education for nurses and other health professionals should be increased.[13]

The American Dietetic Association (ADA) supports nutrition education for the health professions and advocates including nutrition in didactic, clinical, and continuing education programs.[14] Dietitians are uniquely prepared to provide leadership for such programs and to direct nutrition education efforts in schools of nursing, pharmacy, allied health, and social work. There is a shortage of qualified faculty in this area, and funding is sometimes tenuous.

Industry-Based Education

Companies that manufacture medical nutrition products often employ dietitians to provide technical and clinical information to the sales force and other personnel, clinicians, retail pharmacists, and educators of health care professionals. Here, dietitians may educate via telephone, written correspondence, and electronic mail. They may organize educational conferences and disseminate proceedings. They might participate in developing video, audio, and slide programs; technical monographs; newsletters; brochures; and professional and patient education publications on topics of medical nutrition therapy.[15]

Personal characteristics and skills necessary for success in industry-based education include "technical and professional proficiency, ability to critically and objectively analyze issues, attention to detail, high work standards, skill at written and oral communication, adaptability, and ability to tolerate stress."[15] Clearly, such positions require a proficiency in nutritional sciences, practitioner experience, both conceptual and analytic skills, altruistic values, and service ethic.

Worksite Nutrition Education

As increased attention is given to the role of nutrition in health and disease prevention, there will be more opportunities for dietitians in worksite wellness programs. These worksites may include manufacturing plants, insurance companies, or service organizations. Some of these positions will focus entirely on nutrition education and may include screening for nutritional risk, developing programs, giving classes and demonstrations, creating exhibits and displays, and evaluating effectiveness of nutrition education initiatives. Dietitians in these positions may provide valuable experience for dietetic interns or other students.[16]

Worksite education opportunities can also include coordinators of training in large dietetics departments or at the regional level of contract food and nutrition service companies such as Marriott, ARAMark, and Morrisons. Dietitians in such roles may oversee a dietetic internship, coordinate inservice training for food service and other personnel, and direct training for students from affiliating programs. Individuals with the appropriate background may be promoted to director of training and development at the institutional or corporate level.

DIETITIANS IN RESEARCH

Much of the research in nutrition and dietetics is conducted by students and faculty members at colleges and universities. Some of these researchers are RDs, others are food or nutrition scientists. Most faculty members are in research as well as teaching as part of their faculty responsibilities. They may conduct laboratory research such as metabolic studies in human nutrient requirements or in food science to determine utilization of specific food components. Other studies may be conducted in controlled working environments as, for example, in foodservice management productivity studies. Other kinds of research may deal with applied studies in nutrition education and data collection through surveys. Further career opportunities for dietitians in research are described in the following selected types of positions.

Academic Health Centers

Many university affiliated hospitals have centers dedicated to one or another type of clinical research. Others have long-term multidisciplinary research projects that include a nutrition component. The work of research dietitians at a few of these centers is described here.

Some research dietitians work at a general clinical research center (GCRC), usually associated with an academic medical center. There are 78 GCRCs funded by the National Institutes of Health (NIH) located at universities such as Ohio State, Emory, Stanford, Rockefeller, and Iowa. Research dietitians may oversee the metabolic kitchen associated with the GCRC, analyze nutrient intakes, conduct calorimetry studies, assist in development of nutrition-related protocols, and participate in rounds and seminars.

Some GCRC dietitians manage their own research programs. For example, Ann Coulston, MS, RD, senior research dietitian at the Stanford University Medical Center CRC, directs clinical nutrition research projects and collaborates with the medical school faculty on diabetes, cancer, and AIDS research.[17] She has more than 25 research publications to her credit, many coauthored with dietetic students.

There is a Nutrition Research Clinic at The Baylor College of Medicine, Houston, Texas. Nutrition studies at this center first related to the effectiveness of nutrition/behavioral programs designed to reduce cholesterol levels for the general public and to teach the concept of diet modification as a prevention technique. Here, Becky Reeves, Dr PH, RD, FADA, conducts behavioral-oriented nutrition research.[18] She develops and designs nutrition education materials for each protocol. She spends much of her time teaching adults to change their eating and exercise behaviors to reduce plasma cholesterol levels or achieve weight loss.

Madelyn L. Wheeler, MS, RD, CDE, is coordinator of research dietetics at the Diabetes Research and Training Center (DRTC) at Indiana University School of Medicine, Indianapolis.[19] There are six DRTCs funded by the NIH and National Institute of Diabetes and Digestive and Kidney Diseases. In her position, Wheeler is part of a large multidisciplinary group engaged in several different research projects. Early studies were designed to determine if education makes a difference in the patient's ability to self-manage diabetes (it does!). Some studies involved the use of a home-style kitchen for patient education; for other studies, interactive computer programs were used. Wheeler also studied various sweetening agents and how they affect persons with diabetes mellitus. In 1997, she received a grant to study the effect of plant versus animal protein on kidney function and blood glucose levels.

In recent years, several medical centers signed on to participate in long-term studies related to the NIH Women's Health Initiative. Some of these studies are designed to explore the relationship between diet and heart disease, osteoporosis, or cancer. Because each site enrolls large numbers of women, there are numerous opportunities for dietitians to become involved as nutrition counselors, data managers, or project directors.

Nutrition research sometimes involves the use of computerized nutrient databases for functional analysis. Dietitians who are adept at computers are in demand at such sites. For example, Catherine Champagne, PhD, RD, LDN, holds a position as associate professor and nutrient data systems chief at the Pennington Biomedical Research Center, Louisiana State University, Baton Rouge.[20] In this role, Champagne conducts research using MENu (Moore's extended nutrient) database. One such study was to develop new recipes and menus to meet the US Army's strict specifications for specific nutrients. Another study examined nutrient intakes of female soldiers during combat training.

Marlene M. Windhauser, PhD, RD, LDN, is also a research dietitian at the Pennington Biomedical Research Center.[21] Windhauser's research interests lead her to study nutrient content of products targeted toward children and advertised on Saturday morning television programs. Most such commercials focus primarily on flavor, with little attention given to sweetness or nutrient content. For better health of children, these commercials ought to focus more on healthy food choices.

Some clinical research dietitians are affiliated with medical departments to coordinate research projects designed by physicians. Marjorie McCullough, MS, RD, serves such a role in the endocrinology-hypertension division at Brigham and Women's Hospital, Boston.[22] In this capacity, McCullough recruits patients for studies, collects and analyzes research data, helps write research papers, and drafts grant proposals. She sometimes serves as coinvestigator for projects, such as the one related to salt- and calcium-sensitive hypertension.

The need for dietitians in clinical research continues. Efficacious dietetics practice must be based on scientific principles and sound theory. However, there is little evidence to support the value of many approaches to clinical dietetics. Additional knowledge is needed in areas of nutritional status of individuals and populations at risk for disease, identification of nutrient requirements associated with disease conditions, and nutrition interventions as therapy for disease conditions.[23] With the current crisis in health care delivery, the outcomes of nutrition intervention are an important area of investigation.

Food Companies

Many food companies employ dietitians. Roles vary but often include research related to product or recipe development. Roles can also focus on translation of research into meaningful information for the public or development of nutrition education programs for children, adults, and professionals. For example, at the Kellogg Company, Leila Saldanha, PhD, RD, initiated and managed research programs to demonstrate the importance of breakfast and the significant contributions that ready-to-eat cereals make to nutrient intake and health.[24]

Industry

Companies that manufacture infant formulas and medical nutritional products often employ dietitians to conduct research or to monitor clinical investigations at hospitals, nursing homes, and home care settings. Roles might include work related to

- nutritional needs of infants, children, patients, and the elderly
- acceptability of flavors and textures of products designed for oral use
- coordination of intervention studies to determine the effectiveness of new products

- initiation of outcomes research studies to explore cost-effectiveness of medical nutrition therapy

Several research dietitians are employed by companies such as Nestle. For example, at Ross Products Division of Abbott Laboratories, Anne Voss, PhD, RD, is manager of outcomes research. She works with a staff of seven professionals, including four RDs who hold advanced degrees. This group conducts studies to determine the effect of malnutrition, nutrition intervention, or the use of nutrition supplements on drug usage, complications or adverse events, length of hospital stays, unexpected hospital readmission, and health care costs.[25] The studies involve patients with specific conditions such as bone marrow transplants, colorectal cancer, joint replacements, pressure ulcers, or diabetes. They also are studying the cost-effectiveness of adding snacks or supplements to Meals-on-Wheels programs.

Dawn C. Laine, MPH, RD, is another research dietitian.[26] She is manager of clinical development at GalaGen Inc, a small biotechnology company headquartered in Minnesota. Here, Laine oversees protocol development, identifies study sites, manages the active studies including clinical monitoring, and participates in data management and writing final reports. Before joining the research team at GalaGen, Laine was a research dietitian at the University of Minnesota General Clinical Research Center.

Government

There are many opportunities for research dietitians in government-sponsored centers and laboratories. These include positions such as

- nutrition scientist at the USDA Laboratory in North Dakota devoted to the study of vitamins and minerals
- researcher at the US Army Natick Research, Development and Engineering Center in Massachusetts involved in studies related to food behaviors and the acceptance and consumption of military rations
- nutrition epidemiologist at the Centers for Disease Control in Atlanta exploring patterns of nutrition-related diseases throughout the country
- extension specialist at a land-grant university exploring ways to maximize food production, quality, and safety
- life science specialist at the congressional research service in the Library of Congress, answering questions and conducting research for members of Congress and staff on food safety and nutrition issues

CAREER MAPS FOR EDUCATION AND RESEARCH

One or more years practicing in a hospital, nursing home, clinic, or community setting is the first step toward success as a dietitian in education and research. Those with firsthand experience in the field gain a valuable understanding of the practice milieu, and they can draw from their backgrounds for illustrations and examples.

Interest in research can develop early. Fundamental skill development often begins with an undergraduate research course, completion of an honors research study, or summer work in a research laboratory. A few internships, such as the one at NIH, emphasize research; this is a good option for those contemplating a research career. During graduate school, it may also be possible to arrange for field work at a food company, industry, or government research setting.

Nearly all dietitians in education and research have attained at least a master's degree, and many have an earned doctorates. In addition, these individuals tend to be creative, intellectually curious, and self-directed achievers. They love libraries, and they enjoy working at a scholarly level. Because much of their work involves communication and motivating others, they must have good interpersonal skills and a sense of humor.

Often, an interest in university teaching begins with an assistantship during graduate school. During this time, neophytes work directly with a faculty mentor in the college classroom or laboratory and develop basic teaching and research skills. Other early job opportunities in these areas may include

- teaching part time at a community college or technical school
- conducting research while filling a role in clinical dietetics
- volunteering to serve as a research subject for a clinical trial
- lecturing to community groups
- giving classes for medical students and residents, nurses, and other allied health professionals

IMPORTANCE OF EDUCATION AND RESEARCH TO THE PROFESSION

Any profession needs to continually reshape itself to meet ever-changing needs in society. Leaders in dietetics recognized this and took a key role in defining new directions in dietetic practice, education, and credentialing.[27] This new direction positions dietetics professionals to carry out ADA's mission and vision "to shape the food choices and impact the nutritional status of the public." Such a role facilitates dynamic movement of the profession into the twenty-first century and beyond.

To meet the challenges ahead, it is expected that

- Dietetics practitioners will be leaders in the field. They will affect optimal nutritional health of the public by the use of innovative "multitechnology," collaboration with other health professionals, and practice in diverse settings.
- Dietetics educational programs will develop and sustain leaders in the field by adapting curricula to meet changing needs, by linking new research with current practice, and by facilitating lifelong pursuit and application of new knowledge.
- Dietetics credentialing programs will ensure continuing competence of dietetics professionals by setting high standards, developing quality assessment procedures, and supporting methods to safeguard the nutritional health and safety of the public.

Research is essential for advancement of the profession. Not only do dietitians need to engage in research to uncover new knowledge and define new modes of therapy, they need to take a scholarly approach to everyday practice. As Parks et al. pointed out:[28]

> To ensure that our clients receive only the very best dietetics care, we must develop aptitudes and attitudes for scholarship; question underlying assumptions to our knowledge base and to our practice; be curious about how science can be used to make us better practitioners; be eager for collaboration among scientists and practitioners; and have the courage to challenge the very essence of our current knowledge.

Science is ever changing. Dietitians need to avoid the pitfalls of maintaining the status quo, of assuming that current practice is acceptable when based on past and present knowledge only. The field of dietetics needs practitioners who are interested in science as a basis for practice. The profession can maintain its vitality only when infused by new knowledge, scholarship, and research. By continually updating contemporary practice, rooted in science, dietitians can stay ahead of the trends shaping consumer health and food behaviors.

ADA EDUCATION AND RESEARCH PRACTICE GROUPS

Dietitians in education and research have numerous opportunities to unite with colleagues having similar interests (Exhibit 11–1). These ADA practice groups promote networking, mentoring, information exchange, professional enhancement, and leadership opportunities in organized areas of practice. Generally, practice groups offer their members continuing education programs, quarterly

Exhibit 11–1 Purpose of ADA Practice Groups for Dietitians in Research and Education

Nutrition Research Practice Group
   Promotes visibility of nutrition research and communication between research-
   ers and practitioners.
Dietetic Educators of Practitioners
   Unites members of ADA who are interested in or engaged in educating dietitians and dietetic technicians; represents the concerns of dietetic educators to
   the ADA, the government, institutions of higher learning, and the public.
Nutrition Educators of Health Professionals
   Advocates improvement in the quality of nutrition education of medical,
   dental, nursing, and allied health students; provides a forum for communication
   and information exchange between members, especially new educators; offers
   expertise in the development of nutrition curricula for undergraduate and
   graduate education.
Nutrition Education for the Public
   Champions improved well-being of the public by providing leadership in
   nutrition education planning, implementation, and evaluation; provides members with resources and opportunities to enhance both personal skills and
   nutrition expertise.

   Source: Adapted with permission from *Dietetic Practice Group Information,* American
Dietetic Association.

newsletters, forums for exploring practice issues, and innovative products and
services.

ETHICAL AND LEGAL BASES OF PRACTICE

   Like all professionals, dietitians in education and research are expected to
adhere to strict ethical standards. In addition to upholding principles of honesty,
fidelity, and justice, educators and researchers are expected to maintain both
confidentiality and objectivity to avoid favoritism and any type of discrimination.
Exhibit 11–2 outlines some specific ethical and legal considerations.

CASE STUDY OF A DIETITIAN EDUCATOR

   Kay Wolf, PhD, is an assistant professor at a major university where her
primary responsibility is teaching food service management courses for dietetics
students. Wolf is uniquely prepared for this position through education, experience, and linkages (written communication, November 1, 1996).

Wolf received all her degrees from The Ohio State University, Columbus: a BS in medical dietetics, an MS in human nutrition and food management, and a PhD in human resource development and training. She constantly engages in continuing education by attending meetings of the district, state, and national dietetic associations; participating in an annual food service management workshop; reading professional journals; and joining other university faculty at forums to improve teaching.

Ten years as a dietetics practitioner enrich Wolf's teaching. Her past job titles include staff dietitian, administrative dietitian, consultant, and community nutritionist. She spent three years teaching at a community college where she also coordinated the field work of students in a dietetic technician program. To keep current with trends in food service, she continually confers with food service managers and dietitians at practice sites where her students engage in field work experiences.

Linkages are important to any successful educator. Wolf maintains regular contact with dietitians in the community; they provide field experiences for her students, and they often invite her to give inservice programs for staff members at their institutions. Early in her career, she was active in committees of the district dietetic association and now sits on the board and holds elected office at the state level. In addition, she is an active member and attends meetings of the American

---

Exhibit 11–2 Some Ethical and Legal Considerations for Dietitians in Education and Research

Education
- Integrity, respect, and professionalism in dealings with students, administrators, and peers.
- Adherence to laws and norms regarding copyright, plagiarism, and use of intellectual property.
- Truth and objectivity in grading and evaluating students.
- Model healthy lifestyles; avoid taking a moralistic approach toward others based on health practices, personal beliefs, or economic circumstances.

Research
- Ethical treatment of research subjects, both humans and animals.
- Full disclosure and honest interpretation of data.
- Instruction regarding correct laboratory procedures, accurate data collection and recording, principles of research conduct, and guidelines for authorship.
- Avoidance of pressures to fabricate data or falsify interpretation of it.
- Disclosure of potential conflicts of interest that may influence research procedures, results, applications, or presentations.

Source: Adapted from R. Schiller, Ethics in Practice of Dietetics, *Topics in Clinical Nutrition*, Vol. 12, No. 2, pp. 1–11, © 1997, Aspen Publishers, Inc.

Society for Hospital Food Service Administrators and Foodservice Systems Management Education Council. Every year, she presents poster sessions and gives oral presentations at dietetics meetings. She writes articles, submits grant proposals, and shares her expertise with both students and other professionals.

CASE STUDY OF A DIETITIAN IN RESEARCH

Brenda Bossetti, PhD, is director of nutrition research at the Clinical Research Center (CRC) at a major medical center (written communication, November 6, 1996). Bossetti states, "We provide quality nutritional care as well as the highest caliber of science for our investigators. Our expertise enables us to deliver the high quality package for clinical research."[29] Such competence does not just happen—it is the result of a strong academic background, commitment to research, and effective networks in the professional community.

Bossetti received both her BS (cum laude) and MS in medical dietetics. To gain valuable practitioner skills, Bossetti worked three years as a clinical dietitian at Children's Hospital and The Ohio State University Hospital. When a part-time opening occurred at the CRC, Bossetti took it and continued to work part time as a clinical dietitian. Within a few years, the CRC position became full time and Bossetti was a step closer to her "dream" job. As senior dietitian, Bossetti and her staff ensure that food is measured precisely and that records are kept meticulously for accurately administered protocols.

So that she could take a leadership role in designing and conducting studies, Bossetti pursued doctoral studies while continuing her work at the CRC. She received her doctorate in human nutrition and wrote her dissertation on effect of energy restriction on insulin resistance and insulin-like growth factor I (IGF-1) in obese female non–insulin-dependent diabetic (NIDDM) and nondiabetic control subjects. This clinical research study honed her research skills and enhanced her value to other research team members. She also became a certified diabetes educator and works closely with the endocrinology team on various research studies.

Recently, her research responsibilities expanded to include numerous nutrition assessments, such as use of a portable metabolic cart to estimate individual caloric needs, anthropometric measurements, and bioelectrical impedance tests. She oversees a specialized computer program that analyzes food intake, calculates nutrients, recalls past intake, and figures percentages for any nutrient known to science.

In addition to her membership in the ADA and its state and local affiliates, Bossetti is a member of three ADA practice groups: diabetes care and education, nutrition support dietitians, and research dietitians. She also holds memberships in the American Association of Diabetes Educators, American Diabetes Association, American Federation for Clinical Research, American Institute of Nutrition, American Society for Clinical Nutrition, and American Society for Parenteral and Enteral Nutrition. She held several offices in the Central Ohio Diabetes Association and is past-president of the Central Ohio Association of Diabetes Educators.

Bossetti has to her credit several refereed articles, abstracts, and presentations. She received several grants both as principal investigator and in collaboration with other clinical scientists. One study of particular interest was related to type II diabetes in African-Americans before abnormal blood glucose patterns appeared.

Bossetti's career is both interesting and rewarding. She knows first-hand the challenge of getting research subjects to consume carefully controlled diets AND the thrill of participating in studies that push the frontiers of medicine into the future.

CONCLUSION

Opportunities abound for dietitians interested in education and research. Essential personal qualities for such roles are independent thinking, creativity, and strong internal motivation. Advanced training, including a doctoral degree, is important for success at the highest levels of education and research.

Nutrition education for elementary and secondary school children is usually incorporated in other subjects; teaching certification is required. Teaching at the college level can include instruction of those preparing for careers in dietetics, nutrition science, nursing, allied health, dentistry, and medicine. These positions require a comprehensive understanding of nutrition, physiology, biochemistry, pathophysiology, and food science. Previous experience as a health care team member is very useful.

Dietitian researchers may be based in specialized clinical research centers, government agencies, industry, or universities. Roles vary according to the employing institution's mission and purpose. Key areas of investigation relate to nutrient requirements, food and specialized nutritional products, nutrient utilization, and outcomes of medical nutrition therapy.

Both education and research are essential for advancement of the dietetics profession. To begin preparation for such careers, students are encouraged to become associate members of ADA, join relevant ADA practice groups, seek career advice or mentoring from dietitians in education and research, enroll in pertinent elective courses, and begin planning for graduate school.

DEFINITIONS

Academic Health Centers Hospitals, medical centers, or clinics affiliated with a medical school or medical residency program.

ADA Practice Groups Organized special-interest groups within ADA. In 1997 there were 26 practice groups. Some of these are clinical nutrition management, dietitians in business and communications, nutrition education for the public, nutrition entrepreneurs, school nutrition services, and vegetarian nutrition. To belong, one must be a member of ADA and pay dues to the practice group. To learn more about practice groups, visit ADA's website at www.eatright.org.

Career Map Nonlinear career development pathway. Such pathways allow flexibility and they build on personal interests and qualities, work experience, multifaceted skill applications, networking, and both formal and informal training and education.

Medical Nutrition Education Teaching basic and applied nutrition to medical students or residents. This often requires integration of concepts related to food science, nutrition, biochemistry, physiology, pathophysiology, health promotion, and human behavior.

Medical Nutrition Therapy Comprehensive process including nutrition risk assessment, care planning, nutrition intervention, counseling, documentation, evaluation, and outcomes management.

Nutrition Education Teaching children or adults principles of normal nutrition as the basis for optimal health and disease prevention.

Research Systematic investigations leading to new knowledge or new applications of known information. Research may occur in numerous settings, such as laboratories, schools and colleges, hospitals and clinics, libraries, worksites, nursing homes, food companies, cafeterias, grocery stores, and day care centers.

Teaching Certificate State legislated credentials required for teaching in elementary and secondary schools.

REFERENCES

1. Royal Bank Letter, Royal Bank of Canada, 78(2), Spring 1997.
2. Rubin KW. Creative nutrition education for Headstart children of the Seminole Tribe of Florida. *Top Clin Nutr.* 1994;9:73–78.
3. Gates G, McDonald M, Dalton M. Nutrition education in Missouri schools. *J School Health.* 1994;64:410–412.
4. Shannon B, Mullis R, Bernardo V, Ervin B, et al. The status of school-based nutrition at the state agency level. *J School Health.* 1992; 62:88–92.
5. Shupe SD, Sandoval WM. Nutrition education: from the lunchroom to the classroom. *J School Health.* 1987;57:122–123.

6. Juszczak L, Fisher M, Lear JG, Friedman SB. Back to school: training opportunities in school-based health centers. *J Dev Behav Pediatr.* 1995;16:L101–104.

7. Kessler L, Jonas JR, Gilhan MB. The status of nutrition education in ACHA college and university health centers. *J Am Coll Health.* 1992;4:31–34.

8. Kessler LA, Gilhan MB, Vickers J. Peer involvement in the nutrition education of college students. *J Am Diet Assoc.* 1992;92:989–991.

9. Kolasa KM, Lasswell AB. Dietitians as medical educators. *Top Clin Nutr.* 1995;10: 20–28.

10. Tillman HH, Woods M, Gorbach SL. Enhancing the level of nutrition education at Tufts University's medical and dental schools. *J Cancer Ed.* 1992;7:215–219.

11. Reiter SA, Rasmann-Nuhlicek DN, Biernat K, Lawrence SL. Registered dietitians as problem-based learning facilitators in a nutrition curriculum for freshman medical students. *J Am Diet Assoc.* 1994;94:652–654.

12. Weigley ES. Nutrition in nursing education and beginning practice. *J Am Diet Assoc.* 1994;94:654–656.

13. Englert DAM, Crocker KS, Stotts NA. Nutrition education in Schools of Nursing in the United States. Part 1. The evolution of nutrition education in schools of nursing. *JPEN.* 1986;10:522–527.

14. Position of The American Dietetic Association: nutrition education of health professionals. *J Am Diet Assoc.* 1991;91:611–613.

15. Campbell SM. Looking for Wonder Woman: a role for registered dietitians in industry-based education. *Top Clin Nutr.* 1995;10:14–19.

16. Sandoval WM, Mueller HD. Nutrition education at the worksite: a team approach. *J Am Diet Assoc.* 1989;89:543–544.

17. Coulston AM. NRDPG member candidates for ADA offices. *The Digest: ADA Nutrition Research Dietetic Practice Group.* 1990;26(4):1–2.

18. Reeves RS. Spotlight dietitian. *The Digest: ADA Nutrition Research Dietetic Practice Group.* 1992;28(4):1–2.

19. Wheeler ML. Spotlight dietitian. *The Digest: ADA Nutrition Research Dietetic Practice Group.* 1992;28(2):1–2.

20. Champagne CM. Spotlight dietitian. *The Digest: ADA Nutrition Research Dietetic Practice Group.* 1994;30(4):1–2.

21. Windhauser MM. Spotlight dietitian. *The Digest: ADA Nutrition Research Dietetic Practice Group.* 1992;28(1):1–2.

22. McCullough M. Spotlight dietitian. *The Digest: ADA Nutrition Research Dietetic Practice Group.* 1995;31(1):1–2.

23. Coulston AM. Make a career of clinical nutrition research. *Top Clin Nutr.* 1995;10: 29–33.

24. Saldanha L. Spotlight dietitian. *The Digest: ADA Nutrition Research Dietetic Practice Group.* 1993;29(2):1.

25. Gallagher-Allred CR, Voss AC, Finn SC, McCamish MA. Malnutrition and clinical outcomes: the case for medical nutrition therapy. *J Am Diet Assoc.* 1996;96:361–368.

26. Laine DC. Spotlight dietitian. *The Digest: ADA Nutrition Research Dietetic Practice Group.* 1995;31(3):1–2.

27. Parks SC, Babjak PM, Fitz PA, Maillet JO, et al. President's page: Future Search Conference helps define new directions in practice, education, and credentialing. *J Am Diet Assoc.* 1994;94:1046–1047.

28. Parks SC, Schiller MR, Bryk J. President's page: investment in our future—the role of science and scholarship in developing knowledge for dietetic practice. *J Am Diet Assoc.* 1994;94:1159–1161.

29. Phillips, DC. Nutrition: a fundamental for today's clinical research. *Clin Res Link.* 1995;2:3–4.

The Consultant in Private Practice

Donna Alexander-Israel and Carmen Roman-Shriver

"Many dietitians are doing what has not been done before. They embody the entrepreneurial spirit. Their ingenuity, creative verve, and aggressiveness are leading them and the dietetic profession into new fields of experience." KK Helm in *The Entrepreneurial Nutritionist*[1]

Outline—Chapter 12

INTRODUCTION

Traditional roles in dietetics are undergoing change. A number of trends contribute to the changes: the downsizing of business and industry, the early dehospitalization of patients, managed care in hospitals, and the emphasis of technology in food and nutrition service. Cost controls through decreasing the work force as well as through changed ways of operation have led to what many business and industry sources perceive as the wave of the future: contracting for services.[2] Dietitians in private practice are in a unique position to contract their expertise and services in several of or all the areas of practice described in this book and are doing so in increasing numbers.

The 1995 member survey by The American Dietetic Association (ADA) shows that 12 percent of the registered dietitians (RD) surveyed were employed in consultation and business practice, although data were not available for the number of RDs in private practice.[3] The Dietetic Practice Groups (DPG) consultants often join are Nutrition Entrepreneurs, Consultant Dietitians in Health Care Facilities, Dietitians in Business and Communications, and Nutrition Education for the Public.

ENTREPRENEURISM

Demographic Trends

More dietitians are becoming entrepreneurs and for a variety of reasons. Some seek entrepreneurial opportunities out of choice or due to circumstances that make entrepreneurism a very viable option. Examples of the latter might be the loss of . a job or the need to work varying hours due to family responsibilities. Opportunities for women in the business world are increasing, as shown by the fact that nationwide the number of women-owned firms grew by 78 percent between 1987 and 1996 and sales for 1996 from women-owned businesses totaled about $7 billion, with $4.6 billion of that coming from service sector firms.[4] The opportunities, especially for women entrepreneurs, have grown to an unprecedented extent.

Reasons that might account for the growth in women entering the business world are changes in the health care industry with downsizing at all levels, dietitians seeking more independence and new challenges, and a business climate that encourages entrepreneurism.[5] Not all entrepreneurs start a business as such. Some work at home and may combine home and family responsibilities with part-time, contract-type work including consulting, writing, using the computer in various ways, making home visits, etc.[1] Others may open an office, hire assistants, and establish a full-time practice or business.

Personal Characteristics

Cross, a PhD nutritionist and attorney, indicates that the successful dietitian who enters private practice needs to exhibit several personal characteristics.[6] These include determination, initiative, and perseverance. Self-confidence and speed in decision making allows one to make realistic choices, and the ability to organize keeps administrative and managerial responsibilities in financial and legal order. Exhibit 12–1 shows a list of questions that can be used to determine a person's readiness to enter private practice.

Rejent-Scholtz indicates that the successful entrepreneur needs to be self-directed, self-nurturing, action-oriented, highly energetic, and tolerant of uncertainty, as there is always an element of risk.[5]

Beginning a Practice

Two excellent publications are available as guides for the dietitian entering private practice: *The Competitive Edge. Advanced Marketing for Dietetics Professionals,* published by the ADA,[7] and *The Entrepreneurial Nutritionist* by Helm.[1] A wealth of information is provided in these publications for establishing an office, finding capital funding, determining the type of business organization, and deciding on insurance both for the business and for the practice. Professional liability insurance is also available through ADA.[8] Further guides to business and legal considerations are provided by Cross.[6,9,10] Most cities have a small business association or an economic development center, both of which provide assistance to persons in the early stages of establishing a business or a practice. Banks and investment companies provide advice and assistance to entrepreneurs starting a business and often provide services specifically for women.

Networking with other successful dietitians through the DPGs is an excellent way of gaining valuable information about private practice and what is involved in establishing a practice, making contacts, finding funding, etc. Information is provided by each DPG at the annual ADA meeting in 3 arenas:

1. Individual DPG Business Meetings & Continuing Education Workshops
2. ADA Exhibition Hall
3. ADA Product Marketplace

DPG members discuss show and market products and services they have developed. This fall meeting is another source for making contacts and sharing new ideas.

Marketing

Whatever area of private practice is pursued, marketing will be an essential part of the planning. To gain the "competitive edge" in private practice, clients and the

Exhibit 12–1 Questionnaire To Determine Readiness for Private Practice

Are you a self-starter?

3—I do things on my own—nobody has to tell me what or when to get going.

2—If someone gets me started, I keep going by myself.

1—Easy does it! Keep prodding me and I will move along fine.

Are you a risk taker?

3—I'll take a chance, even if I am unsure of success.

2—I'll jump in, if I am fairly sure of succeeding.

1—Uncertainty is not for me—I'll wait until success is guaranteed.

Do you have a positive, friendly interest in others?

3—I enjoy new people and can get along with just about anybody.

2—I am most comfortable with existing friends and don't need anyone else.

1—Meeting new people is not my forte. I prefer being alone.

Are you a leader?

3—I can get most people to go along when I start something.

2—I can give the orders if someone else tells me what we should do.

1—I let someone else get things moving. Then I go along if I feel like it.

Can you handle responsibility?

3—I like to take charge of things and see them through.

2—I'll take over if I have to, but I'd rather let someone else be responsible.

1—I would just rather not have the final responsibility.

Are you a good organizer?

3—I like to make plans and check them off. I'm usually the one to get things lined up when the group wants to do something.

2—I do all right until things get too confused. Then I quit.

1—Things get done as they come. I don't like too much structure.

Are you prepared to put in long hours?

3—I can keep going long and hard for something I want.

2—I'll work hard for a while, but when I've had enough, that's it.

1—It will either happen or it won't, so there is no merit in working yourself to death.

Do you make up your mind quickly?

3—If I have to, I can make up my mind in a hurry and it usually turns out okay.

2—I need time to decide. When I make up my mind too fast, I often think later I should have decided the other way.

1—I simply can't decide without considering all the details and discussing them with others.

Can people rely on you?

3—I say what I mean and I deliver. It's simplest.

2—I try to be on the level, but sometimes I don't know or can't deliver but don't really want to admit it.

1—People never really pay attention, so I just say whatever is easiest.

continues

Exhibit 12–1 continued

Can you withstand reversals without quitting?
3—Once I've made up my mind, nothing stops me.
2—I usually finish what I start—if it goes well.
1—If it doesn't go right away, I see no reason to keep hammering away.

Total your score. If your score is 24–30, you probably have what it takes to be in private practice in nutrition. If your score is 17–23, running a business of your own would likely be an uphill battle. A total score below 16 suggests that you may not be ready to be independent in business. Rare is the person who has an abundance of all the traits essential to business success, or who does not need to improve in one or more areas to be better in business. There are ways to strengthen them both before and after you begin your business. Attend conferences and lectures on aspects of private practice in nutrition and on business operations in general. Experts on business management often have tips gathered through years of experience. Read books and articles to keep up with developments in the field of nutrition and in the business world.

Source: A.T. Cross, Practical and Legal Considerations of Private Nutrition Practice. Copyright The American Dietetic Association. Reprinted by permission from *Journal of The American Dietetic Association*, Vol. 95, pp. 21–29, © 1995.

public will be receptive when they are convinced that the service or product being sold is one they can trust and that they need. Establishing credibility and visibility will therefore be a large part of a successful marketing strategy. It is often more difficult to market a service versus a product. However, the selling process is greatly facilitated by the creation of an image and a message that establishes the most positive aspects of the service to be provided. Dietitians are even aided in "selling" dietetic services in that, first and foremost, good and/or improved health is the outcome.

Many successful entrepreneurs are in nontraditional career paths, creating opportunities for themselves and others where none existed before. This is perhaps why private practice is an increasingly attractive option for many dietitians.

AREAS OF PRACTICE

Practice Settings

The consultant in private practice will usually be located outside an organization but may also be an "intrapreneur," which describes a person within an organization who develops new ideas or services that are used profitably in some way. The work setting is as diverse as the practitioner's interests and expertise as well as the market demands.[11,12] This is illustrated in Exhibit 12–2.

The professional services provided in private practice are influenced by the needs of the consumers,[13] the demands and changing environments of health care,[13] industries and communities, changes in regulatory agencies, increased autonomy, and advances in science and technology.[14,15] As new ideas are disseminated and needs identified, more roles are defined for the private practitioner. Dietitians may also form alliances and networks to provide services. By teaming with other professionals, the ability to market services and products and share business expenses is enhanced. The opportunities, through a wider range of contacts, may also be increased. Examples of such associations are preferred provider organizations to managed care companies, dietitian networks, or dietitian independent practice associations.[16] DPGs in ADA also provide a way for networking to occur among professionals.

Exhibit 12–2 Settings for Consulting in Private Practice

Private office
Private home
Physician or other allied health professional offices
Home health care
Health/fitness centers and spas
Community-based programs
Schools
Hospitals
Day homes
Senior citizen centers
Nursing homes
Contracts with government agencies
Media and communications
Grocery stores
Restaurant and culinary industry (chefs)
Corporate settings or worksites
Business and industry
Food companies
Hotels and resorts
Research centers
Medical education consulting firms
Private specialty clinics (sports medicine clinics, eating disorder clinics, diabetes, renal, oncology, HIV/AIDS)
Rehabilitation centers

Exhibit 12–3 Roles of Consultants in Private Practice

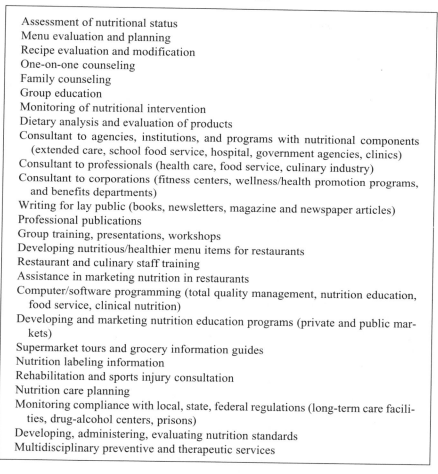

Assessment of nutritional status
Menu evaluation and planning
Recipe evaluation and modification
One-on-one counseling
Family counseling
Group education
Monitoring of nutritional intervention
Dietary analysis and evaluation of products
Consultant to agencies, institutions, and programs with nutritional components (extended care, school food service, hospital, government agencies, clinics)
Consultant to professionals (health care, food service, culinary industry)
Consultant to corporations (fitness centers, wellness/health promotion programs, and benefits departments)
Writing for lay public (books, newsletters, magazine and newspaper articles)
Professional publications
Group training, presentations, workshops
Developing nutritious/healthier menu items for restaurants
Restaurant and culinary staff training
Assistance in marketing nutrition in restaurants
Computer/software programming (total quality management, nutrition education, food service, clinical nutrition)
Developing and marketing nutrition education programs (private and public markets)
Supermarket tours and grocery information guides
Nutrition labeling information
Rehabilitation and sports injury consultation
Nutrition care planning
Monitoring compliance with local, state, federal regulations (long-term care facilities, drug-alcohol centers, prisons)
Developing, administering, evaluating nutrition standards
Multidisciplinary preventive and therapeutic services

Practice Roles

Consultants in private practice reach a variety of clients and consumers in areas ranging from wellness and prevention, medical nutrition therapy, business and industry, education and training, food service and culinary trades to writing and media presentation. A list of activities is shown in Exhibit 12–3 as examples of the types of services that consultants may perform.

Practice roles can often be expanded with more training in business, marketing, and communications and with the development of new skills that cross the boundaries of other health professions without infringing on their practice.[10] For example, dietitians can become proficient at taking blood pressures and body composition measurements in the home care setting; can secure American College of Sports Medicine Exercise Test Technology Certification for performing electrocardiogram monitored stress tests in sports medicine clinics or Clinical Laboratory Improvement Amendment Certification for blood analysis or can use phlebotomy skills in wellness programs.

Emerging roles demand expanding the RD's scope of practice and skills[17] and capitalizing on the talents that set dietitians apart.[18] Among these talents are the ability to:

- apply food and nutrition knowledge
- use nutrition assessment tools
- apply lifestyle-change education to prevent and manage disease
- collect data on positive outcomes of nutrition intervention in quality of life and reduced overall health care costs

Reimbursement for Services

A major consideration for the dietitian in private practice is setting prices and fees and obtaining reimbursement for services in the health care system. A discussion of setting prices and fees may be found in Chapters 13 and 14. The information and references also apply to the consultant in private practice. A comprehensive discussion of a process for setting prices and fees is presented by Hamilton in *The Competitive Edge.*[19]

Several studies have been reported on efforts to obtain reimbursement for nutrition services by the government, insurance companies, and businesses (usually referred to as "third-party payment"). Dietitians in North Dakota, for instance, obtained payment from Medicaid and a large insurance provider for treatment of specified conditions in outpatient clinics.[20] In Ohio, of 296 business and insurance carriers contacted, 108 reimbursed for nutrition services when services were provided in specific locations and for designated types of services.[21]

The ADA has promoted legislation that would provide reimbursement for dietetic services from health care providers for many years. The association is currently lobbying for and monitoring legislation toward securing Medicare coverage for medical nutrition therapy (MNT).[22] For nutrition services to be included in those health care costs that the Medicare program pays for, great effort has gone into collecting cost/benefit data and in showing how nutrition therapy can actually lower costs of treatment for many conditions. Legislation was introduced in 1996 in both houses of Congress and gained support but was not enacted; however, bills are again being introduced in the 105th Congress for MNT.

ADA Network Providers

The nationwide nutrition network is a service offered by ADA through which requests from anyone for nutrition counseling may be referred to dietitian-subscribers to the service. The service is to be expanded to include more business-related areas of dietetic practice, along with increased marketing to business and industry.[23]

Successful Private Practitioners

Accounts of two successful dietitians in private practice and how they established their practice follow. The first, Lisa Dorfman, MS, RD, LMHC (personal communication, June 10, 1997), is a very involved dietitian in private practice in Florida. She lists her titles as sports nutritionist, licensed psychotherapist, and athlete, and in addition, she is a consultant, counselor, educator, and spokesperson. And if that were not enough, she is a champion marathon runner. She says, however, that what she is doing has been possible because she is first and foremost an RD and that her food and nutrition background has enabled her to carve out an exciting and challenging career.

First, she is president of Food Fitness International, Inc., in Miami, Florida. In this capacity, she consults with more than 15 hospitals and clinics in south Florida as well as in a federal correctional institution; with the American College of Sports Medicine; with the USA Triathlon; and with the US Tennis Association. She is also a nutrition professor at Johnson and Wales University. Dorfman has been featured in more than 100 publications in popular lay publications and on television. She is also the author of a chapter on eating disorders for the *Sports Nutrition Manual.*

Professionally, she has been active in several practice groups in ADA including Nutrition Entrepreneurs (former chair and public relations chair); Sports, Cardiovascular and Nutritionists (member and speaker for a symposium); Dietitians in Business and Communications; Dietetics in Developmental and Psychiatric Disorders; and Vegetarian Nutritionists (chair-elect).

Dorfman sets an example of an entrepreneurial dietitian who, through her professional affiliation, participates in an array of activities that promote health and nutritional well-being of her clients and the public as well as a very successful career.

The second dietitian, Donna A. Israel, PhD, RD, LD, LPC, an author of this chapter, is the president of The Fitness Formula, a company she founded in 1982 in Richardson, Texas. This is a health promotion company designed to assist both individuals and employers in achieving self-responsibility for improving the quality of lives at home and at work. The company also provides wellness services for drug and alcohol rehabilitation centers, retirement homes, hospitals, and fitness centers. Besides staffing both public and private wellness accounts, the company works on innovative programs to offer corporate employees wellness and health services under one umbrella including fitness, employee assistance, self-care, safety, and health education.

In 1995, she established a new company, Preferred Nutrition Therapists, Inc. (PNT), with two RD partners. Through the company, dietitians are provided who perform MNT in settings as diverse as home health care, acute and subacute care, managed care clinics, and physician's offices. A distinction for the company was that it was the first home health care company formed by dietitians to be accredited, with commendation, by the Joint Commission on Accreditation of Healthcare Organizations and licensed with the Texas State Department of Health.

Israel has a somewhat different background from many dietitians in that her bachelor's and master's degrees were in sociology and in guidance and counseling. This expertise has added to her effectiveness in having counseled more than 8,000 individuals since beginning her practice in 1982. Her early career included vocational counseling and social work in schools, universities, and hospitals in Texas. She is currently an adjunct faculty member for the Dallas County Community Colleges in addition to her many other activities.

She has been active in professional activities, having served on the board of the Nutrition Entrepreneurs practice group for three years and as content expert for the worksite Wellness Continuing Education Professional Self-Assessment Series with ADA and Pennsylvania State University. This latter program assesses and trains health professionals for skill in developing worksite health promotion programs. She is active as well in Texas and Dallas Dietetic Associations and was awarded the 1996 ADA Foundation Award for Excellence in Consultation and Private Practice.

As an innovator in developing programs tailored for customer needs, she has managed multicounty nutrition services for Early Childhood Intervention programs, teamed with a registered nurse to produce a prenatal program, provided programs for child care centers as a nutrition educator, and developed computer-based courses of study in nutrition/health promotion targeted to specific populations. These include hospitals, utility companies, manufacturing companies, and high-technology business. Her development of multidiscipline self-care packages that she began in 1989 provided participants toll-free counseling by a health professional, a personalized manual review, and follow-up service to track outcomes.

As a role model for what can be accomplished in private practice, Israel has set the pace for many.

CAREER LADDER PLANNING

Although many students and entry-level dietitians are attracted to the area of consultation and private practice,[14] the reality is that experience and the development of expertise in one or more areas of practice are essential for success. Entry-level dietitians at times enter private practice as an assistant to an established consultant. Another way the RD wishing to become a consultant in private practice may start is through intrapreneurship, or entrepreneurship within a practice or business, which can be an initial rung on the ladder. For the dietitian lacking experience but with the drive, desire, and the other characteristics needed to succeed as a consultant, starting in a small way may be the entry to a practice.

Whether starting as an intrapreneur or an entrepreneur, careful planning should be the initial step.[14,18] This may begin with envisioning what is most enjoyable and rewarding to the RD, such as working with individuals, contributing to the nutritional health of others, growing professionally, and benefitting financially. If the plan then includes starting and owning a business, all the considerations as outlined in the earlier references must follow. The RD must determine the type of ownership (i.e., whether it will be a sole proprietorship or partnership operation, determining start-up costs and finding capital funding, setting up an office or working out of the home or other business location, and legal assistance).[1,6] Once established, plans for making contacts, marketing, setting fees, and details of contracting will need to be determined. The dietitian entrepreneur needs to consult the plan regularly and realize that success is not guaranteed; there are risks as well as rewards. For instance, Cross has pointed out that entrepreneurial success is a function of business know-how and personal traits.[6]

By joining DPGs and developing associations for networking and mentoring, the dietitian in private practice will be assisted in identifying business opportunities as well as in providing the services or products. Continuing education needs to be central to the overall plan, along with an awareness of changing trends in the profession and in business.

ETHICAL AND LEGAL BASES OF PRACTICE

One of the most important guides for the dietitian is the ADA Code of Ethics (see Appendix A) and any applicable rule or statute of practice from the state and local authorities under whose jurisdiction the dietitian practices. These documents will clarify disciplinary actions that can be taken by the professional or regulatory agencies on violations of code covering such areas as advertising and practicing medicine versus nutrition. When establishing a business, the advice of an attorney is indispensable relative to business law and limits on the private practice of nutrition and the laws of the state in which the practice is established.[10]

THE FUTURE

According to the Bureau of Labor Statistics,[24] the year 2005 will see a 91 percent change in demand for dietitians in home health care from the year 1992; the federal government will show an 11 percent decrease in demand, and hospitals will show only a 7 percent increase in demand for the RD. The dietetic and health care growth of the future will be outside the hospital setting.[25] When compared with 1994 employment opportunities for dietitians, the year 2005 will be almost completely reversed according to these projections.[26]

To upgrade career ladders for more management opportunities, a working knowledge of what it takes to start and manage a business is crucial. Entrepreneurs of the future are expected to be[5]

- more educated—including advanced degrees
- more experienced—with a variety of experiences leading to entrepreneurship
- more mature—many will start their new careers later in life
- more organized—carefully plan and make decisions

CONCLUSION

Opportunities for dietitians in private practice are rapidly expanding as businesses and especially the health care industry undergo changes. In this and other chapters of this book, successful practitioners in private practice in a variety of settings are presented. They are role models for those with an entrepreneurial spirit and drive and have advanced the profession in whole new areas of practice. Traditional institutional roles for dietitians, especially in clinical dietetics, are still predominant practice settings for many; however, many dietitians are using their clinical background to become entrepreneurs in their own practice. DPGs provide networking and mentoring for the dietitian thinking of entering private practice. RDs who have become successful in their own businesses or practice have written books and guides that provide specific "how-to" information as well. The dietitian who possesses the needed personal attributes plus the initiative and creativity needed for entrepreneurial success may thus find a rewarding new career of his or her own making in private practice.

DEFINITIONS

Consultant Skilled or knowledgeable person qualified to give expert professional advice.

Entrepreneur Person who organizes and manages a commercial undertaking, especially one involving commercial risk. Also describes an innovative, risk-taking individual.

Intrapreneur Person within a corporation or institution who develops new ideas or services, usually for a profit.

Managed Care System of health care usually administered by an entity outside a hospital or other health care institution in which access, cost, and quality are controlled by direct intervention before or during service for purposes of creating efficiencies or reducing costs.

Private Practice Self-employment in which a person does not receive a paycheck or benefits from an employer.

REFERENCES

1. Helm KK. *The Entrepreneurial Nutritionist*. 2nd ed. Lake Dallas, TX. KK Helm Publisher; 1992.
2. O'Brien R. Contracting: the wave of the future. *Wall Street J*. October 22, 1996:C27.
3. Bryk JA, Soto TK. Report on the 1995 membership database of The American Dietetic Association. *J Am Diet Assoc*. 1997;97:197–203.
4. Female business owners catching up: number of female entrepreneurs grows. *Daily Oklahoman*. April 29, 1997.
5. Rejent-Scholtz A. The growth of entrepreneurship. In: Helm KK, ed. *The Competitive Edge: Advanced Marketing for Dietetics Professionals*. Chicago: The American Dietetic Association; 1995:8–10.
6. Cross AT. Practical and legal considerations of private nutrition practice. *J Am Diet Assoc*. 1995;95:21–29.
7. Helm KK, ed. *The Competitive Edge: Advanced Marketing for Dietetics Professionals*. Chicago: The American Dietetic Association; 1995.
8. Do you need professional liability insurance? *ADA Courier*. 1997;36(2):6.
9. Cross AT. Malpractice liability in private practice of nutrition. *J Am Diet Assoc*. 1988;88:946–948.
10. Cross AT. Legal limits of private practice in nutrition. In: Israel DA, Moores S, eds. *Beyond Nutrition Counseling*. Chicago: The American Dietetic Association; 1996: 123–131.
11. Sneed J, Burkhalter JP. Marketing nutrition in restaurants: a survey of current practices and attitudes. *J Am Diet Assoc*. 1991;91:459–462.
12. Laramee SH. Nutrition services in managed care: new paradigms for dietitians. *J Am Diet Assoc*. 1996;96:335–336.

13. Dittoe AB. To learn the secret of success in business, listen to consumer needs: marketing the value of dietitian's services. *J Am Diet Assoc.* 1993;93:397–399.

14. Helm KK. Finding nontraditional jobs in dietetics. *J Am Diet Assoc.* 1991;91:419–420.

15. ADA. Nutrition education of health professionals. Position paper. The American Dietetic Association. *J Am Diet Assoc.* 1991;91:611–613, reaffirmed Feb. 1997.

16. Israel D, Moores S. *Beyond Nutrition Counseling: Achieving Positive Outcomes through Nutrition Therapy.* Nutrition Entrepreneurs Dietetic Practice Group; 1996.

17. Parks SC, Fitz PA, Maillet JO, Babjak P, et al. Challenging the future of dietetics education and credentialing—dialogue, discovery, and directions: a summary of the 1994 Future Search Conference. *J Am Diet Assoc.* 1995;95:598–606.

18. Rinke WJ, Finn SC. Winning strategies to excel in dietetics. *J Am Diet Assoc.* 1990;90:52–58.

19. Hamilton E. How to set prices and fees. In: Helm KK, ed. *The Competitive Edge: Advanced Marketing for Dietetics Professionals.* Chicago: The American Dietetic Association; 1995:178–182.

20. Anderson P, Webb AR. Negotiating nutrition reimbursement. *Top Clin Nutr.* 1996;11: 33–42.

21. Rood RS, Griffith M. The Ohio NSPS statewide survey of third-party reimbursement policies for nutrition services. *J Am Diet Assoc.* 1993;93:181–182.

22. ADA mobilizes grassroots action to secure Medicare coverage for medical nutrition therapy. Legislative highlights. *J Am Diet Assoc.* 1996;96:1241.

23. Nationwide nutrition network subscription offer extended. *ADA Courier.* 1996;35(9):1.

24. Bureau of Labor Statistics. *The National Industry-Occupation Employment Matrix 1992 and Projected Year 2005.* Washington, DC: US Department of Labor; 1993.

25. Parks SC. Creating your future—career opportunities in an era of change. *J Am Diet Assoc.* 1994;94:451–452.

26. Kornblum TH. Professional demand for dietitians and nutritionists in the year 2005. *J Am Diet Assoc.* 1994;94:21–22.

The Consultant in Health Care Facilities/Extended Care

Phyllis Nichols

"We are what we repeatedly do. Excellence, then, is not an act, but a habit." Aristotle

---

Outline—Chapter 13

INTRODUCTION

The role of the consultant in health care facilities and extended care became an important one for dietitians with the enactment of the Medicare/Medicaid regulations by the Health Care Financing Administration (HCFA) in the 1960s. Long-term care facilities (primarily nursing homes) were required to have the services of a qualified dietitian by the legislation, and the demand for consultant dietitians rapidly increased as a result. From a limited employment area with little history, few guidelines, and dietitians "on their own" insofar as job requirements and benefits were concerned, consultation in health care facilities became one in which many dietitians soon found positions. Many were dietitians who had been out of the work force for varying periods of time but returned to practice with this opportunity. At the same time, many needed to be updated in practice knowledge and skills and participated in continuing education to do so. By 1975, 90 percent of skilled nursing homes used the services of a dietitian.[1]

The amount of time a dietitian's services is required is not specified in federal regulations, stating instead that consultant's visits be of "sufficient duration and frequency to meet the food and nutrition needs of the facility."[2] State licensing requirements, however, frequently specify a minimum of eight hours per month. A dietitian contracts with a facility for the amount of time needed, at or above the minimum, to meet the facility's needs.

A study in 1985 showed that licensing standards in many states at that time specified dietetic consulting time requirements ranging from semiannual visits to eight hours every two weeks.[3] Welch et al. reported a study in Illinois in 1988 showing that consultants contracted for an average of eight hours per month but actually worked an average of nine and one-half hours per month in a facility.[4] Many in the survey thought more time was actually needed to perform all responsibilities fully.

Most consultants are employed on a part-time basis in one or more facilities, although the individual time commitment could be full time, depending on the number of facilities in which the consultant works. Some dietitians are full-time corporate dietitians for a multifacility chain or in one large facility.

Regulations

A consultant dietitian must be familiar with state and federal regulations that apply to long-term/extended care facilities. The health department in each state will have copies of the state and federal regulations. The federal regulations may be obtained from the US Government Printing Office. The federal regulations are precise concerning both the physical plant and the operation and staffing of the facility. In general, state regulations follow the federal but may be even more specific in certain areas.

Each facility has its own procedures and set of regulations governing its operation as well. The consultant needs to be familiar with these as well as the purposes and goals of each facility.

The Omnibus Reconciliation Act (OBRA) of 1987 (updated 1991) published regulations for long-term care that are followed in nursing homes and other facilities receiving federal Medicare funds.[5] Detailed regulations implementing the provision were developed by HCFA. Medicare regulations and their effects on dietetic practice were discussed by Johnson and Coulston in relation to reimbursement for nutrition care.[6] In addition, many long-term care facilities seek accreditation from the Joint Commission on Accreditation of Healthcare Organizations (the Joint Commission), which also sets specific regulations for care.[7]

Periodic visits are made to facilities as a means of ensuring that regulations are being met. "The survey," as the visit is often termed, is conducted by the state department of health and/or HCFA surveyors who tour the facility, observe and interview residents, check records, observe a meal service, and in general, become familiar with the daily operation. The survey may last two to three days, after which commendations and recommendations for necessary changes will be made. There may also be a Joint Commission survey if the facility is accredited by that organization. The Joint Commission and the state/HCFA survey is similar except the latter is not announced in advance.

The American Dietetic Association Positions

The American Dietetic Association (ADA) issued a position paper in 1992 (reaffirmed in 1996) stating that quality health care should be available, accessible, and affordable to all Americans. Quality health care was defined to include nutrition services that are integral to meeting the preventive and therapeutic health care needs of all segments of the population.[8] Another position paper in 1996 affirmed that the association supports comprehensive food and nutrition services for older adults as a component of the continuum of care.[9] Because most residents in long-term care facilities are older adults, this is an especially timely statement.

Consultant dietitians usually belong to the Consultant Dietitians in Health Care Facilities Practice Group (CD-HCF), and some will also affiliate with other practice groups. The mission of CD-HCF is continuous improvement of quality care by supporting health care professionals through research, education advocacy, information, and professional development.[10]

AREAS OF PRACTICE

Long-term care facilities include nursing facilities or nursing homes, skilled nursing facilities, subacute centers, adult day care, residential care facilities, and alcohol and drug rehabilitation facilities. Long-term care facilities may be privately owned, city/county owned, owned by religious denominations, or owned by corporations. They may be for profit or not-for-profit. They may range in size from 50 to 200 beds or more.

Consultants may also be hired to visit developmentally disabled clients in their homes, and some state health departments are contracting with consultants to provide services for Women, Infants, and Children (WIC) program participants. Other consultants are in home care, congregate feeding site/senior citizen centers, correctional facilities, group homes for the developmentally disabled, hospice programs, and small rural hospitals.

Opportunities for employment are limited only by the assertiveness and imagination of dietitians as well as their location.

ESTABLISHING A CONSULTANT PRACTICE

Starting a practice requires thought and planning. One may start by reading and talking with other consultants, and joining the national and state practice groups. Mentors may be found and networks established from these contacts. Many suggestions for the initial steps in starting a practice are discussed in Chapter 12. A guide to legal and practical considerations involved in starting a practice is provided by Cross.[11]

Setting fees will require consideration of several factors.[12] Usually, an hourly fee is established, but the amount will vary widely depending on the area and the competition for jobs. A consultant starting in practice may be guided by the prevailing rates among other consultants in the region.

The consultant will need letterhead and business cards as well as working space, such as home or other business office. Equipment required as businesses grow may include a computer, a copy machine, and fax machine. Many consultants carry laptop computers and portable printers as well as cell telephones. Consulting is a business and will require some investment to establish a practice.

Locating positions or "accounts" often occurs through networking with other dietitians. Initiating contacts with facilities aids this process and, if positive, is followed by an interview with the administrator. Meeting the dietary manager and the director of nursing plus the administrator and medical staff should occur early in the interview. Expectations of these persons will be important to know, as will the opportunity to view the facility and observe the daily routines. The number of consulting hours per month and fees will be negotiated with the administrator. Even though state regulations may require a minimum of eight hours per month, there may be compelling reasons for more time. The reasons might include situations in which there are a large number of residents or in which many residents require skilled care due to medical conditions including any evidence of malnutrition.

ROLES AND RESPONSIBILITIES

A consultant dietitian is a generalist and must be able to function in all areas of dietetics. The logo of CD-HFCs contains the words, "Administration, Clinical, Education," which describe the activities of consultants. Because of the range of responsibilities and the independent practice required of consultants, the dietitian with previous experience is usually the most effective. Work as a hospital dietitian is invaluable. Many internship programs also offer a component on consulting, which provides helpful experience. Along with background experience, a good consultant will have a variety of resources at his or her fingertips to find the help needed at any point.

The 1995 Commission on Dietetic Registration Dietetics Practice Audit surveyed both dietitians and dietetic technicians on work settings and activities performed.[13] The findings clearly show that those working in long-term care and combined acute/long-term care provided primarily clinical services but most also had food service and management as a function. These data are shown in Tables 13–1 and 13–2.

Activities To Be Performed

When a consultant begins employment in a facility, one of the first activities should be an assessment of needs in food service and nutrition services for

Table 13–1 Registered Dietitian (RD)/Registered Dietetic Technician (DTR) Involvement in Dietetic Services

Work Setting	Long-Term Care RD (%) (n=305)	DTR (%) (n=169)	Acute/ Long-Term Care RD (%) (n=155)	DTR (%) (n=57)	Home Care RD (%) (n=18)	DTR (%) —	Consulting Firm RD (%) (n=11)	DTR (%) —
Clinical	84	78	92	73	88	—	38	—
Management	51	43	48	29	31	—	40	—
Food service	76	69	59	49	11	—	36	—
Community	39	28	54	27	57	—	48	—
Other	62	51	71	50	62	—	48	—

Source: M.T. Kane et al., 1995 Commission on Dietetic Registration Dietetic Practice Audit. Copyright The American Dietetic Association. Reprinted by permission from *Journal of The American Dietetic Association,* Vol. 96, pp. 1292–1301, © 1996.

Table 13–2 Registered Dietitians Performing Selected Job Functions

Work Setting	Long-Term Care (%) (n=305)	Acute Long-Term Care (%) (n=155)	Home Care (%) (n=18)	Consulting Firm (%) (n=11)
Clinical services	93	96	89	27
Food service	59	43	0	27
Public health	1	3	11	18
Wellness/disease prevention	2	10	6	27
Research	1	1	0	9
Sales/marketing	0	1	11	27
Nutrition information	13	17	33	55
Higher education	1	2	0	9
Other	5	4	17	0

Source: M.T. Kane et al., 1995 Commission on Dietetic Registration Dietetic Practice Audit. Copyright The American Dietetic Association. Reprinted by permission from *Journal of The American Dietetic Association,* Vol. 96, pp. 1292–1301, © 1996.

residents as a guide to further planning and action. Documentation of observations and plans for future visits is very important, beginning with the first visit.

The typical activities a consultant may perform during a visit to the facility include the following:

1. Conference with the dietary manager and the administrator regarding day-to-day operations and any problem areas that need to be addressed during the visit.
2. Perform nutrition assessments of new residents and follow up all others.
3. Check at-risk residents and make recommendations for further nutritional care as indicated. This would include unexplained changes in weight, presence of pressure ulcers, those on tube feedings, and any signs of dehydration or poor nutritional status.[14–16]
4. Observe the meal service and eat a meal to evaluate food quality.
5. Make nutrition rounds, at meal time at least some of the time, to observe the residents' acceptance of food and their food intakes.
6. Conduct educational inservice sessions for employees and exchange information regarding departmental activities.
7. Document all activities with any recommendations for follow-up.

The consultant may also be responsible for developing policy and procedure manuals, for the continuous quality improvement program,[17] for safety and sanitation procedures, or for budget management. The designated diet manual should also be reviewed with and signed by the chief of the medical staff at least yearly.

Consultants may also be involved in teaching dietetic students, dietetic technician students, and conducting classes for dietary managers. He or she may also serve as a preceptor for students in supervised experiences in long-term care.

The federal regulations (OBRA) include specific provisions for the nutritional care of residents.[17,18] Dietitians are held accountable for high-quality nutrition care and the elimination of malnutrition. Quality-of-care provisions include the following:

- care of residents with pressure ulcers to promote healing, prevent infection, and prevent development of new sores
- assistance for patients receiving enteral (by tube) nutrition support to ensure compliance with nutritional needs: for the prevention of diarrhea, vomiting, dehydration, and metabolic abnormalities and, if possible, to resume normal feeding
- care for those who require a therapeutic diet to ensure that optimal nutritional status is maintained unless the resident's clinical condition demonstrates that this is not possible
- assistance for patients to ensure that proper hydration is maintained
- care for patients receiving parenteral (formula feeding directly into vein) fluids or nutrition support to ensure proper treatment in line with assessed needs

The regulations also give residents the right to choose where, when, and what they eat. Residents also have the right to refuse a therapeutic diet. Nutrition assessments must be conducted on admission and periodically thereafter.

The ADA promotes Medical Nutrition Therapy (MNT) as a means of providing health benefits and reduced health care costs.[19] The process is one of assessing and treating illness and injury, thereby reducing hospital stays and treatment costs. Among patients admitted to long-term care facilities, 39 percent have been shown to be malnourished.[20] Pressure sores are often a notable problem for which MNT can speed healing. Optimal nutrition may also prevent ulcers from occurring.[21] Residents on enteral or parenteral feeding benefit from the application of appropriate MNT.

An indication of the important role played by consultants in long-term care facilities in making dietary recommendations for residents was indicated in a study by Ellis and Cowles in 1995.[22] Physicians were asked if they approved recommended changes in nutrition care procedures for residents initiated by the dietitian. Of 524 recommendations, more than 86 percent were approved by physicians. Not only were the dietitians' recommendations accepted for diet change orders but also for enteral feedings, hydration requirements, laboratory tests for assessment of nutritional status, and referral to other health professionals.

Standards for Quality Assurance

The CD-HCF practice group has developed standards for practice as a guide for quality assurance (Exhibit 13–1).[23] The standards follow those developed by the

Exhibit 13–1 Standards of Practice for Consultant Dietitians in Health Care Facilities

Standard 1. The dietetics practitioner establishes performance criteria, compares actual performance with expected performance, documents results, and takes appropriate action.

1.1 Administrative/professional staff believe consultant dietitian functions according to criteria.

1.2 Consultation reports are acknowledged by administration and dietary manager with follow-up and completion dates met.

1.3 Dietetics department complies with applicable state and federal regulations.

1.4 Dietetics department uses forms for efficient operation.

1.5 Food quality is evident by specified criteria.

Standard 2. The dietetics practitioner develops, implements, and evaluates an individual plan for practice based on assessment of consumer needs, current knowledge, and clinical experience.

2.1 A contract specifies a plan for services.

2.2 Menus are coordinated, implemented/evaluated.

2.3 Products/services are coordinated/evaluated.

2.4 A system for environmental sanitation is developed, implemented, evaluated.

Standard 3. The dietetics practitioner, using his or her unique knowledge of nutrition, collaborates with other professionals, personnel, and/or consumers in integrating, interpreting, and communicating nutrition care principles.

3.1 Resident is evaluated for physical condition/food acceptance.

3.2 Nutrition care is evaluated and documented.

3.3 Inter-/intradepartmental communications are developed, coordinated, monitored.

3.4 Dietetics operations manual is developed, implemented, and reviewed annually.

3.5 Nutrition resources are available to all.

3.6 Unique knowledge of nutrition principles is demonstrated.

3.7 Staff education and inservice education are developed, implemented, evaluated.

Standard 4. The dietetics practitioner engages in lifelong self-development to improve knowledge and skills.

4.1 Standards for membership are met in professional organizations.

4.2 Practice is enhanced by improving competency and learning-related skills.

4.3 Self-assessment is conducted.

4.4 A personal development style is adopted.

4.5 High standards of ethics are adhered to.

Standard 5. The dietetics practitioner generates, interprets, and uses research to enhance dietetics practice.

5.1 Daily practice standards implement current nutrition/management research.

continues

Exhibit 13–1 continued

5.2 Resident-oriented research is initiated and evaluated.

5.3 New products and current trends are evaluated/implemented.

Standard 6. The dietetics practitioner identifies, monitors, analyzes, and justifies the use of resources.

6.1 Tangible resources in department operation are identified/justified.

6.2 Current management practices of the facility are analyzed.

6.3 Department costs are monitored and evaluated.

Source: S.A. Gilmore et al., Standards of Practice Criteria: Consultant Dietitians in Health Care Facilities. Copyright The American Dietetic Association. Reprinted by permission from *Journal of The American Dietetic Association,* Vol. 93, pp. 305–308, © 1993.

ADA Council on Practice in 1988 and include six general categories with specific outcome statements pertaining to consultant practice. Through written documentation, consultant dietitians can verify actual performance and implement action to meet the expected criteria. The standards can also help the dietitian develop a workable plan to meet the responsibilities for which they have contracted and to evaluate their own knowledge, clinical experience, and management expertise.

In 1991, guidelines for nutrition screening for older Americans were developed by a group of professional associations, including ADA.[16] The Nutrition Screening Initiative was a collaborative effort of the American Academy of Family Physicians, the ADA, and the National Council on Aging. Risk factors and major indicators of poor nutritional status in older Americans were identified to use in routine nutrition screening in both health and medical care settings.

The Consultant

A consultant functions primarily in an advisory capacity within a facility; however, he or she has ethical and professional responsibilities for the nutritional care of the residents. By developing rapport and using organizational skills, the consultant is able to accomplish the needed tasks. Because he or she is not in the facility full time, the day-to-day supervision is usually provided by a dietetic manager or technician.

There are advantages and disadvantages to consulting. Advantages include setting one's own work schedule and amount of work, as well as the choice of facilities in which to work. Some consultants state they chose consulting because they needed flexibility in work time. A disadvantage is that a consultant works essentially alone and has little contact with peers on the job. A consultant is also responsible for office expenses and travel. In addition, benefits including vacation time, insurances, and retirement are the responsibility of the consultant.

CAREER LADDER OPPORTUNITIES

A consultant may enlarge his or her practice by forming a company and hiring staff and/or other dietitians. Some dietitians have taken this a step farther and developed a management company providing a variety of services to several institutions. The services may include providing menus, food purchasing, financial and documentation forms, and securing staff, in addition to providing all traditional consultant duties. The full management of dietary departments on a contract basis is another approach.

Consultants may acquire advanced education and teach both dietetic and nursing students and provide classes for medical and other allied health students and/or staff. Publishing and marketing materials used in consulting practice and offering seminars and workshops are other ways of enlarging practice. Networking among consultants is common and is a very positive way of obtaining and sharing knowledge of new developments in practice and in gaining competence.

An entrepreneurial dietitian may decide to become a nursing home owner/operator or a manager in one or more homes. Appointment as a case manager in home health care is another managerial position a consultant may hold. Becoming an equipment or kitchen design specialist or developing food production systems are other possibilities. Computer programs providing a full range of dietary and other departmental services including nutrition assessments, care plans, and documentation of all care can be another entrepreneurial approach. There are many possibilities for enlarging practice and increasing services by consultant dietitians.

ETHICAL AND LEGAL BASES OF PRACTICE

A strong personal and professional code of ethics is essential in consulting as in other areas of practice. The ADA Code of Ethics for the Profession of Dietetics (Appendix A) is the guide to ethical practice for the dietitian. The consultant working in several long-term care facilities can be faced with the need to be very attentive in maintaining confidentiality in regard to all operational information as well as information about residents and treatments. Residents are protected by rights to privacy and self-choice through the regulatory agencies that also enforce the regulations.

A consultant must be conscientious in fulfilling contractual obligations regarding time and services in a facility. The contract will specify the number of hours to be spent on site, meaning travel time is not included, nor usually is time spent in preparation for the visit or follow-up time in preparing reports. It is also unethical to contract with more facilities than a consultant can fully satisfy in terms of time and performance.

SUCCESS STORIES

For many consultants, the first position is in a hospital. Then, with marriage and a family, home obligations are paramount and part-time work as a consultant fits best when the dietitian is ready to resume work. Situations differ; however, the following accounts relate the experiences of individuals in successful practice.

Carol Sichterman, MA, RD, LD, Kentwood, Michigan (personal communication, June 20, 1997), first worked part time in a hospital 50 miles from home and had two small children. Medicare regulations had created a real impact in the area, and she was bombarded by local nursing homes to consult. She started with nursing homes on "off" days and after two and one-half years gave up commuting to be nearer to home. The day after leaving the hospital, a growing nursing home corporation called, and she gradually increased her time with them, eventually becoming their corporate dietitian. She formed a company for her own business, which was run by her husband and serviced by several part-time consultant RDs she hired.

Carole Deering, MS, RD (personal communication, June 20, 1997), was working part time in a new acute care hospital after the birth of her first child and was on the city's dietetic association board. Another board member asked if she would be interested in training as a consultant with a small consulting company. She took the offer, was trained for long-term care, and worked for the company for two years. After this, she worked alone as a consultant. Deering now resides in Wallingford, Pennsylvania.

Another successful consultant, Becky Dorner, RD, LD, Akron, Ohio, knew from junior high school that she wanted to have a business of her own. After graduation from college, she tried to start a private practice and quickly discovered she needed experience first. The experience came from working in acute care, home care, and wellness programs doing individual counseling and group classes. After she started consulting in long-term care, her private practice took off rapidly. She loves being an entrepreneur and cannot imagine working for anyone but herself.

Carlene Russell, MS, RD,LD, FADA, Mason City, Iowa (personal communication, June 20, 1997), began her dietetics career as a relief dietitian in a large hospital in Omaha, Nebraska. This position soon developed into an assignment to the cardiac/pulmonary unit including the intensive care unit. Five years later, her husband changed jobs, which resulted in a move to rural Iowa. After her first child, she was interested in working only part time, but in the new location, the nearest hospital was 35 miles away. Not being willing to drive that distance, she began looking for other work options.

She sent letters to the Iowa Dietetic Association and dietitians in the area requesting information about availability of jobs. After several months, the only position available was in a nursing home, which she accepted, and went on to set up contracts with several other nursing homes. The flexibility of working part time was a perfect match with her family needs, and an added benefit was that she discovered she enjoyed working in long-term care. Involvement in the CD-HCF provided support she needed to deliver quality nutritional care. She says

> I look back on the day I was reluctant to accept the position as consultant dietitian to a nursing home. During the 20 years that have since elapsed, it has been very helpful to have my professional goals identified, then the opportunities to achieve the goals. After all this time, my job is not done and there are more goals to set. Currrently, I am expanding my practice into home care and assisted living. Approximately 75 percent of my time is now spent in home care. With the changes in health care and shorter hospital stays, there is an increased need for home care.

THE FUTURE

Balch has pointed out that the trend for the future in health care is *the need to do more and better with less.*[24] The impact of managed care will be felt in all health care organizations in control of costs and also emphasis on quality care. Many health care systems are outsourcing a greater number and variety of services, including food services. Contractors can provide a specialist on demand and can provide models for policy manuals, patient education materials, menus, management support, quality assurance, and others. This frees health care professionals to spend more time providing care or management expertise and also creates opportunities for dietitians to become the specialists.

As the number of older people in the United States continues to grow, the need for dietitians in long-term care will increase, and as managed care becomes more prevalent, the number of patients in nursing homes who need complex care will also grow.[24] Dietitians and other professionals will have to work closely with patients and work quickly and continuously in multidisciplinary teams as well as with patients and their families.

If the legislation for MNT is enacted, residents of long-term care facilities will benefit through the care offered and dietitians will benefit through the reimbursement of nutrition care services not presently covered under Medicare regulations.[19]

CONCLUSION

Opportunities abound for dietitians as consultants in long-term care facilities, and the need may be even greater in the future. The potential for creating entrepreneurial and managerial roles in consulting is a further pathway for dietitians.

The provision of nutritional care for all age groups is critical to health and enjoyment of life. For residents of long-term facilities, the quality of life is greatly dependent on their nutritional status, and because of this, both federal and state regulations governing care include guidelines for the provision of dietetic services. The ADA promotes quality nutritional care for all persons and has initiated programs and initiatives and issued position papers toward this end.

DEFINITIONS

Case Manager Individual who facilitates equitable arrangements between a home health care provider and payers as an outcome of case management.

Client The recipient of services or products.

Consultant Dietitian Registered dietitian who is qualified through education, training, and experience in administrative, education, and clinical skills. The consultant may be in private practice or provide advice and service in a health care organization by guiding the staff for the purpose of providing nutrition care that will result in optimal health and nutritional status to the client/resident.

Consultant Dietitians in Health Care Facilities Dietetic practice group of The American Dietetic Association.

Continuous Quality Improvement Approach to the continuous study and improvement of the process and outcomes of the provision of health care services to meet the needs of those served. Specific structured problem-solving methods are used that rely on data and group process tools.

Continuum of Care Coordinated system of settings, services, providers, and care levels in which health, medical, and supportive services are provided in the appropriate care setting.

Facility Institution such as a hospital, nursing, or group home.

Health Care Financing Administration (HCFA) Federal agency that administers the Medicare/Medicaid programs and sets federal standards for institutions caring for recipients of the funding.

Home Health Care Services delivered to patients in the home setting.

Joint Commission on Accreditation of Healthcare Organizations (the Joint Commission) Accrediting agency that sets standards for health care units and conducts reviews based on the standards for those institutions requesting the accreditation. The standards are identified as essential factors that result in safe, effective, high-yield patient care.

Long-Term Care Assistance expected to be provided over a long period of time to people with chronic health conditions and/or physical disabilities and those who are unable to care for themselves without the help of other persons.

Managed Care System of health care usually administered by an entity outside a hospital or other health care institution in which access, cost, and quality of care

are controlled by direct intervention before or during service for purposes of creating efficiencies and/or reducing costs.

Medicare Federal insurance program that provides hospital and medical services for individuals 65 years of age or older, individuals of any age who have permanent kidney failure that requires dialysis or a kidney replacement, and certain individuals younger than 65 years of age who have disabilities.

Nutrition Assessment Evaluation of an individual's nutritional status based on anthropometric, biochemical, clinical, and dietary information.

Nutrition Screening Use of diagnostic tools and methodology to determine nutritional risk and the necessity of an in-depth nutrition assessment.

Omnibus Budget Reconciliation Act (OBRA) of 1987 Legislation that led to regulations for residents in long-term care facilities. The regulations are developed and implemented by the Health Care Financing Administration.

Resident Recipient of care from a long-term care provider; used interchangeably with *client, customer,* or *patient.*

Subacute Care Services provided in a treatment unit, usually after acute hospital care and before home care or a long-term care facility.

REFERENCES

1. Office of Nursing Home Affairs. *Long Term Care Improvement Study.* 1975. DHEW Publ. No. (05). 76–50021.

2. Skilled nursing facilities: standards for certification and participation in Medicare and Medicaid programs. *Federal Register.* January 17, 1974;39:2238.

3. ADA. *Nursing Facilities: A Comparison of the State Regulations and the Federal Conditions of Participation.* Chicago: The American Dietetic Association; 1985.

4. Welch P, Oelrich E, Endres J, Poon SW. Consulting dietitians in nursing homes: time in role functions and perceived problems. *J Am Diet Assoc.* 1988;88:29–34.

5. Robinson G, Russell C. OBRA regulations revisited. *Diet Curr.* 1996;23:15–20.

6. Johnson RK, Coulston AM. Medicare: reimbursement rules, impediments, and opportunities for dietitians. *J Am Diet Assoc.* 1995;95:1378–1380.

7. Robinson GE. Applying the 1996 JCAHO nutrition care standards in a long-term-care setting. *J Am Diet Assoc.* 1996;96:400–403.

8. ADA. Position of The American Dietetic Association: affordable and accessible health care costs. *J Am Diet Assoc.* 1992;92:746–748.

9. ADA. Position of The American Dietetic Association: nutrition, aging, and the continuum of care. *J Am Diet Assoc.* 1996;96:1048–1052.

10. ADA. *Resource Guide for the Consultant Dietitian: Consultant Dietitians in Health Care Facilities.* Chicago: The American Dietetic Association; 1993.

11. Cross AT. Practical and legal considerations of private nutrition practice. *J Am Diet Assoc.* 1995;95:21–29.

12. Hamilton E. How to set prices and fees. In: Helm KK, ed. *The Competitive Edge: Advanced Marketing for Dietetics Professionals.* 2nd ed. Chicago: The American Dietetic Association; 1995:178–182.

13. Kane MT, Cohen AS, Smith ER, Lewis C, et al. 1995 commission on dietetic registration dietetic practice audit. *J Am Diet Assoc.* 1996;96:1292–1301.

14. Gilmore SA, Robinson G, Posthauer ME, Raymond J. Clinical indicators associated with unintentional weight loss and pressure ulcers in elderly residents of nursing facilities. *J Am Diet Assoc.* 1995;95:984–992.

15. Chidester JC, Spangler AA. Fluid intake in the institutionalized elderly. *J Am Diet Assoc.* 1997;97:23–27.

16. White JV, Ham RJ, Lipschitz DA, Dwyer JY, et al. Consensus of the nutrition screening initiative: risk factors and indicators of poor nutritional status in older Americans. *J Am Diet Assoc.* 1991;91:783–787.

17. Quality management in hospital-affiliated services. In: Schiller MR, Miller-Kovich K, Miller MA, eds. *Total Quality Management for Hospital Nutrition Services.* Gaithersburg, MD: Aspen Publishers, 1994.

18. Gallagher CR. *OBRA: A Challenge and an Opportunity for Nutrition Care.* The Ross Professional Development Series. Columbus, OH: Ross Laboratories; 1992.

19. ADA. Position of The American Dietetic Association: cost-effectiveness of medical nutrition therapy. *J Am Diet Assoc.* 1995;95:88–91.

20. Nelson KJ, Coulston AM, Sucher KP, Tseng RY. Prevalence of malnutrition in the elderly admitted to long-term-care facilities. *J Am Diet Assoc.* 1993;93:459–461.

21. Pinchcofsky-Devin GD, Kaminski MV. Correlation of pressure sores and nutritional status. *J Am Geriatr Soc.* 1986;34:435–440.

22. Ellis JR, Cowles ED. Physician responses to dietary recommendations in long-term-care facilities. *J Am Diet Assoc.* 1995;95:1424–1425.

23. Gilmore SA, Niedert KC, Lief E, Nichols P. Standards of practice criteria: consultant dietitians in health care facilities. *J Am Diet Assoc.* 1993;93:305–308.

24. Balch GI. Employer's perceptions of the roles of dietetics practitioners: challenge to survive and opportunities to thrive. *J Am Diet Assoc.* 1996;96:1301–1305.

The Consultant in Business Practice

L. Charnette Norton

"The consultant's prayer: 'Give me good abstract reasoning ability, interpersonal skills, cultural perspectives, linguistic comprehension, and a high sociodynamic potential.'"[1]

Outline—Chapter 14

- Introduction

- Opportunities in Business Practice

- Practice Qualifications

- Starting a Practice

- Stories of Successful Consultants
  - Success story 1
  - Success story 2
  - Success story 3

- Conclusion

INTRODUCTION

In the past, employment in dietetics in the United States was very stable. Most dietitians could expect to take a position as a clinical dietitian. After several years of hard work, they could move up to the position of clinical nutrition manager.

The next opportunity was to become an assistant director with increased responsibilities, including production, tray line supervision, and purchasing. This would prepare the dietitian to assume the role of department director, in which the dietitian would remain until retirement. Now, however, changes are occurring rapidly in health care including hospital mergers, hospital closings, concerns about health care reform, and the national economy.[2]

The reengineering of health care has changed this typical career track dramatically for many dietitians. The unstable environment of health care has caused many dietitians to be displaced—either by their own choice or that of the institution—and in the prime of their careers.

One of the options open to this group of dietitians is to make the transition from operations to a consultant in business practice. These dietitians have already developed the skills to work in diverse fields. As department directors and managers of units, they have been involved in and made multiple decisions in many areas of practice, such as tray delivery system selection, preparation of documents for the Joint Commission on Accreditation of Healthcare Organizations (the Joint Commission) and the Omnibus Budget Reconciliation Act (OBRA) assessment, menu planning (including recipe development and nutritional analysis), cook-serve and cook-chill applications, cafeteria operations, catering, and vending.

OPPORTUNITIES IN BUSINESS PRACTICE

Only the imagination and desire of the dietitian limit the opportunities for experienced dietitians to be employed in business practice. A dietitian's potential practice areas as identified by the nutrition entrepreneurs practice group of The American Dietetic Association (ADA) is with "individuals, corporations, media, restaurants, food companies, and sports or health facilities." Another practice group of the ADA, dietitians in business and communications, identify their members as "presidents, vice presidents, food service directors, food stylists, researchers, consultants, sales managers, marketing managers, restaurateurs, test kitchen managers, and software specialists." Other areas of employment for the consultant dietitian in business practices include the practice settings identified by the consultant dietitians in health care facilities in its brochure: "long-term care facilities, retirement and assisted living centers, health and hospice agencies, hospital/subacute units, physician's offices and clinics, facilities for the developmentally disabled, health maintenance organization rehabilitation centers, psychiatric facilities, correctional facilities, alcohol and substance abuse centers, food and equipment vendors, and health professional education programs."

A reemphasis on ADA members as food/food management experts was urged by Halling and Hess, who believe innovative opportunities for career expansion abound for dietitians in the foods business.[3] In the early 1990s, through its strategic planning activities, the ADA identified commercial food service as a major market linkage for dietetic services. It was pointed out that to compete in this environment, management of rapid product introduction and of sales among a variety of food products and knowledge of rapidly changing technology and environmental controls is essential.[4]

Several options for a dietetic career have already been identified in other chapters of this book. What is different for the dietitian working as a consultant in business practice? Dietitians who decide to enter a business consulting practice are risk takers. They like to take on new challenges and to become part of a powerful group of innovative thinkers and doers. They are energetic versatile professionals with a wide range of interests and agendas in the business community. They are dietitians on the front lines of nutrition and public health, many of whom have chosen nontraditional career paths.

Although many of the assignments for a consultant may be similar to those of a full-time staff dietitian, one of the main differences is in the duration of the assignment. The consultant in business practices is given a short-term contract with an identified scope. The scope of services is usually an assignment to set up or improve the business practice of the client. It may also be a specific project with a defined beginning and ending, for one month, one year, etc. Examples of activities the consultant may perform are evaluating staffing patterns, establishing an inventory and cost control system, planning a new production or service system, and recommending equipment purchases.

PRACTICE QUALIFICATIONS

The opportunities for the entry-level dietitian as a consultant in business practices are limited because of the depth of knowledge and experience needed to be successful as a consultant. However, older students who have life experience or expertise in another profession have an advantage in this area. Another deterrent to the entry-level dietitian is that most dietitians who are consultants in business practices are sole operators. Many do not employ full-time secretarial staff or other assistants. If they have an overload of work, they simply contract out portions of jobs that they either do not have time to finish or do not have the expertise with which to satisfy the client. Thus, it is difficult for beginning-level dietitians to break into the consulting field.

A limited number of business consulting firms do employ entry-level dietitians for consulting but in a defined scope of responsibilities. The usual requirement is that the dietitian be experienced in another area (e.g., as a clinical dietitian in a health care facility or manager of a food service system). The dietitian may also have worked as an assistant to another dietitian for a food processor, equipment manufacturer, publisher, marketing company, or software specialist.

When dietitians are hired by a consulting firm, they are often assigned as an assistant to a team leader to work on a specific part of a major project. The entry-level dietitian would have minimal client contact and would not be involved in selling services in the same way as the team leader.

The dietitian in the business setting may also have the opportunity to expand into other nontraditional roles such as facility management, accounting, design, sales, or marketing. The range of expanded responsibility is dependent on the scope of the services performed by the company and those that the dietitian can develop on his or her own for the company.

A smaller number of dietitians are now being employed by food service design firms as specialists in management advisory services. These dietitians are usually former food service directors with at least 10 years of continuous experience or experience in several different facilities.

The career ladder for the consultant dietitian is often very short. Many dietitians choosing this career path are the owners or co-owners of their companies. Therefore, they are already at the top of the organization when they begin practice. These dietitians, however, have the freedom to develop their career path as they want. The path becomes one of self-development of highly valued expertise rather than one provided by others. They will have the further ability and drive to develop new skills to enable them to offer expanded services to a targeted client base.

The dietitian who may be thinking of moving into management with the goal of consultation and perhaps his or her own business can benefit from guidelines that have been proposed as follows: Discuss new plans with the immediate supervisor, seek advice from a veteran manager or mentor, react deliberately rather than spontaneously, weigh solutions against the mission of the organization, practice active listening with everyone involved, and investigate the literature for continued information and self-education.[5]

STARTING A PRACTICE

Once a dietitian has made the decision to start a consulting practice, several decisions must be made. If an office is established, appropriate office equipment must be obtained and decisions made about secretarial and/or office manager assistance. Starting with a base of operations, the type of business ownership, the start-up costs, setting a fee structure, and financial accounting will need to be determined.

From the beginning, it is imperative that the services of at least three professional advisors be obtained: a lawyer, an accountant, and a banker. They will guide the dietitian in many business decisions that the dietitian does not have the skills or expertise to make alone. Cross has provided a comprehensive discussion of the practical and legal considerations in establishing a private practice along with some of the characteristics of success.[6] She indicates that success depends on four factors: the personal characteristics required for successful business owner-ship, the type of legal and financial ownership structure under which the business operates, the adequacy of start-up funding, and the appropriate pricing of services.

The dietitian entering consulting practice will also benefit from networks established with other members of dietetic practice groups, with other dietitians, and with small business owners in similar practice. Suggestions for making use of other business management people may also be found in *The Entrepreneurial Nutritionist* by Helm.[7] Consideration should also be given to whether the consultant's practice will be within a geographic area (e.g., a community, a state, nationally, or internationally). If the business is widespread, travel as well as time involvement may be a decisive factor.

Depending on the consultant's business organization—partnership, corpora-tion, sole practitioner, etc.—the consultant dietitian may also have a board of directors. In such cases, the advisors mentioned (i.e., the lawyer, banker, and accountant) should have designated responsibilities as board advisors.

STORIES OF SUCCESSFUL CONSULTANTS

Success Story 1

One reason dietitians may choose to become consultants is that they cannot decide on a particular career path because several appear to be interesting. This author is one such dietitian. I chose not to pursue dietetics on graduation from college at the University of Missouri-Columbia because I decided I did not want to work in patient care in hospitals; however, health care was the primary option available to dietitians in the 1960s. So I changed jobs every three to five years, working in management capacities in a restaurant, long-term care facility, several acute care hospitals ranging from a 100-bed community hospital to an 800-bed university teaching hospital, and a corporate dining facility. In these environ-ments, I managed self-operated food services and worked for contract manage-ment companies. In addition, I taught food-related subjects at the university level.

At one time in my career, I became bored with my job as a food service director and became commissioned as a captain in the United States Army Reserve, offering my dietetic skills to the government.

While working in an acute care hospital in California, I applied for membership in the ADA and successfully passed the registration examination. However, not having gone through an internship, I began to study for advanced degrees.

The opportunity to work with Aimee Moore, PhD, in Food Systems Manage-ment at the University of Missouri-Columbia, was the chance of a lifetime (personal communication, November 15, 1997). Moore was a leader and innova-tor in the field of dietetics. She challenged all her students to become involved in their profession and develop their careers to the fullest. When I began my work toward the PhD, I was counseled by Moore to continue working and not take a break in my career.

As my career progressed, my experience and expertise increased. However, health care administration was becoming more unstable. At the last university hospital where I worked, I had six new bosses in three years. The last one decided that he wanted an entirely new food service team. Rather than move to another hospital and face the same uncertainty, I decided to open my own consulting practice. Because of my varied experiences and the network of contacts I had developed over the years, my practice was financially viable the first year.

The Norton Group, Inc., today offers a wide variety of services. The management services include operational management and financial audits for contract and self-operated food service facilities; operation conceptualization; reengineering development; preparation of request for proposal (RFP) packages for selection of food service contract management firms, and the development of the operation's response to RFPs; operation plan/facility design review and analysis; assisting clients with facility start-up in manual and vending services; assessing existing facility/operations team performance; repositioning for long-established operations; development of transition plans and assistance in conversion from contracted food service to self-operated; establishment of buying programs and prime vendor services; continuous quality management and improvement review for food service; and feasibility studies and cost justification for computerized dietary operations.

In addition, the Norton Group provides technical expertise in several areas: menu planning, including recipes and nutritional analysis; implementation of hazard analysis of critical control points (HACCP) programs; cook-chill implementation; OBRA compliance; clinical nutrition services for day care for adults and children; the Joint Commission and Medicare presurveys; food labeling law compliance; and tray delivery system selection for cook-chill programs.

Finally, the consulting firm provides marketing services such as conducting focus groups and customer preference surveys, developing training and inservice videos, writing articles for newsletters, developing marketing and merchandising programs, writing magazine articles on trends and technology, producing brochures and support materials, and marketing programs for manufacturers.

Success Story 2

Another career track for a consultant in business practice may involve branching out, or leaving, employment with a corporation with other dietitians and then selling his or her services back to the former employer. Many corporations today are outsourcing dietitian's services, so this may be increasingly possible. Not only can the former employee work with the company, he or she can develop additional services for similar companies—sometimes services the dietitian may only have envisioned earlier.

Vi Stancik is one such dietitian (personal communication, November 15, 1996). A graduate of Case Western Reserve University with a bachelor's degree in chemistry/foods and nutrition and a master's degree in public health nutrition, Stancik started out as a traditional clinical dietitian. From 1971 to 1974, she worked as a consulting dietitian in Cleveland, Ohio, in several venues, including health care, schools, and industrial cafeterias.

In health care, Stancik wrote policy and procedure manuals for hospitals and extended care facilities in compliance with state and federal regulations governing dietary departments. She also organized and managed patients' nutritional care, dietary histories, and nutritional assessment for 80 extended care facilities.

Stancik also supervised school lunch programs in five school districts, writing menus and handbooks on equipment handling, and helped the Society for the Blind plan cycle menus, improve the nutritional value of meals, and develop modified diets.

In 1974, Stancik joined the staff of Cleveland Range, Inc., a division of the Welbilt Corporation. Her job at Cleveland was to develop a new method of cooking by using steam. As one of three pioneers in the technology, she helped perfect the technique of steam cooking and developed the recipes and cooking timetable to go with the technology.

The convection steamer was introduced in 1974. After its introduction, Stancik traveled around the world marketing the new piece of equipment. She conducted an education program for steam cooking in every state in the country and continually sought new markets for the equipment.

In 1976, Stancik became manager of the test kitchen in Cleveland. In 1979, she became the first national account manager, then was named vice president of marketing for Cleveland. She was the first female vice president in the company's history.

In 1994, after almost 20 years with Cleveland Range, Stancik decided to take her expertise and branch out on her own. She continues to work with Cleveland Range, but she also consults with several other restaurant-related companies in marketing, customer service, public relations, business operations, recipe and menu development, quantity food preparation, cook-chill preparation and sanitation, and HACCP implementation. She is now a successful consultant in business and a role model for others.

Success Story 3

Many consulting dietitians choose their career paths simply by following their love. For Caren Messina-Hirsch, that love is food. As the founder and president of Food Performance, Inc., Wheaton, Illinois, she works with food and food concepts for food manufacturers, advertising agencies, food service contractors, and restaurants. The company creates recipes, manages food shows, tests new products, and develops menus.

Messina-Hirsch grew up in an Italian family in New Jersey, learning kitchen skills from her mother. When she was in eighth grade, she won a local baking contest with her recipe for German chocolate cake, and her destiny was decided.

Messina-Hirsch received her BS degree in dietetics and food and nutrition from Notre Dame College of Ohio and her master's degree in institutional administration from Oklahoma State University.

From working in the test kitchens at General Mills, Inc., early in her career, Messina-Hirsch learned how to test products, write label directions, and develop recipes and menus by learning first how the products were to be used in the food service setting. She worked in kitchens all over the country, training customers to prepare and merchandise foods for the greatest degree of success.

In 1981, Messina-Hirsch decided to use her experience and knowledge to set up her own food service consulting firm. When asked what it is that keeps her involved with food, she explains that combining nutrition with culinary arts links "the creative, artistic, freedom elements" of the culinary world with "the technical, scientific, more disciplined elements" of nutrition. She believes that the field of dietetics and nutrition offers a myriad of opportunities and much flexibility of choice.

Messina-Hirsch's association with ADA provides her with ample opportunity for networking with other dietitians. She has served as chair of the Dietitians in Business and Communications Practice Group and also as chair of the National Center for Nutrition and Dietetics development committee.

Messina-Hirsch's experience in the field has also taught her that one is never too old to learn. That is why, after 25 years in the business, she opted to attend Kendall College in Evanston, Illinois, to earn a culinary arts degree. Her business and artistic talents will no doubt continue to grow.

CONCLUSION

The 1990s are a time when many changes are occurring in health care, in career options, and in dietetics. The opportunities for dietitians to become consultants in their own business practice are open for the person with determination, initiative, and perseverance, and experience in food service management. Commercial food service, health care facilities of all types, food and equipment companies, the communications industry, and other businesses are potential clients for dietitian consultants. Establishing the expertise and versatility needed to function in the business world can lead to a satisfying, lucrative, and successful career as evidenced by the career histories of the three dietitians in this chapter.

DEFINITIONS

Consultation Advice and guidance provided by a skilled, knowledgeable, qualified person.

Continuous Quality Improvement Specific, structural, problem-solving methods that rely on data and group process tools.

Contract Foodservice Facility An organization providing foodservices administered by a contract management company.

Entrepreneurial Pertaining to the characteristics of a person who organizes and manages a commercial undertaking that is usually an innovative undertaking involving risk.

Hazard Analysis of Critical Control Points (HACCP) A system for quality control in food and foodservices starting with food products from suppliers and ending with consumption of the food by customers.

Joint Commission on Accreditation of Healthcare Organizations The accrediting agency that sets standards for healthcare units and conducts reviews based on the standards for those institutions requesting the review. The standards are identified as essential factors that result in safe, effective, high-yield patient care.

Omnibus Budget Reconciliation Act (OBRA) of 1987 Legislation that led to regulations for the care of residents in long-term care facilities. The regulations are developed and implemented by the Health Care Financing Administration.

Operation Conceptualization Processes primarily involved in forecasting and planning for a business organization or entity.

Outsourcing A process by which services are sought or contracted for outside an organization.

Reengineering Development The re-design of a business process.

REFERENCES

1. Bolles RN. *What Color Is Your Parachute?* Berkeley, CA: Ten Speed Press; 1995.

2. Davidhizar R. When you lose your job in health care management. *Health Care Supervisor.* 1996;14:42–46.

3. Halling JF, Hess MA. Vision vs reality: ADA members as food/food management experts. *J Am Diet Assoc.* 1995;95:169–170.

4. Lechowich KA, Soto TK. Opportunities in commercial foodservice: the industry perspective. *J Am Diet Assoc.* 1995;95:1163–1166.

5. Davidhizar R. Evaluating creative management solutions. *Health Care Supervisor.* 1996;14:46–49.

6. Cross AT. Practical and legal considerations of private nutrition practice. *J Am Diet Assoc.* 1995;95:21–29.

7. Helm KK. *The Entrepreneurial Nutritionist.* 2nd ed. Lake Dallas, TX: Helm Publishers; 1991.

The Dietitian in Business and Communications

Susan Calvert Finn

"The assumption that we will have only one job or one profession throughout our careers is no longer valid; nor is the assumption valid that institutionally based positions will dominate our professional membership. All indicators point to a new workplace for members of our profession."[1]

Outline—Chapter 15

- Introduction

- New Pathways

- Climbing the Career Ladder
  - Power of mentoring
  - Networking connection
  - Strategic skill building

- Requirements for Successful Practice

- Looking Ahead

- Case Studies
  - Case study 1
  - Case study 2
  - Case study 3

- Conclusion

INTRODUCTION

Following a career path in business and communications has long been considered a nontraditional choice for dietitians—and a career path that has its pros and cons. (See Exhibit 15–1.) The American Dietetic Association (ADA) membership surveys conducted between 1990 and 1995 show about 4 percent of dietitians working in the for-profit corporate sector[2] (IA Bryk, personal communication, 1996). It is important to note, however, that while this percentage has remained constant, the *absolute* number of dietitians working in business and communications has increased along with an increase in number of dietitians overall.

In a study of employment trends for dietitians in business and industry, most current employers (72 percent) as well as prospective employers (62 percent) indicated that the trend toward hiring dietitians is, in fact, increasing. More than 40 percent of employers said their organizations were creating new positions for dietitians.[3] Among the major reasons cited for adding a registered dietitian (RD) to the staff were to increase the company's credibility, to promote the health and nutrition of customers, and to increase the understanding of customer needs.[3] Often, these positions are not directly related to dietetics. RDs are being hired for positions in sales, marketing, and communications as well.

This trend is likely to continue as consumers become increasingly interested in health promotion and disease prevention. Food Marketing Institute research shows that more than 60 percent of food shoppers are very concerned about nutrition. And 45 percent say they are taking more responsibility to ensure that what they eat is nutritious. Although taste remains the number 1 criterion when choosing food, nutrition is also cited by more than 7 out of 10 shoppers as very important in food selection.[4]

But an ADA survey shows that although 80 percent of Americans recognize the importance of good nutrition, only 35 percent are doing all they can to eat a balanced diet. The other 65 percent say perceived obstacles of taste, time, and confusion deter their efforts toward improved eating habits.[5] The ADA survey also indicates that consumers look to dietitians as their most valuable source of reliable nutrition information.

In the light of this knowledge–action gap and the high regard in which the public holds dietitians, it is clear that the mission of the ADA—"to serve the public through the promotion of optimal nutrition, health and well-being"—cannot stop at the threshold of so-called traditional dietetics.

NEW PATHWAYS

There are as many different paths to a career in business and communications as there are dietitians to take them. For example, after graduating from the

Exhibit 15–1 What Do Dietitians in Business and Communications Like (and Dislike) Most about Their Jobs?

Pros
Fast pace
Variety of projects and individuals
Challenging work
Learning opportunities
Team work
Opportunities for creativity
Translating science into something individuals can use
Remuneration
Visibility

Cons
Fast pace
Stressful
Long hours
Red tape and paperwork
Too much information to digest
Lack of administrative support
Managing rather than doing
Battles for project funding
Company politics

Source: Based on an informal survey of dietitians working in business and communications, February 1996.

University of Illinois with a degree in nutrition and medical dietetics, Jean Ragalie, RD (personal communication, February 5, 1996) expected to work in food service and dietary management. "But I followed my strengths and passions," she says, "and they led me into nutrition communications." Ragalie is currently vice president, food and nutrition communications, at McCarroll Marketing, Inc., in Mt. Prospect, Illinois, where she develops marketing and public relations programs for a variety of food and nutrition clients.

Ragalie's first job was in outpatient counseling and community work. Later, she joined the Chicago Heart Association, working in the community and with the media. An association volunteer told her she belonged in public relations and advised her about an opportunity at Burson-Marsteller, one of the world's largest public relations firms. After four years at Burson-Marsteller, Ragalie joined the NutraSweet Co. in worldwide health communications. A year and a half ago, she moved from NutraSweet to McCarroll Marketing, where she is responsible for the "soup to nuts" of any program involving food and nutrition.

When Janet Helm, MS, RD, graduated from Kansas State University with a degree in mass communications and home economics, she was not sure what to do. "Looking back now, I can see that my life has had a lot of repeating themes," she says (personal communication, January 31, 1996). "I always intended to combine my majors into a job like being a food editor. At the time, dietetics seemed very limiting to me. But after I learned more about the profession, I discovered just how important the RD credential is."

Helm worked at a hospital as a diet technician and returned to school to earn the undergraduate credits she needed to enter Kansas State's MS program. After graduation, she did a six-month qualifying experience at the hospital where she had worked and at the NBC affiliate in Kansas City as a health reporter. She subsequently landed a job at the Dairy Council, which included a monthly spot on the NBC affiliate's noon news. "The Dairy Council was very adept at public relations," says Helm. "The job was a great learning experience, like a mini-agency atmosphere."

After three years, Helm moved to New York to work for Ketchum Public Relations at the behest of a woman who had been one of her mentors during college. At Ketchum, she worked on two commodity group accounts—the Egg Nutrition Center and the National Livestock and Meat Board. During her three-year stay at Ketchum, she also worked on a public service announcement sponsored by McDonald's. Later, when the fast-food giant created a communications position for an RD, Helm got the job.

"After several years, I felt I had done what I could do at McDonald's and that it was time to move on," says Helm. She worked for a former client, the Meat Board, for a year and a half, then joined Bozell Worldwide as vice president of consumer marketing, where she heads up a couple of teams specializing in food marketing, notably the public relations effort behind "Milk, What a Surprise!"—also known as the "milk mustache campaign." "My early Dairy Council experience and national program experience were instrumental in my joining Bozell," Helm says.

Like Helm, Martin M. Yadrick, MS, MBA, RD, has also followed a nontraditional path, whose repeating themes are bringing him full circle. "I changed my major a lot," Yadrick remembers (personal communication, February 1, 1996), "from foreign language, to business, to nutrition. The health and wellness aspect of nutrition especially appealed to me, as opposed to clinical dietetics. But one of my teachers advised me to get a clinical background and to pursue an RD."

After Yadrick earned an MS in clinical nutrition at the University of Kansas Medical Center, he intended to do clinical work. While pursuing his master's, he also worked in long-term care, in a veterans' hospital, and in cardiac rehabilitation. About 18 months after getting his MS, he began work on an MBA. "It was the mid-80s," he says. "Everyone was doing it and I wasn't sure of my opportunities without additional training."

Yadrick subsequently took a job at the University of Kansas Medical Center in food service financial administration. "It was a great transition position combining dietetics and accounting," he says. Yadrick taught himself to use some very basic software and started to learn about computers.

After three years, he decided to head west. He moved to California—jobless, but not for long. Networking with members of the practice group SCAN (he was chairman in 1993–1994) and with his ADA Ambassador Program colleagues (he has been an ADA spokesperson since 1989), Yadrick found a job at Computrition, a dietary software company, where he now trains customers who purchase the company's long-term care or hospital-use software. He is also project manager for a new risk assessment module that encompasses the entire health care continuum. Yadrick says that he sees a long-term opportunity for global sales of Computrition's software products. That college work in foreign languages may come in handy after all.

Elizabeth Hiser, MS, RD, wanted to be a writer and a teacher—and she is, although not exactly as she planned. After graduating from the University of Rhode Island with a BA in English, Hiser taught for six years and worked for a newspaper. She then decided to go back to school, made up the necessary undergraduate credits, and earned an MS in nutrition from the University of Vermont.

"After I had been working for 10 years in clinical research at the university," she remembers, "my medical director 'volunteered' me to consult for *Eating Well* magazine—free of charge. The next thing he knew, I was gone!" Hiser has been with *Eating Well* for several years and is now the nutrition editor. She is responsible for ensuring that all the nutrition information in the magazine is accurate and timely (personal communication, February 6, 1996).

Hiser says that her experience in research and with patients has really helped her. In addition to her work at *Eating Well,* she also teaches cardiac rehabilitation. She is on the board of the American Association of Cardiopulmonary Rehabilitation and is nutrition editor of the *Journal of Cardiopulmonary Rehabilitation*. In 1996, at Hiser's urging, *Eating Well* launched a newsletter for cardiac rehabilitation patients.

Delia Hammock, MS, RD, is nutrition editor for *Good Housekeeping* magazine. In addition to writing a monthly editorial, she is nutrition consultant for the entire magazine as well as its media liaison. She also reviews all food advertising.

"School teacher, nurse, secretary. Those were the career choices for women in the small town I come from," says Hammock. "I had no idea what I was going to do. I fell into dietetics as a way to support myself." After earning a BS in home economics with a specialty in dietetics, Hammock worked at New York Hospital for two years, eventually specializing in renal care. She then earned her master's in nutrition at Boston University. She went on to work at New York University Medical Center for six years but soon became bored.

"By this time, I knew clinical dietetics wasn't for me," she remembers. "But when I started, RDs were only in hospitals. My boss said I could do anything I wanted as long as I did my job, too. So I looked for opportunities for experience wherever I could."

Hammock started with some freelance writing. A friend from graduate school gave her a job doing some nutrition-related direct mail work. "I started to work up a portfolio," Hammock says. "But it was very hard to move from clinical dietetics into public relations." She joined a public relations group sponsored by the New York Dietetic Association, networked with New York University educators, and made contacts that led to jobs such as doing food demonstrations at Bloomingdale's department store.

When the New York Heart Association needed an educator for a pilot course in the continuing education program, Hammock's networking paid off. She was hired to write the course and also taught it for several years. "It was little pay but great experience," says Hammock, "and it forced me to become a real food person and to learn presentation skills. The course led to other teaching assignments as well."

In 1982, Hammock had her first article published in *Good Housekeeping*. "I had gone for a job interview," she recalls, "and they asked for a sample article. They bought the article, but I didn't get the job." Hammock continued with her freelance work and teaching. After about six years, she moved to Philadelphia but soon returned to New York and relentlessly pursued any opportunity that offered the chance to learn new skills. "When the right job came along," she says, "I wanted to be more qualified than any other candidate."

In 1988, she interviewed at *Good Housekeeping* again. "From the time I'd come for my first interview six years earlier, I knew that's where I wanted to work." This time, she got the job.

CLIMBING THE CAREER LADDER

Dietitians traveling a nontraditional path agree that having a mentor, networking, developing a strategic skill set, and keeping up-to-date with research and consumer trends (see Exhibit 15–2) are four factors necessary to building a successful career.

Power of Mentoring

The *Wall Street Journal* reports that 9 of 10 workers who have received job coaching or mentoring think it is an effective development tool.[6] Some companies have established "inplacement" programs modeled on outplacement techniques to help plan the careers of employees they do not want to lose.[7]

Exhibit 15–2 What Do Dietitians in Business and Communications Read?

Newspapers: major metropolitan and national dailies
Magazines: news, health, culinary, women's service
Newsletters: nutrition, health, fitness
Trade publications: food, food manufacturing/technology, retail food, food service, managed care, advertising, public relations
Professional journals: nutrition, medical
Books: cookbooks, diet, fitness

Source: Based on an informal survey of dietitians working in business and communications, February 1996.

Cathy Miller, MS, RD, is director of research and development at Tulsa-based National Steak and Poultry, a company that sizes, marinates, and freezes meat products for chain restaurants. Her key responsibility is to develop new products for existing or potential customers. Miller has two mentors who have been with her since the early days of her career—her internship director and the owner of a consulting firm she worked for. "Both are RDs and both have followed nontraditional paths," says Miller (personal communication, February 6, 1996). "They encouraged me not to settle for an entry-level job but to stretch. I learned from them how to be professional. I still rely on them today."

Karen Kafer, PhD, RD, director of communications for Kellogg USA, says one of her managers at Kellogg has been a very important mentor to her. "She's helped me grow as a person and to see my strengths and weaknesses," Kafer says (personal communication, January 29, 1996). "She also has provided insight into policies, procedures, and the unspoken policies of the company." Kafer joined Kellogg in nutrition communications. Initially, she wrote brochures for both consumers and health professionals. She later moved into public relations and marketing. "My mentor helped give me mobility in the company," Kafer says. "She championed my advancement." Kafer now oversees marketing communications and public relations for new products, research programs, and cross-merchandising efforts.

As vice president of advertising and promotion at the National Cattlemen's Beef Association in Chicago, Mary Adolf, MS, RD, LD, says (personal communication, January 30, 1996) she has been fortunate to have some excellent bosses who have molded positions to fit her strengths. "Having a mentor is important," she says. "It's a 'been there, done that' kind of thing. A mentor can really help a young person when his or her choices are not obvious."

Mentoring is, however, a two-way street. Martin Yadrick of Computrition says young dietetics students and dietitians write or call him for advice (personal communication, February 1, 1996). "I learned a lot from my colleagues in ADA's

Ambassador Program, and I had one boss in particular who urged me to move forward," he says. "It's only right to return the favor when someone comes to you for help." Carolyn O'Neil, MS, RD, LD, executive producer and correspondent for CNN's "On the Menu," agrees (personal communication, January 29, 1996). "I am very conscious about how I can share what I'm doing with young professionals. We need each other's support."

Networking Connection

One of the best ways to find a mentor is to network both inside and outside the boundaries of dietetics. Rita Storey, MS, RD, is director of nutrition services for the food service division of ConAgra Frozen Foods in Omaha. In addition to giving technical support to the sales force and working in product development, Storey heads up outreach to professional health and food service associations. "Networking is at the top of my list," she says (personal communication, February 1, 1996). "I have two huge three-ring binders filled with business cards. I use my network for projects and information gathering and also to connect other people with each other."

Jean Ragalie of McCarroll Marketing says she is "huge in networking" and would not be where she is today without it. "When I left NutraSweet, I got on the phone and had a job offer the next day," she recalls (personal communication, February 5, 1996). "After the ADA annual meeting, I had eight different job leads." Ragalie says that networking with RDs and public relations professionals is also important because no one can be an expert on everything. "That is why I belong to a number of ADA practice groups," she explains. "Their very focused look into an area of practice helps me keep current."

Tama Bloch, RD, LD, nutrition coordinator for the Nestle Frozen, Refrigerated and Ice Cream Co. plays a leadership role in the nutrition science behind new and existing products. She also spearheads the nutrition strategy involved in labeling, product positioning, and advertising. Like Jean Ragalie, Bloch uses her network for expert input. "There are other RDs in my department, in sales, and in Nestle USA," she says (personal communication, January 31, 1996). "I joined the American Heart Association and work with RDs there, too. I also stay in touch with current thinking by networking with clinical RDs in hospitals, outpatient clinics, and private practice. They are on the front lines."

Mary Adolf of the National Cattlemen's Beef Association says she networks with other dietitians, especially at ADA's annual meeting and through the ADA Dietitians in Business and Communications practice group. "I also network with people in other professional associations," she says. "For example, the food service members of the International Foodservice Manufacturers Association (IFMA) are a source of ideas for me. Theirs may be products totally different from mine, but our marketing challenges are the same."

Strategic Skill Building

The ability to communicate well, a strong clinical background, and business savvy are three of the strategic skills behind a successful career. In a 1989 ADA study assessing employment trends for dietitians in business and industry, both employers and dietitians ranked communication skills as essential for success.[3] "Being good in math and science won't mean much if communication skills are poor," says ConAgra's Rita Storey. "No matter what setting we are in, dietetics is about teaching and communicating."

Martin Yadrick prides himself on being able to communicate well with people of different backgrounds and levels of expertise. He attributes much of this skill to some experience acting and to his work with the media, both of which forced him to deliver clear succinct messages. Mary Adolf explains that one reason strong communication skills are important in her job is that she is directly responsible to the beef producers who comprise her association. "I have to communicate what we're doing on their behalf and why," she says. "Luckily, I was forced to do a lot of presentations during my education, and I have worked with some first-rank communicators along the way."

Although dietitians in business and communications may have followed a nontraditional path, that in no way diminishes the importance of their clinical education and experience. "If your job requires evaluating research and working with research and development, a good grounding in science is important," maintains Rita Storey. Delia Hammock says her years in clinical dietetics have been very helpful. "Young RDs want to skip the clinical part," she says. "But I prefer to hire dietitians who have a couple of years of clinical experience. They have to be able to understand research before they can report on it." Jean Ragalie agrees: "The fundamentals of nutrition therapy are important. That's where you learn what people's needs and habits are."

A sound clinical background is important, but a good business education also helps. Martin Yadrick values his MBA courses in organizational behavior. Both Karen Kafer and Rita Storey wish they had taken more classes in finance, and Storey also notes the need to be savvy about technology. Marcella Gelman, MS, RD, supervisor of consumer affairs for Vons Companies, Inc. (the nation's ninth largest supermarket chain), laments that her education included only one class in computers. "The curriculum has probably changed," she notes (personal communication, February 6, 1996), "but taking courses late in your career, as I have had to do with computers, is not the same as the immersion you experience as a young student."

REQUIREMENTS FOR SUCCESSFUL PRACTICE

A career in business and communications demands a value system that balances personal, professional, and business ethics. "ADA's code of ethics is really applicable everywhere," says Marcella Gelman. "The RD's ethics are very high. In my dealings with other dietitians, I always know what to expect."

"I am first and foremost a nutrition professional, not a public relations person or magazine editor," says *Good Housekeeping*'s Delia Hammock. *Eating Well*'s Elizabeth Hiser reinforces Hammock's sentiments: "You have to always keep the client or reader at the center, despite any pressures that advertisers may bring to bear. I talk to food industry PR people all day every day," Hiser continues. "But I can't be influenced by special interests."

As CNN's Carolyn O'Neil points out, dietitians in communications must also follow journalism's code of ethics: to seek out the truth. "There's a lot of conflicting information out there," she explained. "I have to be very careful how I report on quackery and must avoid getting involved in product endorsements." O'Neil is responsible for producing five food and health segments plus one 30–minute "On the Menu" show each week.

Dietitians on public relations side of communications must look closely at the motivation behind their PR campaigns. "Make your efforts 100 percent science-based," says Bozell Worldwide's Janet Helm. "The milk mustache campaign, for example, is very much a nutrition education effort—using the media." Mary Adolf, at the national Cattlemen's Beef Association, admits that marketing beef can be a challenge. "Honesty and integrity are critical," she says. "We are trying to help consumers understand how beef can be a part of a balanced diet. Our positioning strategy goes back to ADA's code of ethics—information based in science and fact."

At Nestle Frozen, Refrigerated and Ice Cream Co., Tama Bloch makes sure every promotion she advises on is based on sound science. "As a result," she says, "I have earned my colleagues' trust and Nestle keeps its customers' trust." At Kellogg USA, concern for ethics is the very reason the company hires nutrition professionals. "Our code of ethics is very similar to ADA's," says Kellogg's Karen Kafer. "We're interested in making sure that our nutrition communications are honest and accurate."

LOOKING AHEAD

What will dietitians do in the future? Virtually anything they want to do, predicts Rita Storey. "But it's becoming a very competitive marketplace," warns Jean Ragalie. "Dietitians must jump in and seize the opportunities. Our skills are transferable to the business world." For example, Ragalie sees a bright future for dietitians in food marketing and sales. "Anywhere food is, we can go!" she asserts.

As Janet Helm points out, however, most nontraditional jobs will not have RD at the top of the job description. "But having an RD may be enough to close the deal," she says. "It can be the value-added extra that makes you stand out from other candidates. You have to package yourself."

Often this positioning effort means demonstrating to employers exactly what a dietitian's skills are. For example, when Cathy Miller started at Jack in the Box (where she eventually became director of R&D), she had to overcome some preconceived notions. "I was their first and only RD," Miller recalls. "During my interviews, people expressed concern that I could only do nutrition-related projects. Maybe I'd take all the fat out of everything! I had to explain I am a food person first and that my nutrition expertise was an added benefit to them."

Rita Storey advises dietitians seeking a career in business to determine why their skills would be an asset to a certain company. "Don't expect the company to fit you," she explains. "Know the company's products and services and what they are looking for. Then translate what you've done to meet those needs."

Mary Adolf concurs: "You have to help the person doing the hiring know how the skills you've acquired through education and experience can help the organization. Do your homework. Know the company's products and the barriers to increasing product usage. Use your communications skills to sell yourself."

It is also important to go the extra mile. "No one is going to hire you just because you're eager," says Delia Hammock. "You have to pay your dues, and you have to give it away, if necessary, to get started." Cathy Miller suggests that dietetics students start getting experience as soon as they can. "Pursue internships, practicums, or volunteer work," she advises. "Meet as many people as you can. A person I met at a summer job helped me get my first position in recipe development after graduation. Also," she advises, "take advantage of student rates to join professional groups and keep your options open."

Adds Martin Yadrick, "Don't allow the expectations of others to define you. Be willing to step out of the box and assume responsibility you never imagined. As the connection between nutrition and disease is made even clearer, the value of the RD will grow exponentially." Whether in a traditional or nontraditional job, the dietitian is still the guardian of accurate nutrition information. "This is the real value of the profession," says CNN's Carolyn O'Neil, "to have this knowledge and to communicate how to apply it in daily life."

CASE STUDIES

Case Study 1

Helen Hranchak, MBA, RD, is director of field services for Audits International, a 14-year-old company based in Highland Park, Illinois, that conducts safety and sanitation inspections for fast-food restaurants and evaluates retail food products for food manufacturers. "We are the people who count the chocolate chips in cookies and count how many cookies are broken in the bag," says Hranchak (personal communication, January 30, 1996). Audits International uses the services of about 650 RDs worldwide. Hranchak identifies and trains the company's auditors and helps to implement studies.

> My original intention was to be a clinical dietitian, and I worked in that area for a number of years while I was getting an MBA. Eventually, I decided to leave the clinical world for the business world. I joined the sales force of a food service equipment and supplies company. It was a rude awakening to step out of the hospital and into the cutthroat world of sales. Later, a friend of mine told me about Audits International. I joined the company about seven years ago. When I started, there was only one full-time RD with the company. Now, we have three full-time RDs corporately in addition to our cadre of field dietitians. Dietitians seem to work very well for us.
>
> Looking back on my education from where I am now, I think my food safety and sanitation classes were valuable, as were my MBA classes in management and marketing. Undergraduate programs today should offer some more practical experience. We're seeing dietitians in a variety of positions now—food technology, food manufacturing, food styling, and facility food safety inspections. And I firmly believe no one should be allowed to graduate without a class in computers.
>
> I network with other RDs every day. Recruiting dietitians across the United States as auditors is part of my job. I probably don't network with other professionals in other fields as much as I should. It's one of my goals to better understand food technology and restaurant/hotel management. Networking with others in those fields will help.
>
> Being versatile is a very valuable trait these days. Resourcefulness, diligence, attention to detail, organization and diplomacy are also important skills for a good manager. Some of these skills you are born with, others you learn along the way—and not necessarily in school.

Case Study 2

EC Henley, PhD, RD, is director of nutritional science for Protein Technologies International, a subsidiary of St. Louis–based Ralston Purina. Protein Technologies International is a worldwide leader in research, product development, manufacturing, and marketing of soy protein and soy polysaccharide fiber products. Among the tasks of the nutritional science department are initiating and facilitating basic and clinical research in the health benefits of the company's products; developing nutrition profiles for products; assisting in developing marketing strategies that emphasize nutrition and health benefits; maintaining a worldwide network of scientific advisors; and communicating scientific findings about company products to scientific audiences, businesses, and consumers. Henley has been instrumental in facilitating research on phytochemicals, which she believes are likely to be the "third wave" in nutrition.

> I enrolled in prearchitecture (engineering) at the University of Mississippi with the intention of transferring to Auburn University to complete my degree. Due to a lack of student housing at Auburn, I remained at Ole Miss and switched my major to art ad interior design. Along the way, I got acquainted with home economics and took a couple of nutrition courses. During the summer before my senior year, I took a job in a hospital dietetics department. By this time, it was too late to change my major and graduate on time. After graduation, I moved to Houston. Over the next 15 years, I completed course work in dietetics, a three-year preplanned work experience at Rice University for ADA membership, and earned a master's and a doctorate. Jobs I have had include designing and operating a restaurant, private practice, and directorships of both school food service and hospital dietetics.
>
> After earning my PhD, I joined the University of Texas School of Allied Health Sciences in Houston. As the first chairperson of the nutrition and dietetics department, I founded the university's coordinated undergraduate program in community dietetics as well as the graduate nutrition program in the University of Texas Graduate School of Biomedical Sciences in Houston.
>
> After seven years at the university, I moved to industry. My first job was as director of operations for a chain of 32 weight loss clinics in the Southwest. From 1985 to 1990 I headed up a software development venture—The Institute for Futuristic Health Care Delivery—that developed online, interactive, real-time clinical management programs. I remember thinking at the time that a "byte" was something you ate at a table and found myself having to write specifications for a computer-based information system after only three months on the job! So I described the outcome we wanted from a clinical and educational viewpoint and looked for the best solution-based answer.
>
> Eventually the software venture spun off from its parent, was acquired and acquired again. After two years as president, I left, but not before I'd learned to work with venture capitalists and write proformas. I learned that marketing is really key. I was educated in facts and research but came to understand that perception is more important than reality to most people. In 1991, I joined Protein Technologies International.

I think my liberal arts education, especially my design background, has helped me in my career, perhaps by seeing situations differently or thinking creatively. The business courses I subsequently took have helped me in evaluating and assessing business opportunities, but there were times early in my career when I felt lacking in the ability to put together business proposals and financial statements. I picked up these skills on the job.

I have been fortunate to have many mentors, starting early in my career—two professors, a colleague, a boss, and one of my students. I think it's important to remember that a mentor need not be older than you are. Younger people see the world from a totally different perspective. I also network all the time, with other dietitians as well as with physicians, scientists, and business professionals all over the world. I miss teaching, but I do some professional education and am involved working with our customers. I also read constantly, not only professional journals but also the popular press so I know what consumers are being exposed to.

Through the school of hard knocks, I've learned how important it is to listen carefully, analyze critically, and communicate well both orally and in writing. You also must keep an open mind, both as a student and later as a working professional. Understanding the political culture of one's workplace is paramount.

A dietitian's education is still geared toward clinical practice, food service management, community dietetics, and health and wellness. But dietitians must learn the culture of business, too. In the future, I think we'll see more RDs using the skills of food science and nutrition to respond to consumer interest in health. More companies will be hiring dietitians and RDs will be using their research skills in new ways. Dietetics is an incredible field. People are always going to eat! (personal communication, February 1, 1996)

Case Study 3

Janis M. Verderose, MS, RD, DCN, is the administrator of the Demand Management Programs and Nutrition Services for the Community Health Plan (CHP)/Kaiser Permanente Northeast Division, a Latham, New York–based management care organization. With 53 centers in four states, 4,000 affiliated physicians and health care providers serve 500,000 subscribers. Verderose is responsible for program management and administration, and planning of preventive and health improvement services, including clinical pathways, education, coding, and reimbursement—in short, wherever nutrition fits into the medical model. She negotiated a contract that opened up nutrition services for subscribers to the plan and led to the publication of Medical Nutrition Management Protocols.

I entered the dietetics program at Immaculata College (Troy, New York) knowing I wanted to be a clinical RD. Upon graduation, I started working at a community hospital doing inpatient nutrition, but I didn't like the lack of follow-up. So in the late 1970s, I started an outpatient nutrition service at that hospital. When the administration said I had to make money, I set it up like a counseling business. Our 10-week weight-reduction program was so well received that it was covered on local television.

Eventually, I noticed we were getting referrals from CHP so I called a physician there and suggested they needed an RD. I recommended a friend for the job and later joined her. Together, we built the department. People told us we were crazy, that HMOs would never make it. While working at CHP, I went to night school to earn an MS.

I really carved my own career path by looking for opportunities where nutrition would fit—and where I would fit. I've had to justify my ideas and convince others they would work. Early on, the best training I had was during the summer in college when I worked for a food service management company. They really made me take charge.

Looking back on my education, I regret not having more business training. Lately I have been attending seminars on business, strategic thinking, and marketing communications. I have always been very customer-centered, and that's how I train my staff. And I'm careful to ensure that my clinical professional standards always supersede "good business" if there's a conflict.

I do a lot of networking both within ADA and in my company. Serving on ADA's reimbursement team has given me the opportunity to meet many interesting people who are really the pathfinders when it comes to nutrition services in managed care. And participating on various teams at work keeps me in touch with other health professionals as well as community leaders. I'm hoping to establish a network of dietitians in the northeast that can contract with managed care organizations. Acting as a group, RDs will have more clout.

I've had to work on building my self-confidence and diplomacy skills over the years. Success has helped me do this, and mistakes have taught me a lot, too. I try to listen and learn. I see a much larger role for dietitians in managed care. Obviously, for someone in my position, it is critical to know behavioral and clinical outcomes and the cost-effectiveness of nutrition services, and how it all fits into the medical model. And you need to know how to write a business plan and how to market, too (personal communication, January 30, 1996).

CONCLUSION

Dietitians in business and communications represent a small percentage of the total membership of The American Dietetic Association, however, this is a growing area of opportunity. As both businesses and consumers recognize the importance of promoting good health measures, especially good nutrition, the role of the dietitian gains in visibility and impact.

DEFINITIONS

Mentoring Advising, teaching, tutoring, or coaching between a mentor and another.
Networking Activities directed toward making connections with others through varied contacts.
Nontraditional Job Job or position outside the usual or most common areas of practice.
Value System Set of principles guiding actions that adhere to professional and ethical practice.

REFERENCES

1. Parks S. President's page: creating your future—career opportunities in an era of change. *J Am Diet Assoc.* 1994;94:451–452.
2. Bryk JA, Soto TK. Report on the 1993 membership database of The American Dietetic Association. *J Am Diet Assoc.* 1994;94:1433–1438.
3. Kirk D, Shanklin CW, Gorman MA. Attributes and qualifications that employers seek when hiring dietitians in business and industry. *J Am Diet Assoc.* 1989;89:494–498.
4. *Trends in the United States: Consumer Attitudes and the Supermarket 1995.* Washington, DC: Food Marketing Institute; 1995.
5. ADA. *Executive Summary: Nutrition Trends Survey 1995.* Chicago: The American Dietetic Association; 1995.
6. Buddy system. *Wall Street J.* December 12, 1995:A1. Business Briefings.
7. "Inplacement" programs. *Wall Street J.* December 14, 1995:A1. Business Briefings.

The Dietitian in Health and Wellness and Sports Nutrition Programs

Martin M. Yadrick

"The ancient Greeks attained a high level of civilization based on good nutrition, regular physical activity, and intellectual development."[1]

Outline—Chapter 16

- Introduction

- Sports, Cardiovascular, and Wellness Nutritionists

- Sports Nutrition
  - Practitioner in sports nutrition

- Cardiovascular Nutrition
  - Dietitian in cardiovascular nutrition

- Wellness and Health Promotion
  - Practitioner in wellness and health promotion

- Disordered Eating
  - Story of a specialist in disordered eating

- Conclusion

INTRODUCTION

Wellness, health promotion, corporate fitness, and sports nutrition programs were virtually unheard of 20 years ago. Although both sports and dietetics as professions or areas of interest have existed for centuries, the combination of the two as a career specialty is a relatively recent development. The growth of wellness and fitness programs has been rapid as the relationship between nutritional status and maintenance of health and prevention of disease becomes more evident.[2]

Diet is a known risk factor for the development of the three chronic diseases that are the leading causes of death in adults in the United States: cancer, cardiovascular disease, and stroke.[3] Additional health problems of adults are also closely associated with diet and eating behaviors: obesity, diabetes, high blood pressure, and osteoporosis. Numbers of deaths and medical care costs can be significantly altered by changes in diet and lifestyles. Billions of dollars are spent per year on schemes and gimmicks to reduce body weight and prevent cancer, not to mention the money spent in treating adults with these diseases and their complications.

In addition, recent reports from the National Health and Nutrition Examination Survey III indicate alarming increases in the prevalence and severity of obesity in young children, older children, and adolescents as well as adults.[4-6] All these statistics and research point to the need for programs in health promotion, wellness, fitness, and prevention and treatment of obesity, which greatly expands career options for dietitians. Some dietitians have developed their own programs through practice and research and now market or license them to other dietitians and health professionals around the country and internationally. Others continue to work in hospitals, ambulatory care centers, clinics, rehabilitation centers, and private practice in providing counseling and other medical nutrition therapies aimed at preventing and treating obesity.

Even with or perhaps because of the increasing prevalence of obesity, many dietary fads, drugs, and questionable dieting programs have escalated and consume enormous amounts of money per year. This emphasizes the need and opportunities that exist for dietitians and other health professionals in this area.[7-9]

Many research programs are under way across the country to test and evaluate programs designed to improve or change food behavior, dietary intake, and physical activity. These programs target adult chronic diseases that science has shown have their beginnings in childhood.[10] Therefore, many of the career opportunities for dietitians in this area would be working with children and their parents or caretakers. Some programs are school based (e.g., the Child and Adolescent Trial for Cardiovascular Health[11] and the Dietary Intervention Study in Children[12]); others are community based—Health Ahead/Heart Smart based on data from the Bogalusa Heart Study;[13-15] still others combine physical education and/or health curricula—"Slice of Life"[16] and "Know Your Body."[17] In all these, dietitians are participating as primary investigators or on staff helping to implement and evaluate the program.

SPORTS, CARDIOVASCULAR, AND WELLNESS NUTRITIONISTS

Interest in sports and cardiovascular nutrition among members of The American Dietetic Association (ADA) led to the formation in 1981 of the Sports and Cardiovascular Nutritionists (SCAN) dietetic practice group, a specialty group of nutrition professionals within the ADA. In 1993, SCAN changed its name to "Sports, Cardiovascular and Wellness Nutritionists" to reflect the importance of wellness and health promotion as a growing area of dietetic practice. In 1994, SCAN welcomed dietetic professionals with an interest in disordered eating into its fold, recognizing the frequent presence of eating disorders among athletes and the critical role that the identification and treatment of disordered eating has in maintaining health and wellness. Nearly 5,300 ADA members were members of SCAN in 1996.

SPORTS NUTRITION

Dietetic professionals with a specialty in sports nutrition can be found in a wide variety of settings from sports medicine clinics to professional football teams, from high school athletics to the Olympics, and from universities to fitness centers.[18] Many incorporate sports nutrition into their more general practice of nutrition consultation or private practice. In the late 1970s, a few entrepreneurial dietitians with interest in sports began offering their services to professional sports teams, often free of charge.[19] Today, several professional teams include dietitians as paid consultants whose expertise serves to enhance the players' performance and endurance. A few professional athletes have employed their personal dietitian primarily to help maintain appropriate body weight and ratio of fat to lean body mass.

In some instances, dietitians are serving as nutrition trainers to college athletes and teams, especially in the areas of wrestling and swimming.[20] Several sports nutritionists have chosen to specialize in the sport or sports in which they have the greatest personal interest, including swimming, wrestling, baseball, cycling, and others. According to Christine Rosenbloom, PhD, RD, LD, associate professor and didactic dietetics program director at Georgia State University, interest in sports nutrition has also helped to increase the number of men entering the profession of dietetics.

The duties and work settings of a sports nutritionist are many and varied and often require irregular work hours such as evenings and weekends. For example, a swimming tournament may be held all day on a weekend, or a fitness center may offer nutrition classes to its members several evenings a week. A dietitian may occasionally need to travel with a sports team, and this travel may not always be funded by the team. Few full-time positions for sports nutritionists actually exist but are gradually becoming more common. Many dietetic professionals working in the area of sports nutrition also work as clinical dietitians for acute care facilities, as outpatient dietitians, or in private practice as nutrition consultants. In addition, some dietitians are employed to supervise the food production and training table in college athletic dormitories. Some professional athletes seek information on eating during off-season to maintain body weight and strength. As part of his or her daily routine, a sports nutritionist may counsel athletes one-on-one regarding their food intake and appropriate nutrients or their use of dietary supplements as ergogenic aids.[21] He or she may also conduct group classes on low-fat eating at a fitness center or work with a high school team to suggest healthful choices for eating on the road. Several sports nutritionists serve as part-time staff at health clubs, available to answer questions members may ask on nutrition or to conduct classes on eating for competition and good health.

An additional career for some dietitians with experience in sports nutrition and fitness has emerged in writing and developing nutrition education materials (videos, slides, etc.) appropriate for athletes of all ages. They also enjoy speaking, writing for the media, and consultative arrangements with any number of organizations.

Many dietetic professionals seek to enhance their education and expertise by entering graduate programs in exercise physiology, counseling psychology, or business administration. In addition, although few college or university programs in sports nutrition currently exist, many graduate students choose to conduct research for their thesis or dissertation on a topic directly related to sports nutrition. By enhancing a strong foundation in foods and normal and clinical nutrition with study of a related area, the dietetic student can better prepare him- or herself for practice in sports nutrition.

Credibility is a critical issue when practicing in the area of sports nutrition. The dietetic professional should look the part, which includes maintaining a healthy lifestyle by not smoking, by maintaining a desirable weight, and by participating in regular exercise. The sports nutritionist need not be an elite athlete in the sport in which he or she counsels but should be aware of any terms unique to the sport and should stay abreast of current issues related to all sports (i.e., he or she should display an obvious interest in a wide variety of sports and sporting events). The dietetic professional who is working with football players to help them eat more healthfully may lose his or her credibility if it becomes clear that he or she is unfamiliar with the basic terminology or rules of the game.

Practitioner in Sports Nutrition: Ellen Coleman, MA, MPH, RD (written communication, April 14, 1996)

As a dietetics major in college, I became interested in sports nutrition because I participated in endurance sports. I sought information on dietary strategies to improve my performance in distance cycling (100- to 200-mile bike rides), distance runs (26.2-mile marathons), and the Ironman Triathlon in Hawaii (2.4-mile swim, 112-mile bike ride, and 26.2-mile marathon). As a result of my nutrition background and personal experience, I began advising other active individuals and lecturing to athletes and health professionals working with athletes. Lecturing gave me the opportunity to reach more people.

I counsel active individuals and athletes both at my home and, on a fee-for-service basis, at The Sport Clinic, a sports medicine facility in Riverside, California. I write monthly columns for a professional sports medicine journal and regularly write articles for several sports magazines. I have authored three continuing education correspondence courses on nutrition and exercise, as well as two sports nutrition books targeted at the consumer. I am frequently invited to give lectures on sports nutrition to athletes, dietitians, athletic trainers, and physicians.

I really enjoy providing sports nutrition information that is up-to-date, valid, and beneficial. Nothing gives me greater pleasure than hearing that my information helped someone to perform better or to feel better. Due to the prevalence of nutrition quackery in sports, I also feel good about supplying information on the safety and effectiveness of nutritional regimens and dietary supplements that are frequently used by athletes.

My involvement in sports nutrition started out as an avocation rather than a profession. I loved learning about sports nutrition and sharing this knowledge with others. I never planned to make a living as a sports nutritionist—this was a fortunate outcome after years of involvement. Registered dietitians usually don't "get a job" as a sports nutritionist working for an athletic team. Instead, they specialize in sports nutrition as part of their private consulting practice. Fortunately, the sports nutrition field has numerous opportunities that are open to individuals who have the desire and persistence to create their own niche.

CARDIOVASCULAR NUTRITION

With the abundance of research continuing in the area of diet and heart disease, as well as the fact that heart disease remains the number 1 cause of death for Americans, careers in cardiovascular nutrition offer abundant options.[2,3] Most acute care facilities whose services include open heart surgery have cardiac rehabilitation programs in place. These typically include inpatient and outpatient components, both of which offer nutrition counseling and education as part of the program. Cardiac rehabilitation programs offer multidisciplinary teams who deal with all aspects of risk factor reduction, as well as education of the patient and family. Team members may include a medical director, cardiac rehabilitation nurse clinicians, exercise specialists, a physical therapist, a social worker, an occupational therapist, and a dietitian. Education of the patient and family is often conducted in a variety of ways, from individual instruction to group classes. The dietitian may also design and conduct classes on low-fat cooking and other food preparation techniques.

Dietitians who specialize in cardiovascular nutrition may be employed by lipid research clinics. These professionals are responsible for teaching clinic patients how to change their eating habits to lower total fat and saturated fat or to comply with a research feeding protocol. In this setting at a university, they may conduct research on the latest cardiology protocols. Opportunities also exist with pharmaceutical companies as sales representatives or in the public relations departments of large food companies that market products to patients with cardiovascular disease and their families.

Dietitian in Cardiovascular Nutrition: Cindy Conroy, MA, RD, LD (written communication, April 1, 1996)

The career of dietetics first interested me as a way to combine a love of the sciences and math with teaching adults. It is especially rewarding to teach adults the information and skills necessary to improve their nutritional status and state of wellness—whether it be for prevention or the secondary treatment of coronary artery disease. I was a clinical dietitian specializing in cardiology at a large metropolitan hospital for more than nine years before joining the Iowa Heart Center. Currently, I am the Lipid Clinic Coordinator, working with a group of 27 cardiologists, 5 cardiac surgeons, and a total staff of over 200.

My daily routine includes (1) reviewing all lipid profiles received by the office with the patient first, followed by the attending cardiologist or lipidologist, (2) educating those patients with elevated lipid levels about the Dietary Guidelines, exercise, and lifestyle management to control their lipids and other risk factors for coronary artery disease, (3) educating those patients requiring lipid lowering medications about their prescription including goals of treatment, side effects, and follow-up lab tests, (4) monitoring ongoing research studies involving patients with elevated lipids and various medications used to treat elevated lipids, (5) continuing development of a computerized lipid tracking system for utilization in the office and in a research-oriented network of cardiology practices in the Midwest, (6) educating patients with congestive heart failure (over 100 patients in the CHF Clinic currently) and nursing personnel about sodium-restricted diets, and (7) presenting wellness lectures at local businesses following health screens.

The most rewarding part of my current position is the opportunity to assist patients with learning life skills and modifying behaviors that will help reduce the risk for coronary disease by lowering their lipids. It is especially rewarding when an individual modifies his or her diet and lifestyle enough to lose significant amounts of weight and/or lowers their lipids enough to be able to discontinue lipid-lowering medications.

Cardiovascular nutrition is an expanding specialty within dietetics and the health care field because of increasing evidence that lowering lipid values, controlling diabetes, and maintaining appropriate weight are major factors in preventing the onset and progression of coronary disease. As consumers search for ways to reduce health care costs, it will be even more important for nutrition educators to actively participate on the health care team to assist in minimizing the progression of disease and monies spent for lipid medications.

WELLNESS AND HEALTH PROMOTION

The opportunities for dietitians that exist in the area of wellness and health promotion are numerous and diverse. Dietitians who specialize in wellness may have their own private practice or consulting business and negotiate contracts with industry, communities, or health clubs. Others are employed by medical centers or corporations to manage their on-site wellness and health promotion programs, which may include conducting classes for employees, developing incentives to foster a greater interest in exercise and nutrition, and increasing productivity by helping to reduce the incidence of employee illness.[22] Because nutrition is just one "piece of the wellness pie," dietitians specializing in wellness and health promotion may also be involved in programs of smoking cessation, meditation and yoga, stress management, exercise, back safety, and employee relations.

Corporations and large institutions initially began providing worksite wellness programs for their employees because of research and reports that these programs improved the health of the employee, increased productivity, and decreased absenteeism and lost work days due to illness.[22] As these programs developed and increased in numbers across the country in businesses of all sizes, data began to accumulate on the economic benefits of worksite wellness programs. With health care costs soaring and major changes occurring in health care and insurance coverages, employers were eager to explore wellness and health promotion programs that would save the corporation money or affect the "bottom line." The common method for defining economic benefits is through the benefit/cost ratio in which the "cost" is the actual dollar cost of providing the program and "benefits" are expressed in dollars saved from less absenteeism, reduced disability expenses, and lowered medical costs. Benefit/cost ratios range from less than a dollar to greater than three dollars.[23] In other words, a ratio of less than one would mean that for each dollar saved, more than a dollar was expended in the program. Ratios greater than one would indicate benefit dollars exceeding the cost dollars.[24] Some report benefit/cost ratios greater than 5.5 with comprehensive health promotion programs including nutrition education and counseling, weight management, physical activity, stress management, smoking cessation, etc.[25] Others have pinpointed the cost of the sedentary nonfit employee. All this indicates the need for the dietitian employed in worksite wellness programs to be flexible and knowledgeable about physical activity and stress management as well as nutrition.[26]

Ability to work as a facilitator and to conduct classes in a group setting are important characteristics of the successful wellness professional. Counseling skills are also necessary, as dealing with high-risk persons may be a regular aspect of the job. In addition, the dietitian must be prepared to analyze and evaluate enormous amounts of "nutrition information" available to the employees and clients through all media routes: television, newspaper, magazines, and the Internet. This counseling may take place in groups, individually, at health fairs, or even over the telephone.

Wellness and fitness programs are emerging for the aging and retired population as well as the younger employed groups. Research is indicating that even though chronologic aging is inevitable, biologic aging can be delayed through appropriate nutrition and exercise.[27] As the number of senior citizens increases, this will provide another career opportunity for dietitians specializing in health promotion. Fitness programs including nutrition, exercise, and lifestyle changes are developing that improve the quality of life and encourage wellness in this age group.

Practitioner in Wellness and Health Promotion: Linda Zorn, MA, RD (written communication, April 4, 1996)

What first interested me in wellness was the knowledge that as a dietitian I was only dealing with one element of a person's health and well-being. As I began to investigate wellness and health promotion, I began to realize that I wanted to expand my work to encompass total health: mind, body, and spirit. Around this time (1980), wellness and health promotion was emerging as a profession. There were no classes or degree programs in this area. I began to read all I could and attend special workshops on wellness and health promotion. In looking at the dimensions of wellness—environmental, intellectual, emotional, spiritual, physical, social, occupational, financial, and time—I began to feel that in helping clients with only nutrition, I was missing a big part of what makes people healthy. I began to learn about all of these areas and explore how I could integrate the principles into my practice as a dietitian. I first branched out into exercise physiology and sports nutrition. After that, I received additional training in stress management.

Currently, I have two positions: director, Pacific Wellness Institute, and wellness promotion manager for Mercy Cardiology and Diabetes Center at Mercy Medical Center. At the Pacific Wellness Institute, I am responsible for the management and coordination of all activities and programs of the institute, which is a program of the California State University at Chico. This includes responsibility for the administration of the Schools as Wellness Communities Grant, fund development, external contracts and grants, and corporate training and development.

The mission of the Pacific Wellness Institute is to promote wellness and to prevent illness in Chico, northern California, and beyond. The institute works in partnership with other community organizations to plan, conduct, and evaluate projects that affect local communities and that can be replicated elsewhere. A major focus of the Pacific Wellness Institute is Healthy Chico Kids 2000, a communitywide campaign to promote the highest possible level of health and well-being of Chico children and youth by the year 2000. Healthy Chico Kids 2000 is part of a nationwide movement to emphasize disease prevention and health promotion as a key approach to solving the major health care crises facing this country in the 1990s.[28] Specific end-of-decade health objectives have been developed for Chico in the following 10 areas of health and wellness: nutrition, physical fitness, emotional well-being, social well-being, living safely, responsible sexual behavior, substance abuse prevention, dental health, living lightly on the earth, and preventive health care.

On a day-to-day basis, my job offers a lot of variety. I attend community meetings as part of community, county, and state coalitions on all areas of wellness and health. For example, I am involved in a Chico–Butte County Coalition on substance abuse prevention in which we were allocated dollars to implement three prevention activities in the spring of 1996. I spent a lot of my time investigating funding sources, developing partnerships, and creating new ideas for and writing grants. I also write proposals for wellness programs and for joint ventures with the local hospitals. I teach conflict and stress management classes, as well as staff inservices on a variety of wellness topics. Since we are university based, I take care of all the mandatory paperwork and reporting. Since we are funded completely by grants and contracts, I write quarterly reports to our funding agencies on the progress we have made toward our goals. I allocate time each week to work on planning for the future of the Pacific Wellness Institute. I work on developing new ideas and talking with community- and school-based personnel on the feasibility of and interest in these ideas. Summing it all up: writing, meeting, partnering, teaching, creating, and reporting.

At Mercy Medical Center, I am responsible for teaching all nutrition and wellness classes, outpatient lifestyle counseling on diabetes and lipids, physician relations and education, and general marketing of all wellness services. Currently, I am on the board of directors for the Association for Worksite Health Promotion in the capacity of international conference vice-president. Prior to moving to Chico, I was co-executive director of the National Wellness Institute in Stevens Point, Wisconsin. In that capacity, I was responsible for the management of the National Wellness Institute, with primary responsibility for the coordination of the National Wellness Conference, regional conferences, retreats, and special topic conferences. In addition, I was responsible for directing all marketing activities, catalog production, new product development, product and conference marketing and sales, consultation on wellness program de-sign, and other special projects.

The best parts of my job are the variety and the knowledge that I have helped integrate dietetics and wellness. Since I am the director of the Pacific Wellness Institute, I can do what I want, when I want. I work hard but also take time to relax and recharge. I have been successful at obtaining grant dollars primarily because we have a nationally recog-nized program. The most rewarding aspect of my position is providing school-based wellness services and seeing the difference in the Chico youth with whom we work. Teaching classes and having a positive impact on people's lives, plus the positive feedback we receive from the schools and corporations we assist, gives me great satisfaction and enjoyment. To me, the definition of wellness is the complete integration of body, mind, and spirit and the realization that everything we do, think, feel, and believe has an effect on our state of well-being. Wellness is a choice, a decision we make to move toward optimal health and maximum life. Wellness means that every choice you make is one toward a more positive lifestyle and excellence in all things.

Several national organizations provide excellent and accurate information for the dietitian seeking up-to-date knowledge on wellness and health promotion programs and concepts. In addition, all have information on the Internet. The major organizations are listed with Internet addresses:

- The American Dietetic Association (www.eatright.org)
- International Food Information Council (ificinfo.health.org)
- NIH National Cancer Institute-5 a Day Program (www.dcpc.nci.nih.gov/5aday)
- President's Council on Physical Fitness and Sports (www.os.dhhs.gov)
- CDC National Center for Chronic Disease Prevention and Health Promotion (www.cdc.gov/nccdphp)
- American College of Sports Medicine (www.acsm.org)
- American Alliance for Health, Physical Education, Recreation, and Dance (www.aahperd.org)

Material found on the Internet must be evaluated by the dietitian for its relevance to nutrition science. Already much misinformation, food fads, and fallacies are showing up on the Internet in the areas of health promotion and fitness. The Internet also offers the registered dietitian opportunities and challenges for placing his or her own nutrition and fitness messages electronically for the public to read.

DISORDERED EATING

Dietitians who specialize in disordered eating work in a variety of settings, including residential treatment centers, hospitals (both medical and psychiatric), outpatient clinics, managed care organizations, university health centers, and private practice. The specialty of disordered or problematic eating encompasses several areas in which nutritional, physical, and psychological issues are intertwined with eating behavior, such as obesity, chronic dieting, anorexia nervosa, bulimia nervosa, compulsive eating, and binge eating disorders.[29–32] Complications of these disorders are potentially life-threatening. Many have their origin or manifestation in childhood or adolescence. Although most of these disorders affect adolescent females, there have been a few reports of similar behavior in males.[33] Effective treatment of disordered eating requires knowledge and skills in counseling, cognitive behavioral therapy, family systems theory, addiction, and psychopharmacology.[34,35]

Because of the biopsychosocial nature of disordered eating, the role of the dietitian on the treatment team is vital. The dietitian educates the client about food, physical activity, and body size and shape and guides him or her in developing a sound eating style and physical activity pattern. Clients may share their thoughts and feelings about food, weight, and physical activity with the dietitian. They may also share life situations and events that are stressful for them, such as job change, marital problems, school problems, relationships, and burnout. The dietitian helps clients identify how stress affects their eating style and how they feel about food, their body size and shape, and physical activity.[36] Ongoing communication with the treatment team therapist, psychiatrist, and physician is essential so that the dietitian can discern which issues are nutrition-related and which are psychological or medical. It takes years of experience for the dietitian to most effectively complement his or her skills and expertise with other members of the team.[33]

Because of the prevalence of disordered eating during adolescence, many schools are beginning to provide programs aimed at preventing eating disorders and obesity and maintaining healthy weights and lifestyles.[37] One of the most comprehensive programs has been designed by the Centers for Disease Control and Prevention entitled School Health Programs to Promote Lifelong Healthy Eating.[38] Registered dietitians helped to develop the program and continue to serve as technical consultants to the national project. The published guidelines for this program provide an opportunity for dietitians to develop, implement, and participate in this high-profile program of health promotion, which emphasizes nutrition and eating behaviors.

Engaging in peaceful, nonrestrained, health-enhancing eating and physical activity is a goal, not only for the client, but for the dietitian as well. Just as many psychotherapists choose to undergo therapy themselves, dietitians who are disordered eating experts often make the decision to participate in counseling to assess their own body image, exercise patterns, and other food and weight issues before counseling others.

Dietitians working in programs to treat disordered eating benefit from regular supervision from a mental health professional who specializes in problematic eating. This provides a forum for discussion of specific cases, as well as helping to clarify which issues are appropriately addressed in nutrition therapy versus psychotherapy. Furthermore, many dietitians are seeking continuing education in areas such as women's issues, cognitive behavioral therapy, family counseling, psychotherapeutic counseling skills, and psychopharmacology. The intention is to sharpen counseling skills, enhance understanding of sociologic and psychological aspects of disordered eating, while consistently staying within the scope of practice of the dietetic professional.

Story of a Specialist in Disordered Eating: Nancy King, MS, RD, CDE (written communication, April 9, 1996)

In high school, I competed in basketball and volleyball, and even though I was in tremendous cardiovascular condition, by the end of the first half of every basketball game I "crashed," suddenly feeling shaky, weak, dizzy, and irritable—even if we were winning! My physician diagnosed me with fasting hypoglycemia and told me to eat more frequently. I did so and began to feel relief from those "crashes" for the first time since about age seven. Unfortunately, without more specific guidance, eating more frequently resulted in a higher intake of calories. Subsequently, I found I was gaining weight and remember feeling discouraged as I realized that the result of feeling better and not "crashing" was going to affect my performance on the court. Determined not to let this happen, I began dieting and soon became preoccupied with my weight. I diligently tried a number of fad diets, not knowing any better. I was not prepared for the results. My blood glucose level became much more erratic, my eating style more confused, and my weight fluctuated up and down, as did my energy and sense of well-being. I tried desperately to find the happy medium where my weight would stay down and my glucose levels would remain normal. It wasn't for lack of trying, because I tried everything I could think of. However, I never found that balance. It was somewhere in this sea of distress and confusion that I realized, "If only there was someone who really understood all this who would sit down and work with me until I get this thing right." Looking back now, I know that person I wished for was a registered dietitian, preferably one in private practice who could take as much time with me as I needed. With my physical problems still unresolved, I headed off to college to study physical therapy. It wasn't until I was in my fourth year of college in a basic nutrition class that I began putting together my newly acquired knowledge in exercise physiology with principles of nutrition. Thrilled with my discoveries, I began to combine sound exercise physiology and nutrition principles and apply them to myself. Whatever I was doing was working, and by the time I was graduating with a bachelor's degree in exercise physiology, I knew my calling was to be that exceptional person that could sit down with an individual, really understand what they are going through, work out a lifestyle to manage their problem, and not leave them until they "got it right."

Knowing I needed some kind of credential or certification to do this kind of work, I sought advice from my nutrition course instructor. It wasn't until that conversation that I learned about registered dietitians. By the end of our discussion, I had set my sights on a master's degree in nutrition. As I look back, the feelings I had by the end of that meeting were the first sparks of the excitement and passion I still have today, more than 15 years later, for the work that I do. In my work, my responsibilities and opportunities are extensive and diverse. Two days a week, I work from 8:00 AM until 8:00 PM. One day a week, I start at 6:30 AM, to accommodate business professionals who commute out of the area, and finish at 5:30 PM. These early appointment slots are extremely popular, and my clients greatly appreciate them. It is one of the services we have chosen to offer that sets us apart from other practitioners. Sessions with clients range from 30 to 75 minutes; in a day, I see 10 to 15 clients. My office is a counseling setting, as opposed to a medical office or clinic. My clients seem more relaxed in this environment and have repeatedly told me so over the years. On any given day, I do the following: nutrition assessments, anthropometric assessments, eating disorder assessments, body composition analyses, counsel clients, place calls to and receive calls from physicians and therapists, refer clients to health care professionals, identify drug nutrient interactions, design and send treatment plans, chart and graph client status and progress, manage staff (full-time administrator and part-time dietitian), and update business accounts and financial reports. At the request of a physician, I also assess hospitalized clients for eating disorders. In addition, I author journal articles, speak locally and nationally, do media interviews, and design handouts and teaching materials. As owner of my business, I deal with profit and loss statements, financial planning, spreadsheets, budgeting, labor costs, insurance, state and federal taxation, and employee development.

A rewarding aspect of my work is that I know I am making a difference in the lives of individuals and families on a daily basis. This is what I set out to do, and I'm doing it. Some days I feel more satisfied than others, but after more than 10 years, I wouldn't want to give it up. I also recognize how fortunate I am that I really like and believe in what I do. I know many people are not fulfilled in their work. The fact that I have built my own successful, thriving business and reputation is another source of satisfaction to me. My business is primarily my responsibility. I have taken risks in going from having no employees to hiring a full-time administrator, who has been invaluable in my business. I have moved my office three times, each time obtaining a larger space. Being in my own business has taught me that I do have the authority and responsibility for its success. If I take a risk and it fails, I have to answer to myself. I figure out what didn't work, and make adjustments.

I make good money. Busy, established private practice dietitians can pay themselves $50,000 annual salary and higher. In addition, there seems to be too little time in a day and in my life to take advantage of all the opportunities in dietetics. Individuals who are self-directed, like to work independently, have an affinity for leadership, and can turn a vision into a mission statement, will likely find this same "problem" of too much opportunity and too little time.

CONCLUSION

Dietitians with expertise in worksite wellness, sports and cardiovascular nutrition, and disordered eating are increasingly in demand in nontraditional settings. They must be creative and adept in the promotion of healthy eating behaviors.[39] This includes the ability—which is frequently lacking in health care professionals—to translate scientific information into "user-friendly" terms.[40]

In addition, the nutrition education must be presented in a manner that is sensitive to the client's age, cultural background, and level of education. This area of dietetics is truly multidisciplinary, and offers the entrepreneurial dietitian a number of opportunities limited only by his or her imagination.

DEFINITIONS

Anorexia Nervosa Type of eating disorder in which preoccupation with dieting and thinness leads to excessive weight loss.

Bulimia Nervosa Eating disorder involving frequent episodes of binge eating, and nearly always followed by purging.

Cardiovascular Nutrition Application of medical nutrition therapy for those with heart and blood vessel conditions or to prevent the diseases.

Health Promotion Education and preventive measures directed toward basically healthy populations to foster wellness.

Sports Nutrition Area of nutrition specific to the needs of those who participate in sports activities.

Wellness State of optimal health and the absence of disease.

REFERENCES

1. Simopoulos A. Declaration of olympia on nutrition and fitness. *Nutrition Today.* 1996;31:250–252.

2. Public Health Service. *The Surgeon General's Report on Nutrition and Health 1988.* Washington, DC: US Department of Health and Human Services; 1988. DHHS publication PHS 88-50210.

3. National Research Council, National Academy of Sciences. *Diet and Health: Implications for Reducing Chronic Disease Risk.* Washington, DC: National Academy Press; 1989.

4. Ogden CL, Troiano RP, Briefel RR, Kuczmarski RJ, et al. Prevalence of overweight among preschool children in U.S. 1971–1994. *Pediatrics.* 1997;99(4). http://www.pediatrics.org/cgi/contents/fuill.

5. Troiano RP, Flegal KM, Kuczmarski RJ, Campbell SM, et al. Overweight prevalence and trends for children and adolescents: the National Health and Nutrition Examination Surveys, 1963–1991. *Arch Pediatr Adolesc Med.* 1995;149:1085–1091.

6. Kuczmarski RJ, Flegal KM, Campbell SM, Johnson CL. Increasing prevalence of overweight among US adults. *JAMA.* 1994;272:205–211.

7. Maloney MJ, McGuire J, Daniels SR, Specker B. Dieting behavior and eating attitudes in children. *Pediatrics.* 1989;84:482–489.

8. Serdula MK, Williamson DF, Anda RF, Levy AS, et al. Weight control practices in adults: results of a multistage telephone survey. *Am J Public Health.* 1994;84:1821–1824.

9. Heaton AW, Levy AS. Information sources of US adults trying to lose weight. *J Nutr Educ.* 1995;27:182–190.

10. Serdula MK, Ivery D, Coates RJ, Freedman DS, et al. Do obese children become obese adults? A review of the literature. *Prev Med.* 1993;22:167–177.

11. Luepker RV, Perry CL, McKinley SM, et al. Outcomes of a field trial to improve children's dietary patterns and physical activity: the Child and Adolescent Trial for Cardiovascular Health (CATCH). *JAMA.* 1996;275:768–776.

12. Van Horn LV, Stumbo P, Moag-Stahlberg A, Obarzanek E, et al. The Dietary Intervention Study in Children (DISC): dietary assessment methods for 8 to 10 yr. olds. *J Am Diet Assoc.* 1993;93:1396–1403.

13. Downey AM, Virgilio SJ, Serpas DC, Nicklas TA, et al. "Heart Smart"—a staff development model for a school-based cardiovascular health intervention. *Health Educ.* 1988;19:64–71.

14. Kirby D. Comprehensive school health and the larger community: issues and a possible scenario. *J School Health.* 1990;60:170–177.

15. Killip DC, Lovick SR, Goldman L, Allensworth DD. Integrated school and community programs. *J School Health.* 1987;57:437–444.

16. Perry CL, Klepp K-I, Halper A, et al. Promoting healthy eating and physical activity patterns among adolescents: a pilot study of "Slice of Life." *Health Educ Res.* 1987;2:93–103.

17. Walter HJ. Primary prevention of chronic disease among children: the school-based "Know Your Body" intervention trials. *Health Educ Q.* 1989;16:201–214.

18. Berning JR. Sports nutrition: a career for the nineties. *Nutrition Update.* Nabisco, Inc. 1991;1:1–3.

19. Grandjean AC. Diet of elite athletes: has the discipline of sports nutrition made an impact? *J Nutr.* 1997;127:874S–877S.

20. Tipton CM. Sports medicine: a century of progress. *J Nutr.* 1997;127:878S–885S.

21. Applegate EA, Grivetti LE. Search for the competitive edge: a history of dietary fads and supplements. *J Nutr.* 1997;127:869S–873S.

22. Kaman RL, ed. *Worksite Health Promotion Economics: Consensus and Analysis.* Champaign, IL: Human Kinetic Publishers; 1995.

23. Messer J, Stone W. Worksite fitness and health promotion benefit/cost analysis: a tutorial, review of literature, and assessment of the state of the art. *Assoc Worksite Health Promotion Worksite Health.* 1995;2:34–43.

24. Shephard RJ. Worksite fitness and exercise programs: a review of methodology and health impact. *Am J Health Promotion.* 1996;10:436–452.

25. Pelletier KR. A review and analysis of the health and cost-effective outcome studies of comprehensive health promotion and disease prevention programs at the worksite: 1991–1993 update. *Am J Health Promotion.* 1993;8:50–62.

26. Milliman and Robertson, Inc. The cost of unhealthy behavior. (In: Workplace prevention: the state of the nation.) *Business Health.* 1995;13:S20–25.

27. Evans WJ, Cyr-Campbell D. Nutrition, exercise, and healthy aging. *J Am Diet Assoc.* 1997;97:632–638.

28. Public Health Service. *Healthy People 2000: National Health Promotion and Disease Prevention Objectives.* Washington, DC: US Department of Health and Human Services; 1991. DHHS publication PHS 91-50212.

29. Seymour M, Hoerr SL, Huang YL. Inappropriate dieting behaviors and related lifestyle factors in young adults: are college students different? *J Nutr Educ.* 1997;29:21–26.

30. Zuckerman DM, Colby A, Ware NC, Lazerson JS. The prevalence of bulimia among college students. *Am J Public Health.* 1986;76:1135–1137.

31. Kriepe RE, Golden NH, Katzman DK, et al. Eating disorders in adolescents: a position paper of the Society for Adolescent Medicine. *J Adolesc Health.* 1995;16:476–480.

32. Smith C, Steiner H. Psychopathology in anorexia nervosa and depression. *J Am Acad Child Adolesc Psychiatry.* 1992;31:841–843.

33. Carlat DJ, Camargo CA. Review of bulimia nervosa in males. *Am J Psychiatry.* 1991;148:831–841.

34. Ammerman SD, Shih GH, Ammerman J. Unique considerations for treating eating disorders in adolescents and preventive intervention. *Top Clin Nutr.* 1996;12:79–85.

35. Fisher M, Golden NH, Katzman DK, et al. Eating disorders in adolescents: a background paper. *J Adolesc Health.* 1995;16:420–437.

36. Mellin LM. Responding to disordered eating in children and adolescents. *Nutr News.* 1988;51:5–7.

37. Neumark-Sztainer D, Butler R, Palti H. Eating disturbances among adolescent girls: evaluation of a school-based primary prevention program. *J Nutr Educ.* 1995;27:24–31.

38. Centers for Disease Control and Prevention. Guidelines for school health programs to promote lifelong healthy eating. *MMWR.* 1996;45.

39. Contento I, Balch GI, Bronner YL, et al. Nutrition education for school-aged children. *J Nutr Educ.* 1995;27:298–311.

40. Lytle L, Achterberg C. Changing the diet of America's children: What works and why? *J Nutr Educ.* 1995;27:250–260.

CHAPTER 17

Dietitians in the Government and the Military Services

Esther A. Winterfeldt

"If Dietetics is your profession, politics is your business."[1]

Outline—Chapter 17

Part 1—The Government

- Introduction

- Government Programs in Food and Nutrition

- Dietitians in Government Programs
  - Federal programs
  - State programs

- Role of The American Dietetic Association in Policy Formation
  - Washington office
  - Legislative symposium
  - Position papers
  - Legislative Network Coordinators

- Policy Issues in Dietetics
  - Medical Nutrition Therapy
  - Health care reform
  - Women's Health Initiative
  - Nutrition and aging
  - National Screening Initiative

Part 2—The Military Services

- Introduction

- Educational Opportunities

- Careers in the Military Service

- Benefits in Career Areas

- Conclusion

PART 1—THE GOVERNMENT

INTRODUCTION

Dietitians and nutritionists are employed in government activities and programs at the federal, state, and city or local levels. In the 1995 member database by The American Dietetic Association (ADA) 27.6 percent of the membership worked in government agencies and programs.[2] As discussed in this chapter, all dietitians have vital interests in government activities because of their impact on professional practice in many areas in food, nutrition, and health and because dietitians are involved in public policy formation.

Dietitians play a leading role in reaching the public about nutrition and nutrition-related issues. To do this, the dietitian relies on his or her base of knowledge as well as on new and continuing information coming from research, from the foods industry, and from the government. Congress passes legislation, and government agencies issue guides and regulations that add to the bases of dietetic practice. For example, the Food and Nutrition Board of the National Research Council develops the recommended dietary allowances (RDA), the Food and Drug Administration develops food labeling regulations, and the US Department of Agriculture (USDA) develops eating guides such as the food pyramid. These guides are important adjuncts to dietetic practice and nutrition education.

GOVERNMENT PROGRAMS IN FOOD AND NUTRITION

The USDA and the Department of Health and Human Services (DHHS) are the two largest agencies of government with the responsibility for the adequacy and safety of the food supply and for the health of all citizens. These objectives are realized through nutrition research, education, and food-related programs. The

USDA has traditionally had the responsibility for food production, food consumption, and normal human nutrition, and DHHS deals with the metabolic effects of dietary consumption patterns, particularly as related to chronic disease.[3] There is overlap in these functions, but the agencies collaborate as well as conduct their specific programs and are concerned with the nutritional health of all citizens.

The number of programs funded and administered by the government is extensive, and they deal with a broad range of activities concerned with the food suppply, nutrition surveillance and monitoring, and recommendations for the public based on food surveys and research. The major programs in food and nutrition may be categorized as the following:

1. *National food and nutrition surveys.* The USDA conducts surveys to determine food intakes of individuals and families and to show trends in food consumption over time. The DHHS collects data on dietary, physical, and biochemical parameters of individuals to determine nutritional status of the population.
2. *Nutrition research.* Both the USDA and the DHHS conduct research regarding nutrient composition of foods, nutrient intakes, and the role of nutrition in treatment and prevention of disease.
3. *Food assistance and nutrition programs.* The USDA is responsible for school feeding programs and food distribution for needy groups in the population. The DHHS conducts group feeding programs for the elderly.
4. *Food legislation and regulation.* Food safety, food labeling, and regulations about food additives are examples of these activities by both USDA and DHHS.
5. *Dietary guidelines for the public.* The food guide pyramid, the RDA, and the dietary guidelines for Americans are issued by governmental agencies.
6. *Nutrition education.* Nutrition education and training in schools and for individuals and families through the Cooperative Extension Service is conducted by the USDA. From the DHHS, education programs regarding nutrition and heart disease, cholesterol control, and other diseases are provided. Guidance is also provided for use of the various dietary guidelines.

Further descriptions of these programs may be found in references 4–9.

DIETITIANS IN GOVERNMENT PROGRAMS

Federal Programs

Many dietitians are employed in government agencies and in programs funded and administered either fully or in part by the government—federal, state, or local.

Examples of programs located in states or districts but under federal government directives are the school lunch and breakfast programs; the food stamp program; the Women's, Infants and Children's (WIC) program, and the Expanded Food and Nutrition Education Program. Dietitians in these programs may be considered to be employees of both the federal and state governments.

Dietitians are located in departments and agencies in both the legislative and executive branches of government as well as in agencies such as the National Research Council and the International Life Sciences Institute, which are semi-governmental agencies.

Congress passes legislation directly or indirectly concerned with the health and well-being of the public. Legislative activities dealing with changes in the welfare system, health care, Medicare, family assistance, and food and agricultural policy are examples. Dietitians on congressional staffs provide information to legislators and also help promote and draft legislation.

Donna Porter, PhD, RD, is one of the influential dietitians in the legislative branch of government who provides information to Congress in the drafting of legislation. She is a Specialist in Life Sciences at the Congressional Research Service (CRS) in the Library of Congress in Washington, D.C., where she has worked since 1980. Her office is located near the US Capitol building. In this job, she is responsible for answering questions and conducting library research for members of Congress and congressional staff on food safety and nutrition research issues. She began her career as a clinical dietitian at the Ohio State University hospitals. She stayed at Ohio State to acquire a PhD, where she majored in human nutrition with a minor in political science. Her dissertation was titled *Nutrition Policymaking in the U.S. Congress, 1966–1978*. Following completion of the degree, she served a year as a fellow with the National Nutrition Consortium in Washington, D.C., where she made contacts and gained firsthand experience in food and nutrition policy, working with both congressional and agency staffs. She was also a congressional science fellow assigned to the science policy research division of CRS.

She served as project director for the 1990 study by the Institute of Medicine's committee on the nutrition components of food labeling that issued the report *Food Labeling: Issues and Directions for the 1990s,* for which she received the FDA Commissioner's Citation Award in 1991. She has recently been involved in the effort to reform the regulation of dietary supplements and has spent consider-able time examining the regulation of dietary supplements in industrialized countries. She often makes presentations on nutrition policy at ADA and state dietetic association meetings.

Porter states: "It has been a real privilege to serve the profession of dietetics and the US Congress as a nutrition policy analyst. Over several decades I have had the opportunity to observe the evolution in the knowledge of nutrition science as it relates to chronic disease and assist in translating that science into nutrition policy for the country. I have been fortunate enough to have participated in policymaking that has effected changes in such important areas as food labeling, nutrition monitoring research, and dietary supplement regulation."

Christine Lewis, PhD, RD, is another dietitian working in the government. She is a special assistant for policy in the Food and Drug Administration. She describes her career as follows:

My career was not "planned" and is best described as just happening. But this is not to say I did not work hard nor make every effort to turn out high-quality projects. When I completed my PhD at Pennsylvania State University, my thoughts were to go into teaching but I felt I needed additional practice and real-world experience first. A Food and Drug Administration (FDA) nutritionist who was a colleague of my major professor indicated that positions were available for nutritionists at FDA for long- and short-term assignments. When I explored the option further, I found that FDA's Center for Food Safety and Applied Nutrition in Washington, D.C., offered the opportunity of research in combination with technical support for policy and food-related regulations. This combination of a supportive environment for research as well as the possibility of seeing one's work immediately applicable within the public health arena held a great deal of appeal for me. My undergraduate work had been in food microbiology, my master's work in nutrition science, and my PhD combined applied nutrition and statistics, so I was well suited to the kind of work FDA does. Although once working inside FDA, I discovered that the work of the agency—because it always has been the link to legal defensibility—is unlike any work that one would experience elsewhere. It is this link to legal statutes and precedent as well as the mission to protect the public health that makes the work at FDA both challenging and rewarding.

During my initial few years at FDA, I worked "quietly" on issues of dietary consumption and risk assessment and assisted in the nutrition monitoring of the US diet. My career within the agency was changed by an act of Congress, literally. In 1990, the Nutrition Labeling and Education Act was passed; legislation that required the FDA to develop an entire framework for the mandatory nutrition labeling of food, for nutrient content claims, health claims, and many related activities. All nutritionists working at FDA—not many—were immediately reassigned to this task. We worked as a team along with lawyers, food chemists, economists, and others to develop a set of regulations that responded to the law, assisted the public, and was scientifically and legally defensible. At the end of this long process, FDA created a new office, the Office of

Food Labeling. I was made director of technical evaluation in the new office, a management and policy position. I remained in this position until 1996 when pressing policy issues within the FDA's Office of Special Nutritionals required a move from food labeling work to the more urgent work that surrounds the issues of dietary supplements, medical foods, and infant formula. In this capacity, I serve as a special assistant to the director and oversee a number of nutrition and regulatory activities.

My advice to students would be to make certain they have a strong scientific and technical basis, even if they do not plan to be "nutrition scientists." My career is now in public health, but it is not possible to determine good policy without first understanding the science behind public health. The most valuable tool I have had in moving through my career has been my formal education and strong grounding in nutrition sciences and epidemiology. It taught me critical thinking and the importance of putting structure on issues. No matter at what level a professional operates, these scientific details are critical and universal (personal communication, June 24, 1997).

A third dietitian working at the national level is Susan M. Krebs-Smith, PhD, MPH, RD, a research nutritionist in the National Cancer Institute. In her position, she conducts research emphasizing monitoring trends in intake of food and nutrients, especially fats, fruits, and vegetables; identifying food sources of nutrients; and assessing factors associated with the intakes of foods and/or nutrients. In the research, she uses data from the National Nutrition Monitoring and Related Research Program. She also conducts research toward the development of a food guidance system to assist consumers in making food choices to implement the dietary guidelines.

Krebs-Smith has a wealth of experience in dietetics, having worked as a hospital clinical dietitian, in public health nutrition, and in the USDA. After completing her PhD at the Pennsylvania State University, she conducted research in nutrition education in the Human Nutrition Information Service, providing nutrition and food guidance. Her activities also included planning and directing research programs in several related areas: nutrient content of the US food supply; the USDA food plans including the thrifty food plan, which forms the basis for food stamp allowances; factors associated with food and nutrient intakes of different population groups; and the USDA food grouping system.

In public health nutrition, she developed a dietary scoring system that was adopted in Iowa and Wyoming as a means of assessing eligibility for the WIC program. Earlier, she was a member of the team that developed a food guidance system for the American Red Cross, resulting in a course of study later adapted for inclusion in the dietary guidelines and the food guide pyramid.

As an author of many publications and an accomplished public speaker, Krebs-Smith is an outstanding example of a dietitian/nutritionist who has advanced in her profession and is now an influential practitioner and researcher. She serves on the board of editors of the *Journal of The American Dietetic Association* and is also active in the American Public Health Association as well as the Society of Nutrition Education.

The role of nutrition in treatment and prevention of cancer continues to become clearer, and she is already in the forefront of those both conducting the research and helping translate the findings into food and nutrition advice for the public.

State Programs

At the state level, dietitians in public health nutrition are employees of state health departments and are involved in nutrition and health programs in the community. Dietitians in the Indian Health Service work in state programs administered from the federal Office of Indian Affairs. The Veterans Administration oversees a network of treatment centers throughout the United States, and dietitians in Veterans Administration hospitals are considered government employees. A more complete discussion of dietitians in public health and other community dietetics programs is found in Chapter 10.

State agencies administering school food service, the nutrition education training program, nutrition for the elderly, and food stamp programs will vary from state to state; however, the programs are all similar and meet the same national standards. The Expanded Food and Nutrition Program is administered through the Cooperative Extension Service from state land-grant colleges and universities. Some dietitians have the title *Nutrition Specialist in Cooperative Extension* and work directly with the public in food and nutrition education. There is a large network of federal, state, and local extension personnel who "extend" research and technical information from the government and the educational institutions to the public.

ROLE OF THE AMERICAN DIETETIC ASSOCIATION IN POLICY FORMATION

Washington Office

The ADA became active in governmental and legislative affairs in the 1960s and now has a sophisticated network in place. In the 1980s, a Washington office was established and staffed with persons registered as lobbyists on behalf of the association. At present, this office is staffed with a government relations team of eight people who monitor legislative developments in nutrition-related issues and work closely with the Department of Government and Legal Affairs in the Chicago headquarters office to promote the association's priorities for action (T Ketch, personal communication, March 1, 1997). A volunteer legislative and public policy team, appointed by the board of directors, works with both these offices to gain information from states and members and, in turn, transmits information back to members and state networks about pending Washington actions. The association has also established a political action committee whereby members may make contributions that are donated to specific legislators who promote nutrition issues.

Legislative Symposium

ADA conducts a legislative symposium each March in Washington to inform members of pending legislation, to help them become knowledgeable about the political process, and to make contacts with legislators and other government officials. Information is also provided members through a "Legislative Highlights" page each month in the *Journal* and also publishes reaction statements when issues of particular importance to members are being considered.

Position Papers

Another important way the association provides policy input is through position papers. A position paper represents a consensus of viewpoints and professional interests and is used in many ways such as in media contacts, in contacting legislators, and with the public. A former president of ADA stated the purpose of a position paper: "A statement of the Association's stance on an issue that affects the nutritional status of the public; is derived from pertinent facts and data and is germane to the ADA's mission, vision, philosophy and values."[10] ADA has issued approximately 40 positions, and new ones are accepted each year at meetings of the House of Delegates. Papers are periodically updated or deleted if the information is out of date or no longer relevant.[11] The list of current papers is shown in Appendix G.

Legislative Network Coordinators

Each state designates a legislative chair and a legislative network coordinator (LNC), who in turn coordinates legislative activities among ADA members in the state. The LNC members helps prepare other volunteers who use talking points from the Association in contacts with legislators, both state and national. He or she is the communication link between the Washington and Chicago staff and the state dietetic association. In addition, Grassroots Liaisons (GRL) are designated in each state, who are assigned to one or more legislators and work with them directly. The GRL is a registered voter in the legislator's district. Working relationships are thus established with the congressman or state legislator and his or her staff in lobbying for ADA positions.[12]

POLICY ISSUES IN DIETETICS

The ADA develops policy positions based on prioritization of issues according to whether the particular issue is one that "would not otherwise be addressed except by ADA and is of vital importance in terms of time and money."[13] In 1996, ADA determined, as an outcome of strategic planning, that legislation and public policy was its highest priority. The top issues identified were (1) expanding access to nutrition services and achieving reimbursement for cost-effective comprehensive nutrition services including Medical Nutrition Therapy (MNT) as well as health promotion and disease prevention services, (2) influencing policy to ensure inclusion of nutrition services and national standards in food and nutrition programs, and (3) becoming a primary participant in making food and nutrition policy for the nation.[13]

Medical Nutrition Therapy

MNT has been a focus of major legislative activity by the association since the emphasis on health care reform began in the 1990s. But even long before this, ADA promoted the inclusion of nutrition as part of paid services in medical treatments. Through collection of cost/benefit data and working with other health care providers, third-party payers, government agencies, and legislators, the association aims to convince policy makers that nutrition services are important in health care outcomes, are cost-effective, and should be a reimbursable component of comprehensive health care.[14] In the era of "managed care," this becomes a critical issue because the emphasis is on health care at less cost and the national interest is in decreasing overall health care costs.[15–17]

MNT refers to the use of nutrition in the management of illness or injury. The treatment is based on an assessment of the nutritional status of patients at risk, which may include diet modification as well as use of specialized nutrition therapies such as supplementation with medical foods and/or enteral or parenteral nutrition.[14] Exhibit 17–1 shows definitions and descriptions of MNT as defined in the ADA 1995 position paper.[14] Through many studies, it has been shown that

Exhibit 17–1 Definitions and Descriptions

Medical Nutrition Therapy Medical Nutrition Therapy involves the assessment of the nutritional status of patients with a condition, illness, or injury that puts them at risk. This includes review and analysis of medical and diet history, laboratory values, and anthropometric measurements. Based on the assessment, nutrition modalities most appropriate to manage the condition or treat the illness or injury are chosen and include the following:

- Diet modification and counseling leading to the development of a personal diet plan to achieve nutritional goals and desired health outcomes.
- Specialized nutrition therapies including supplementation with medical foods for those unable to obtain adequate nutrients through food intake only; enteral nutrition delivered via tube feeding into the gastrointestinal tract for those unable to ingest or digest food; and parenteral nutrition delivered via intravenous infusion for those unable to absorb nutrients.

Nutrition screening The process of identifying characteristics known to be associated with nutrition problems. Its purpose is to pinpoint persons who are malnourished or at nutritional risk. Intervention takes place after screening occurs. The nutrition screening can be done by a health care team member.

Cost-effectiveness analysis Compares two or more alternatives to achieve the same objective.

Cost-benefit analysis This extends cost-effectiveness analysis by placing a dollar value on the outcomes.

Source: Cost-effectiveness of Medical Nutrition Therapy, Position of The American Dietetic Association. Copyright The American Dietetic Association. Reprinted by permission from *Journal of The American Dietetic Association,* Vol. 95, pp. 88–91, © 1995.

---

appropriate MNT leads to improved health outcomes and results in economic benefits and improved quality of life for patients.[18,19]

A report prepared for the Nutrition Screening Initiative in 1996 concluded that nutrition care could produce over $1.3 billion in Medicare savings through use of selected nutrition intervention in a wide range of conditions.[20]

A bill was introduced in the House of Representatives in 1995 and reintroduced in 1996 for MNT and, although it gained support, was not enacted. Plans are under way to introduce bills again in the 105th Congress in 1997.[21]

Health Care Reform

The issue of health care reform became a national initiative in 1992, and although the legislation did not pass Congress, the issue is an important one that is certain to be reintroduced.[22] The ADA took the following position regarding health care reform: "It is the position of The American Dietetic Association that quality health care should be available, accessible, and affordable to all Americans. Quality health care is defined to include nutrition services that are integral to meeting the preventive and therapeutic health care needs of all segments of the population."[23] A White Paper was also issued in 1992 stressing that cost-effective nutrition services can decrease the use of more expensive services in acute care, long-term care, and home health care settings.[24]

Women's Health Initiative

The Women's Health Initiative was started by the National Institutes of Health as a 15-year study on the major causes of death and disability in older women of all races and socioeconomic strata.[25] ADA became part of this effort when President Susan Finn introduced the "ADA's Nutrition and Health Campaign for Women" in 1993. The campaign conducts and supports both research and advocacy in regard to management of the five major diseases affecting women: cancer, diabetes, heart disease, obesity, and osteoporosis.[26,27]

The ADA and the Canadian Dietetic Association (CDA) issued a joint position paper in 1995 and said: "It is the position of the ADA and the CDA that because of the biological, social, and political factors, women are at unique risk for major nutrition-related diseases and conditions including cardiovascular diseases, certain cancers, osteoporosis, diabetes, and weight-related problems. ADA and CDA strongly encourage health promotion activities, health services, research and advocacy efforts that will enable women to adopt desirable nutrition practices for optimal health."[28] ADA is also funding research that documents outcomes of nutrition services in management of these diseases.[29]

Nutrition and Aging

ADA sponsored a conference on nutrition and aging in 1995 at which recommendations were developed regarding nutrition for older persons.[30] The policy recommendations were sent to the White House Conference to be used in producing national policy relating to aging during the next decade and into the 2000s. Fifty-one resolutions were adopted in two main categories: ensuring comprehensive health care including long-term care and promoting economic security.[31]

A position paper on aging was released by ADA in 1996,[32] and a new campaign was announced titled "Nutrition and Health for Older Americans: A Campaign of The American Dietetic Association."[33] Six goals were announced, including one on policy issues that affect older Americans.

National Screening Initiative

Another important initiative in which ADA is a participating partner is the "Nutrition Screening Initiative," designed to detect and prevent malnutrition in the elderly.[34] With the American Academy of Family Physicians and the National Council on Aging, this collaborative effort is aimed to incorporate nutritional awareness into both community health and social service systems at all levels and to establish links to medical services when further assessment and care are needed.

PART 2—THE MILITARY SERVICES

INTRODUCTION

Military service is another area of practice for dietitians in the government. Dietitians are employed in the three major areas of military service: the Army, Navy, and Air Force, where they function in very similar activities as in many other areas of dietetics. Most work in hospitals throughout the United States and in other countries and have positions in clinical dietetics, food service management, and community nutrition. Others are in research, in personnel recruiting, and in health promotion.

Dietitians in the military service meet the education and experience requirements of ADA and are registered. They also receive basic military training, as in a field hospital, for readiness in the event of war or military action. They are commissioned officers and can expect to progress in rank and salary as well as in positions.

About 135 active-duty dietitians and 100 full- and part-time civilian dietitians (as federal government employees) are employed in the Army. Dietetic interns and dietitians are members of the Army Medical Specialist Corps (http://www.acs.amedd.army.mil/amsc/amschom.htm).[35] In the Air Force, dietetic interns and dietitians are members of the US Air Force Biomedical Sciences Corps. In the Navy, most work as staff in hospitals in the United States and in Germany and Korea, where military personnel and their families are located. At the entry level, duties include providing nutrition assessments and counseling for inpatients, consultation with child care centers and schools located on military installations, and nutrition/health promotion for the military community. Other job duties may include supervising food production and service. The entry-level dietitian is often responsible for personnel management of a small military staff and from 3 to 30 civilian staff depending on the position. Senior dietitians are involved in establishing policy that affects the nutritional health of soldiers and their families.

EDUCATIONAL OPPORTUNITIES

The Army offers dietetic internships at the Walter Reed Army Medical Center in Washington, D.C., and at Brooke Army Medical Center in San Antonio, Texas. The Air Force has an internship at Malcolm Grow Air Force Hospital at Andrews Air Force Base in Maryland.[35] The internships prepare dietitians for generalist practice in dietetics. Admission to the internships requires a college degree and completion of ADA educational requirements. In the Army, additional requirements are less than 33 years of age, US citizen or permanent resident, and meeting the medical fitness standards of the military. In both services, the student is commissioned as a Second Lieutenant on acceptance to the internship. Students receive a salary and other benefits during the internship.

After designated periods of service, dietitians may be granted leave to enter graduate school for both the master's and the doctoral degrees at government expense. All dietitians participate in ADA-approved continuing education and are often active in state and district dietetic associations and dietetic practice groups. Some belong to other specialty groups such as the American Society for Parenteral & Enteral Nutrition, The American Diabetes Association, and others (T Dillon, personal communication, April 10, 1996).

CAREERS IN THE MILITARY SERVICE

Major Teresa Dillon, MS, RD (personal communication, July 22, 1996), and Major Vicky Thomas, MS, RD (personal communication, May 15, 1996), are dietitians with distinguished careers in the Army Medical Specialist Corps. Thomas completed her internship at the Brooke Medical Center and her MS degree at Auburn University. Following assignments in North Carolina, Virginia, Alabama, and Texas, she is currently a career-planning officer stationed in Washington, D.C. In her position, she makes personnel assignments in the United States and overseas for some 350 officers. Thomas has found great opportunities as well as challenges in her Army career and says it has provided professional satisfactions including advanced education and promotions.

Dillon's career started with basic training at Fort Sam Houston followed by the internship at Walter Reed Medical Center (T Dillon, personal communication, 1996). Her first assignment as a registered dietitian (RD) was in a small community hospital at Fort Dix, New Jersey, where she was responsible for both inpatients and outpatients plus community service for soldiers and their families. After six months, she moved to management of food production and service and supervision of 35 employees. The next assignment was at Fort Irwin, California, in a small hospital followed by two different assignments again to Walter Reed Medical Center where she was an intern preceptor on the clinical staff. At the largest medical center for the Army with 1,000 beds, she received in-depth clinical experience in critical care of patients as the leader of the hospital's pediatrics support team.

Between these assignments, Dillon received her master's degree at the University of Maryland. Next, she went overseas to Heidelberg, Germany, to a small hospital as chief dietitian working with multinational personnel speaking five different languages. While there, Desert Storm occurred and she went to Saudi Arabia to a combat support hospital where patients were fed in remote and austere conditions. When the war ended, she returned to Fort Gordon in Georgia for a time as chief clinical dietitian.

Dillon's next assignment was very different. She moved to Dallas in the Army and Air Force Exchange Service and managed overseas school lunch programs in 11 countries, traveling around the world to school sites.

In 1996, Dillon was assigned again to Heidelberg as the consultant to a medical brigade with field hospitals in Hungary and Bosnia. This involved responsibility for all feeding at military locations in these countries. She describes it as a new job and a new beginning.

Dillon, reflecting on her varied and widespread career, says she would follow the same path again if she were starting in dietetics as she feels she is continuing to meet her professional expectations and is still achieving. The military life is a very people-oriented career, and she says people skills, counseling skills, and the ability to speak to groups are most important. The dietitian in the military service should also be prepared to function primarily as a generalist due to the varied assignments. Her advice is: "If you like challenges, like to meet other people and see many places, the military is a great choice" (T Dillon, personal communication, 1996).

BENEFITS IN CAREER AREAS

Army dietitians, as commissioned officers, are paid and promoted based on their military rank. The starting salary for a dietetic intern or entry-level dietitian is approximately $27,000 per year. At the rank of Captain, with four years of military service, the salary is approximately $41,000. Air Force salaries are similar. Housing and food allowances and a cost-of-living allowance are also provided based on geographic location.

Promotions are dependent on education (advanced degrees), military education (the Army has a series of officer/leader development courses), and job performance. An advantage of the military promotion system is that a dietitian may change job position or geographic location without a loss of seniority.

Thomas indicates that military dietitians can expect to relocate every two to four years and with each move, there are opportunities for varied positions.

Continuing education to maintain RD eligibility as well as for continued self-development is highly encouraged.

In a study of the quality of work life among US Army and Navy dietitians, Woods[36] found a high level of satisfaction among those surveyed. Most planned to stay in military service until retirement. The perceptions of self, of coworkers, of the organizational environment, and of the current job were all rated highly by respondents.

CONCLUSION

Dietitians are employed in the government at national, state, and local levels. They help draft legislation and issue guidelines and regulations. They participate in food and nutrition research and provide nutrition education for the public. They are commissioned officers in the military services providing nutritional care and food services for military personnel and families.

Activities of the ADA on behalf of dietitians include promotion of policy issues important to the profession and education of dietitians in legislative activities. Dietitians are involved in policy making through contacts with legislators and in support of association activities that further the profession of dietetics.

DEFINITIONS

Department of Health and Human Services (DHHS) Federal agency responsible for research and programs related to the health and well-being of all persons in the United States.

Dietary Guidelines Guidelines issued jointly by the US Department of Agriculture and the Department of Health and Human Services that provide general directives regarding nutrition and disease prevention and that are updated each five years.

Food and Drug Administration (FDA) Agency in DHHS responsible for regulating food safety and quality of foods and drugs for human consumption in the United States.

Food Guide Pyramid Guide for recommended intakes of food groups by importance (in terms of nutrient content) as depicted in a pyramid; developed by the US Department of Agriculture.

Medical Nutrition Therapy (MNT) Application of nutrition in the management of illness or injury.

Recommended Dietary Allowances (RDA) Standards established by the Food and Nutrition Board of the National Research Council for nutrient intakes adequate to meet the known nutrient needs of practically all healthy persons in the United States.

US Department of Agriculture (USDA) Federal agency responsible for programs and research related to food and agriculture in the United States.

REFERENCES

1. Washington Report. *ADA Courier*. 1996;35(9):1.
2. Bryk JA, Soto TK. Report on the 1995 membership database of The American Dietetic Association. *J Am Diet Assoc*. 1995;95:197–203.
3. Sims LS. Research aspects of public policy in nutrition generating research questions to determine the impact of nutritional, agricultural, and health care policy and regulations on the health and nutrition status of the public. In: *The Research Agenda for Dietetics*. Conference Proceedings. Chicago: The American Dietetic Association; 1993:25–38.
4. *The Surgeon General's Report on Nutrition and Health*. Washington, DC: Department of Health and Human Services; 1988.
5. National Research Council. *Diet and Health: Implications for Reducing Chronic Disease Risk*. Washington, DC: National Academy Press; 1989.
6. Escott-Stump S, Mahan LK. *Krause's Food, Nutrition and Diet Therapy*. 9th ed. Philadelphia: WB Saunders Co; 1996.
7. US Department of Agriculture, Agricultural Research Service, Dietary Guidelines. *Report of the Dietary Guidelines Advisory Committee on the Dietary Guidelines for Americans*. Report to the Secretary of Health and Human Services and the Secretary of Agriculture; 1995.
8. Food and Nutrition Board, Commission on Life Sciences, National Research Council. *Recommended Dietary Allowances*. 10th ed. Washington, DC: National Academy Press; 1989.
9. *The Food Guide Pyramid*. Washington, DC: US Department of Agriculture, Human Nutrition Information Service; 1992. Home and Garden Bulletin 252.
10. Derelian D. President's page: positions—an important means of fulfilling our mission and vision. *J Am Diet Assoc*. 1995;95:92.
11. Position paper update for 1997. *J Am Diet Assoc*. 1997;97:194.
12. ADA's grassroots network: the crucial link between nutrition professionals and Washington policy makers. *J Am Diet Assoc*. 1996;96:17.
13. Chernoff R. President's page: legislation and public policy. *J Am Diet Assoc*. 1996;96:511.
14. Position of The American Dietetic Association: cost-effectiveness of medical nutrition therapy. *J Am Diet Assoc*. 1995;95:88–91.
15. Chernoff R. President's page: managing managed care—a mission impossible? *J Am Diet Assoc*. 1996;96:715.
16. Position of The American Dietetic Association: nutrition services in managed care. *J Am Diet Assoc*. 1996;96:391–395.
17. Johnson RK, Coulston AM. Medicare: reimbursement rules, impediments, and opportunities for dietitians. *J Am Diet Assoc*. 1995;95:1378–1380.

18. ADA urges Congress to expand Medicare coverage for Medical Nutrition Therapy. *J Am Diet Assoc.* 1995;95:88–91.

19. Edelman RD, Johnson RK, Coulston AM. Securing the inclusion of Medical Nutrition Therapy in managed care systems. *J Am Diet Assoc.* 1995;95:1100–1102.

20. *The Clinical and Cost-Effectiveness of Medical Nutrition Therapy: Evidence and Estimates of Potential Medicare Savings from the Use of Selected Nutrition Interventions.* Summary Report. Prepared for the Nutrition Screening Initiative Barents Group, Washington, DC, June 1996.

21. Looking ahead at public policy and the 105th Congress. *J Am Diet Assoc.* 1997;97:17.

22. What's the outlook for health care reform? *J Am Diet Assoc.* 1995;95:649.

23. Position of The American Dietary Association: affordable and accessible health care services. *J Am Diet Assoc.* 1992;92:746–748.

24. White paper on health care reform. *J Am Diet Assoc.* 1992;92:749.

25. The Women's Health Initiative: be part of the answer. *J Am Diet Assoc.* 1995;95:1375.

26. Kumanyika S. Nutrition and health campaign for women. *J Am Diet Assoc.* 1995;95:299–300.

27. Outcomes management: Women's health. *ADA Courier.* May 1996, no. 5, 35:4.

28. Position of The American Dietary Association: women's health and nutrition. *J Am Diet Assoc.* 1995;95:362–366.

29. Six receive women's health research grants. *ADA Courier.* September 1996, no. 9, 35:2.

30. ADA sends nutrition policy recommendations to the White House Conference on Aging. *J Am Diet Assoc.* 1995;95:534.

31. Nutrition focus added to national policy resolutions developed by the White House Conference on Aging. *J Am Diet Assoc.* 1995;95:854.

32. Position of The American Dietary Association: nutrition, aging, and the continuum of care. *J Am Diet Assoc.* 1996;96:1048–1052.

33. Chernoff R. President's page: nutrition and health for older Americans. *J Am Diet Assoc.* 1996;96:1053.

34. Dwyer J. Strategies to detect and prevent malnutrition in the elderly: the Nutrition Screening Initiative. *Nutr Today.* 1994;29:14–24.

35. ADA. *Directory of Dietetic Programs.* Chicago: The American Dietetic Association; 1997.

36. Woods SG. *A Quality of Work Life Assessment of the United States Army and Navy Dietitians.* Stillwater: Oklahoma State University; 1992. Unpublished master's thesis.

CHAPTER 18

International Dietetics

Esther A. Winterfeldt

"It may be that the most significant of all the 'recent advances in international nutrition' is the very evident mobilization of the thoughts and concerns of all of us—in government, industry, academic circles, and professional groups such as The American Dietetic Association—toward the problems of the world community."[1]

Outline—Chapter 18

- Introduction

- Dietitians in Other Countries

- Where Dietitians Work

- International Activities of The American Dietetic Association
  - Affiliation with International Committee of Dietetic Associations (ICDA)
  - Reciprocal agreements
  - Member benefits
  - Joint papers and conferences
  - Future activities

- International Opportunities for Dietitians
  - World Hunger
  - Foods and food companies
  - International standards in education and credentialing
  - Dietetic practice
  - Health promotion

INTRODUCTION

Dietetics is becoming increasingly global because of worldwide concern for access to adequate food for the world's population and for nutritional health in the prevention of disease and early mortality. In the United States and in other developed countries, the abundance of food and the wide range of food choices have led to concerns about obesity and related health problems, but in many less developed countries, the major problems are that of having enough food or the economic means to fulfill the nutritional needs of the countries' people.

The growth of free trade and of worldwide communications means that the economies of the world are increasingly interdependent. At the same time, the sharing of research and knowledge is becoming easier, thus allowing for free interchange of strategies and approaches that can lead to alleviation of hunger and to the prevention of diseases related to nutritional deficiencies.

DIETITIANS IN OTHER COUNTRIES

Dietitians are employed worldwide. The International Committee of Dietetics Associations (ICDA) estimated in 1994 that about 100,000 members were located in the 30 member countries.[2] Estimates are not available for countries not belonging to the ICDA, and thus, the actual total is probably higher.

In 1992, the United States had the highest number of registered dietitians (RD) (47,705), with Denmark, Canada, and Germany reporting 5,300, 4,500, and 3,600, respectively. Japan, the United Kingdom, and Korea each had 2,500 to 3,000 members.[2] Currently, more than 400 The American Dietetic Association (ADA) members who live in other countries throughout the world belong to the American Overseas Dietetic Association (AODA), formerly the American European Dietetic Association.[3] They have the same privileges as all ADA members and are represented by a voting delegate in the ADA House of Delegates.[4] The membership of the AODA is made up of dietitians living in Europe (55 percent), Australia (13 percent), North America (13 percent), the Middle East (10 percent), and Africa (4 percent). Some 52 countries are represented in the membership.

Several other dietetic associations have been formed of members in regions of the world. Among these are the European Federation of the Association of Dietitians (EFAD), the Asian Forum of Dietetic Professionals (AFDP), the Caribbean Association of Dietitians, Eastern Central and Southern Africa including Israel, and Confelanyd, a consortium of South American countries. Many other countries are organized internally but do not affiliate with the international or regional associations.

The AFDP, one of the largest, was formed in 1991 by dietetic representatives from eight countries for the purpose of improving the nutritional status of the population, promoting development of the profession, and establishing research and education activities in Asia. The first Asian conference of dietetics was held in 1994 in Indonesia.[5]

The EFAD, with a membership of about 2,000 in 22 countries, was founded during the 1970s to promote collaboration between dietetic associations in European countries. The first European forum for dietitians was held in The Netherlands in 1995.[6]

The Dietitians of Canada, with 7,000 members, is one of the largest in the world and is closely allied with the ADA.[7] The two countries have had reciprocal credentialing eligibility of members for many years and share other activities such as the adoption of position papers and joint meetings.

The Confelanyd, the Latin American Confederation of Nutritionists and Dietitians, is an umbrella organization of 12 South American nutrition and dietetics associations. Every three years, the association conducts a symposium, most recently in Peru in 1995. Professional associations in Argentina, Chile, Colombia, and Venezuela have between 2,000 to 3,000 members and belong to regional groups.[7]

WHERE DIETITIANS WORK

As in the United States, most dietitians worldwide work in hospitals. In Europe and Asia, about half are in clinical dietetics, with community nutrition and public health the next highest areas of employment. In Africa and the Middle East, most are in private practice.[8] Dietitians in the American European Dietetic Association are employed in military and local hospitals, in nutrition education in schools and the community, in university research, in clinical and educational institutions, in food service facilities, and in consultation and private practice.[4]

In South America, 50 percent of the dietitians in Brazil are in food services, and in Argentina, 70 percent are in hospitals and companies that provide services to hospitals. In Venezuela, almost all are in public health assistance programs. In Canada, more than half are clinical dietitians, and smaller numbers are in community health, food services, business and industry, and private practice.[7]

Many countries have no dietitians, and in others, dietitians have different titles and a wide variety of responsibilities. In some countries, dietitians may cook and serve therapeutic meals, whereas in others, many health care institutions do not employ dietitians.[8]

INTERNATIONAL ACTIVITIES OF THE AMERICAN DIETETIC ASSOCIATION

Affiliation with International Committee of Dietetic Associations (ICDA)

The ADA became a founding member of the ICDA in 1952 and has participated in activities of the association continuously since that time. The mission of the ICDA is to support dietetic associations and their members through the use of communications systems, to enhance the image of dietitians, and to raise awareness of ways to improve the standards for dietetic practice.[9] Currently, 26 countries are members of the ICDA.[10]

The ICDA plans the International Congress of Dietetics, which is held every four years in different countries of the world. The international meeting of the association was held in Washington, D.C., in 1969, with the United States as the host country.[11] The most recent meeting was the twelfth in Manila in 1996, and many ADA members participated on the program.[9]

Worldwide contacts are made possible through membership in the ICDA, as the committee is affiliated with the International Union of Nutritional Sciences, which in turn has a liaison with the World Health Organization (WHO), the Food and Agriculture Organization of the United Nations (FAO), the United Nations Children's Fund, and many others.[5]

Reciprocal Agreements[5]

Reciprocity refers to the recognition of the certifying requirements in dietetics between countries by an agency or board in each country. In the United States, this is the Commission on Dietetic Registration. Graduates of educational programs in the cooperating countries are eligible to take the national qualifying examination in either country to become certified for practice.[10] Reciprocity between the United States and Canada has been in effect since 1984, and more recently, reciprocity has been established between the United States and The Netherlands, the Philippines, and Ireland. Similar reciprocal agreements with other countries are also under discussion.[10]

Member Benefits

- *Newsletter.* ADA publishes the ICDA newsletter "Dietetics and Nutrition around the World" approximately twice yearly. The newsletter was initiated in 1994.[5] Plans are being made to distribute this newsletter through a Web page on the Internet in the future, thereby expanding communications between countries.[3]

- *Journal distribution. The Journal of The American Dietetic Association* is distributed to at least 96 other countries.

- *Research collaboration.* Communication among researchers and also librarians worldwide is conducted through the Internet and electronic mail, thus assisting collaboration between countries.

- *Nutrition award.* An international nutrition award has been established by the ADA by which outstanding contributions internationally may be recognized.

Joint Papers and Conferences

The United States and Canada held a joint conference in 1996 titled "Food and Nutrition beyond Borders: Creating Strategies for the Dietetics Professional in North America." Participants, including representatives from Europe and Mexico, discussed issues such as standards of education and accreditation, technology-based practice, food safety, dietary standards, and consumer education.[12]

The United States and Canada have issued joint position papers. These are "Nutrition Intervention in the Care of Persons with Human Immunodeficiency Virus Infection," "Nutrition for Physical Fitness and Athletic Performance for Adults," and "Women's Health in Nutrition."[13]

Future Activities

Parks in 1994 recommended long-term possibilities for international involvement to include the following:[2]

1. Determine how ADA can make the greatest contribution toward improving world health.
2. Develop and maintain international alliances.
3. Serve our international members and colleagues.
4. Define and shape new practice roles.

5. Develop new educational models to help students and faculty become more aware of the multicultural nature of society both domestically and abroad.
6. Foster respect and understanding of how to work effectively with professionals of other cultures.
7. Cooperate with scholars and researchers in other parts of the world.

INTERNATIONAL OPPORTUNITIES FOR DIETITIANS

World Hunger

The ADA affirmed, in a 1995 position paper, the following: "It is the position of the ADA that access to adequate food is a fundamental human right. Hunger continues to be a worldwide problem of staggering proportions. The Association supports programs that combat hunger, allow for self-sufficiency, and are environmentally, economically sustainable."[14]

The extent of the hunger problem is indicated in statistics showing that about 1 billion individuals worldwide are energy-deficient and 2 billion suffer from inadequate intakes of micronutrients, especially iodine, iron, and vitamin A. In 1992, about 3 percent of the world's population lived in countries affected by famine or severe food shortages. It is estimated that about 36 percent of preschool-aged children in developing countries are moderately or severely malnourished based on weight for age.[14]

Woolery,[15] speaking at the annual meeting of the ADA in 1996, said that the knowledge and technology needed to end world hunger is available today but that further actions are needed to make it happen. The actions include (1) a global surveillance network, (2) a response mechanism with trained teams to go into areas where starvation exists, (3) research and development involving health promotion and disease control, and (4) promotion of nutrition as a major defense against disease along with access to clean water, sanitation, and housing.

The opportunities for the dietetics community in alleviating hunger and malnutrition are many and are crucial to efforts worldwide. The pace of global change and the spirit of cooperation among world governments through international trade agreements mean that a climate of increasing collaboration is possible. The opportunities include the following:

- collaboration with health and agriculture organizations and agencies dealing with food production and food distribution as well as with disease prevention and control
- appointments to health teams with other professionals

- participation in international conferences such as those sponsored by the FAO and the WHO that focus on the problems of hunger, malnutrition, and diet-related diseases and that explore ways to extend international cooperation in food and nutrition
- information and research sharing through the ICDA and directly with other dietetics associations; besides conferences, encouragement of full use of communications technology to promote sharing in a more extensive and faster way
- involvement in relief, development, and education activities in the developing world including support for food assistance programs

Foods and Food Companies

Many food companies are expanding their markets abroad, thereby presenting new opportunities for the food and nutrition professional in promotion and marketing of products and in consumer education. Dietitians may also be instrumental in determining new markets as well as expanding those already existing. Some companies producing foods and pharmaceuticals for health purposes develop and sell products specifically for a country based on known deficiencies among the population. An example is vitamin- and mineral-fortified drinks and foods for lactose intolerance because approximately 75 percent of adults worldwide have this condition.[16]

The person trained in food and nutrition can assist food and beverage companies selling abroad in important ways: in assessing social and cultural factors affecting food choices, in determining food consumption patterns, and in providing information to consumers about characteristics and use of the products. Dietitians with an interest in international opportunities will find Exhibit 18–1 a source of potential contacts.[17]

International Standards in Education and Credentialing

The education of dietitians varies among countries of the world from training in technical food service delivery (often referred to as catering) to four-year degree programs with an applied experience component.[6] The United States and Canada have worked together closely in establishing and recognizing each other's educational standards through reciprocity. As mentioned earlier, reciprocal agreements were also signed by the United States with The Netherlands in 1992, the Philippines in 1993, and with Ireland in 1996. The mutual agreements are based on a minimum of a baccalaureate degree, a supervised practice experience meeting

Exhibit 18–1 Suggested Business Opportunities for Dietitians in the International and National Marketplace

Opportunity	*Examples/suggestions*
American food companies with offices overseas	Kellogg, McDonalds, Coca-Cola, Pepsi
Pharmaceutical companies	Sandoz in Basel, Switzerland
Management positions in international food service companies	ARAMARK
American health care companies	Those with offices and facilities abroad
Food label development	American food company exported products
U.S.-based hotels and resorts	Referrals by physicians for nutrition services
International airlines	Menu planning/workshops on food and health
Specialized travel groups	Medical nutrition therapy needs
Cruise lines	Nutrition presentations and workshops
Educational materials preparation	New language designs and translations
International sports nutrition	Consultant to Olympic committees
Peace Corps	Living and working abroad as a volunteer
Health spas	Focus on food behavior, nutrition, fitness
International food brokerage companies	Nutrition and wellness classes for employees

Source: Reprinted from A.B. Dittoe, The Dietetics Professional in the International Arena, *Topics in Clinical Nutrition*, Vol. 11, pp. 7–13, © 1996, Aspen Publishers, Inc.

each country's standards, and successful completion of a national certifying examination. Further reciprocity agreements will no doubt be considered as more countries find it advantageous to strengthen and coordinate their education and credentialing standards for dietitians.

Increasingly, dietetics leaders envision a world credentialing standard for dietitians (M Sharp, personal communication, October 21, 1996). Some professional groups have already achieved this. The fast rate of change occurring through world trade, faster communications, and emphasis on the quality of goods and services provides impetus for the dietetics community to also establish common standards. The EFAD started this process at a forum in 1995 with an objective to lay the foundation for a Pan-American standard for the profession. An Asian conference and the 1996 International Congress of Dietetics in Manila featured several forums on the education and training of dietitians around the world. The United States recognized this need through a 1994 recommendation to review and assess US and other national requirements and to promote the development of international standards.[6]

One way of supporting educational standards is through offering educational opportunities by exchange programs and applied experiences for students. Distance education by worldwide communication means greater program-sharing opportunities as well as the dissemination of research.

Dietetic Practice

When the dietitian is recognized as the food and nutrition specialist, his or her role in disease prevention and treatment as well as in food services becomes broader. International efforts that address nutrition policies and support food assistance programs help alleviate hunger and malnutrition. One such program is the World Alliance in Nutrition and Human Rights established in 1994 as a network linking nutrition to a human rights perspective.[18]

Dietitians have much to offer in areas of food security, food safety, public health, world hunger, and development of food and nutrition policy. Common dietetic practice standards may not be feasible or possible at present; however, the potential benefit of international collaboration by dietetics professionals can only be positive for the public.

Health Promotion

Following the international conference in Rome in 1992, the "World Declaration on Nutrition and Global Plan of Action for Nutrition" was issued, by which the goal of a healthier, better nourished global population and a more informed, empowered public was envisioned by the year 2000.[18] One of the recommendations to governments and other groups that participated in the 1992 conference was to provide dietary guidelines relevant for different age groups and lifestyles appropriate for each country's population.[19] The global plan addressed the enormous problems of hunger and malnutrition but also the prevalence of diseases related to overconsumption and sedentary living that are on the rise in some countries. Over 150 countries will present their national plan, thus beginning a major dialogue and action plans among the world nutrition community.

Recommended dietary allowances are the standards used in at least 40 countries of the world to establish nutrient needs of the population. However, the recommendations vary from one country to another due to the lack of a common science base and differing philosophic approaches. Guthrie and Dwyer,[20] speaking at the XIIth International Congress of Dietetics in Manila, stated that there is a need to synchronize these recommendations among countries to facilitate foods programs and health needs.

Food Composition Data

Another area of international collaboration is in the development of food composition data important in research and in food planning. The International

Network of Food Data Systems was formed in the 1980s to coordinate efforts toward improvement of food composition data around the world.[21] International agencies dealing with food assistance, national governments regulating food supplies for internal and export use, researchers, and individuals need the information. The system is being developed to overcome the complexities of data collection and to provide a common database that may be accessed worldwide.

Quality Control in Food Services

The safety and quality of foods and food services are a focus of the International Organization for Standardization.[22] A process has been established by which quality control procedures for food purchasing, storage, handling, production, and service are monitored. A "Seal of World Approval" is issued, denoting that standards have been met, and some 70 countries worldwide have adopted the standards. The countries are thus linked through the use of a common standard of quality. Dietitians can play a vital role in raising public awareness of this standard for a wide array of food services.

PREPARING FOR INTERNATIONAL OPPORTUNITIES

When US dietitians seek employment in other countries, there are often skills over and above professional knowledge and experience that may be needed.[17] These include a cultural understanding of food and lifestyles in the country of employment, communication skills including both language and nonverbal communication, flexibility, and open-mindedness. Computer skills and experiences abroad such as through international travel are valuable assets. Another dietitian points out that other countries often have government regulations pertaining to practice and professional credentials that must also be considered.[23]

In a recent survey, AODA members residing in more than 50 countries were asked about both obstacles and opportunities they have encountered in finding employment in other countries.[24] The researchers point out that "realistic expectations, flexibility, and adequate planning can facilitate the transition to living in a foreign country and help make living overseas a fascinating and enriching experience."

The recommendations from the AODA survey are listed in Exhibit 18–2.

Each country of the world is different; yet dietitians have commonalities that bridge many of the differences. Included among these are knowledge about food and cultural practices, nutrition science, and the goal of reaching and maintaining good health for persons of all groups and ages.

Exhibit 18–2 Recommendations from the American Overseas Dietetic Association

---

American-trained dietitians who are thinking about moving overseas should:

- Learn as much of the native language as they can before moving overseas or as soon as possible after entering the country. It takes extensive language skills to conduct an in-depth interview. Sound grammar and vocabulary training permit rapid progress to full fluency in the foreign language.
- Get in touch with AODA as soon as possible. Networking opportunities within AODA can help facilitate the transition and alleviate the professional isolation one might feel in the beginning. AODA is the international affiliate of The American Dietetic Association (ADA) serving all ADA members living outside the United States.
- Become locally involved! Volunteer in nutrition, dietetics, or food-related areas. Service as an officer, chair, or committee member in AODA, American women's clubs, and international schools can aid in professional growth.
- Use electronic technology (i.e., E-mail and fax machines) to network and maintain professional contact and to take advantage of distance education.
- Learn skills to promote yourself with international companies, world health organizations, and unfamiliar environments.
- Have realistic expectations, be flexible, and plan in advance as much as possible.

Dietetics students interested in international dietetics should:

- Learn a foreign language. It widens your choice for international studies.
- Seek out and request coursework in cultural diversity. The more one understands and appreciates the diversity of cultures, the more one becomes tolerant of variations in eating habits.
- Investigate possibilities for exchange programs around the world through universities.

ADA should:

- Promote ADA members living overseas for job opportunities.
- Promote and develop the International Dietetic Network of AODA members.
- Help AODA members find resources for graduate-level distance learning around the world.

Source: U.G. Kyle, M. Cerny-Van Camp, and R.J. Stemler, Profile of American-Trained Dietitians in the International Setting: Survey of the Members of the American Overseas Dietetic Association. Copyright The American Dietetic Association. Reprinted by permission from *Journal of The American Dietetic Association*, Vol. 97 pp. 789–791, © 1997.

Dietitians with Positions in Other Countries

Using her background and skills, a dietitian who moved to Vienna, Austria, in 1991 with her husband and two children, describes her present practice. Sara

Rhodes, MS, RD, has an academic background in journalism and nutrition and was instrumental in establishing ADA's book publishing division in 1982. She then taught nutrition at Boston University and Northeastern University and wrote as well as edited medical and nutrition articles. After moving abroad, she continued to edit papers for physicians and also developed skills in new professional areas. For example, she taught a class in weight reduction to English-speaking women and served as a consultant to Coca-Cola's software documentation department in Vienna. This year, she is coauthoring a book on nutrition and acquired immunodeficiency syndrome to be published soon and is working full-time as editor-in-chief at Immuno, Austria's largest pharmaceutical company.

Ursula G. Kyle, MS, RD, is a native of Switzerland who returned to her home country after 23 years in the United States. She completed her bachelor's and master's degrees, received the RD, and worked for 10 years in the United States before returning. Having grown up in the German-speaking part of Switzerland, she had to make adjustments when her husband's job took them to the French area of Switzerland. She is now a research dietitian at the Geneva University Hospital, Geneva, Switzerland.

She describes her job search and present position as follows:

> While I now have a wonderful job, the path to get there was not without obstacles and frustrations. My first year in Switzerland, I worked as a secretary and during the year, learned French and also became computer-literate. Both of these skills are indispensable and help me now in my job as a research dietitian. At the beginning of our second year, I found a job as a dietitian at the University Hospital but found out quickly that the job did not exactly meet my expectations. For four hours each day, I shuffled diet cards and watched the patients' trays go by on the tray line but this was traumatic for me because half the time I couldn't read the handwriting and the other half I didn't know what the foods were! (Currently, both these jobs are no longer the responsibility of the dietitian.) Luckily three months after starting to work at the university hospital, I met the nutritionist (MD specializing in nutrition) and we began an informal collaboration for journal articles and staff training. Several months later, he was able to obtain grant money to hire me as a research dietitian.
>
> For the past six and a half years, I have done the data collection for some of his research projects, have become the coordinator for our body composition database and projects, and have written several articles for publication. I was lucky to have found a mentor willing to invest in me and help expand my professional skills to include indirect calorimetry, bioelectrical impedance, writing for publication, and statistics. I see

patients as part of the research projects, but rarely do nutritional counseling. For some of our research projects, I do calculate food intake and evaluate lab results or make recommendations for nutrition support. In order to do so, I had to become familiar with the local food habits, recipe ingredients, foods available, and the cultural differences. I also had to make the transition to meters, centimeters, kilos, and lab results reported as mmol/L rather than mg/dl. It's been a tremendous learning experience and exciting adventure!

Because dietetic practice differs in different European countries, we cannot always expect to obtain traditional jobs as we might expect in the US. However, if we just look around, we can exchange information and learn from our colleagues around the world. The American-trained dietitian who wishes to work in the international setting must, above all, learn the local language in order to be able to communicate with physicians, colleagues, teachers, patients, and the public (personal communication, July 10, 1997).

CONCLUSION

Dietetics is becoming more global as the need for alleviating hunger and improving nutrition practices grows throughout the world. Dietetics associations in many countries are making strides toward improving food and nutrition practices and the role of the dietitian becomes increasingly important in this process.

The development of international standards for the education and credentialing of dietitians would establish uniformity and facilitate employment and understanding of the role of dietitians. Joint activities and the sharing of research and technology are aids to dietetics practice internationally.

Opportunities for dietitians in the international arena are many. They range from direct involvement in foods programs internationally, development of food and nutrition policy, linkages with health and agriculture organizations, to sharing of information and exchange programs for education and training.

DEFINITIONS

Distance Education Learning that takes place in a location other than the classroom that is usually conducted using communications technology.

Food and Agriculture Organization (FAO) International organization for food and agriculture programs that promote health and prevent disease through food assistance and education programs worldwide.

International Organization for Standardization (ISO) Organization that sets standards in all aspects of food services that aims to improve the quality of food services in countries meeting the standards.

Multicultural Term referring to different cultures as among countries and populations.

Reciprocity Process of giving and receiving of similar privileges; in dietetics, the mutual recognition of credentialing or other standards between dietetic associations.

World Health Organization (WHO) International agency dealing with programs to promote health and prevent disease.

REFERENCES

1. Gortner WA. International facets of USDA nutrition research. *J Am Diet Assoc.* 1967;50:279–283.

2. Parks S. President's page: challenging the future—an evolving global perspective for the profession. *J Am Diet Assoc.* 1994;94:782–784.

3. International affiliate changes its name. In: Dietetics around the world. *Newslett ICDA.* May 1997:7.

4. American European Dietetic Association. Flyer issued at ADA Annual Meeting, San Antonio, TX, 1996.

5. The history of the International Congress of Dietetics. In: Dietetics around the world. *Newslett ICDA.* July 1994:2.

6. Successful forum hosted by European Federation of the Associations of Dietitians (EFAD). In: Dietetics around the world. *Newslett ICDA.* October 1995:2–3.

7. Derelian D. The work of dietitians in the Americas. Presented at XIIth International Congress of Dietetics; 1996; Manila, Philippines.

8. Kennedy R. Trends in dietetics: Africa and the Middle East. Presented at XIIth International Congress of Dietetics; 1996; Manila, Philippines.

9. Helm KK. International Dietetics Congress. *Top Clin Nutr.* 1996;11:81–83.

10. Gilbride JA, Lechowich KA. International opportunities for the dietetics profession. *Top Clin Nutr.* 1996;11:1–6.

11. Cassell JA. *Carry the Flame: The History of The American Dietetic Association.* Chicago: The American Dietetic Association; 1990.

12. Banff meeting sets the stage for future collaboration. *ADA Courier.* 1996;35:1,3.

13. Position paper update for 1997. *J Am Diet Assoc.* 1997;97:194.

14. Position of The American Dietetic Association: world hunger. *J Am Diet Assoc.* 1995;95:1160–1162.

15. Woolery CP. Celebrating successes: future feeding of the world's hungry. Presented at annual meeting of the American Dietetic Association; October 1996; San Antonio, TX.

16. Levine B. About lactose intolerance. *J Nutr Educ.* 1996;31:78–79.

17. Dittoe AB. The dietetics professional in the international arena. *Top Clin Nutr.* 1996;11:7–13.

18. *World Declaration on Nutrition and Plan of Action for Nutrition.* Geneva, Switzerland: World Health Organization; 1992.

19. Schwartz NE. Communicating nutrition and dietetics issues: balancing diverse perspectives. *J Am Diet Assoc.* 1996;96:1137–1139.

20. Guthrie H, Dwyer J. Recommended dietary allowance: current status and emerging issues. Presented at XIIth International Congress of Dietetics; 1996; Manila, Philippines.

21. Rand WM, Windstrom CT, Wyse BW, Young VR. *Food Composition Data: A User's Perspective.* Tokyo: United Nations University; 1987.

22. Gatchalian MM. Linking the world through ISO 9000: focus on foodservice. Presented at XIIth International Congress of Dietetics; 1996; Manila, Philippines.

23. Soloff-Coste CJ. An American dietitian in France. *Top Clin Nutr.* 1996;11:14–20.

24. Kyle UG, Cerny-Van Camp M, Stemler RJ. Profile of American-trained dietitians in the international setting: survey of the members of the American Overseas Dietetic Association. *J Am Diet Assoc.* 1997;97:789–791.

CHAPTER 19

The Future in Dietetics

Sara C. Parks

"The dogmas of the quiet past are inadequate for the stormy present and future. As our circumstances are new, we must think anew, and act anew." Abraham Lincoln

INTRODUCTION

As the profession enters into the next century, the daunting challenges alluded to by one of our nation's early leaders brings a message that is true even today. The new millennium will bring a "hypercompetitive" health care environment, greatly altered by new information technologies, new business practices, new managed care and integrated health care systems, and changing consumer demands. Clearly, the dietetic profession, like all health professions, is entering a time of unprecedented volatility and change.

A growing number of driving forces will dramatically reshape the profession. Among the most significant trends are changing demographics, growing globalization, increasing consumer expectations, emerging knowledge economy, technological revolution, and a restructured work force. To be competitive in a rapidly changing environment will require an unprecedented understanding of changing health care markets, the need for developing new global competencies and capabilities, and a shift from tangible assets to an appreciation of the value of knowledge and technology. Professions aspiring to make a difference in the lives of individuals will be playing an altogether different game—competing for the future.

MACRO TRENDS

Changing Demographics

Demographic factors define health care markets from three perspectives: composition, accessibility, and mobility. The two most significant demographic influences on health care delivery are the aging population and ethnic diversity. The next 15 years will be characterized by a rapidly increasing number of elderly who will dramatically shift the focus of health services from acute to chronic care. In addition, no change will so profoundly alter the nature of health care as the 76 million aging Baby Boomers who are interested in health promotion and disease prevention. Further, the twenty-first century will be characterized by growing ethnic diversity. From 1980 to 1992, our nation's Asian-American population experienced a 123 percent growth rate and our Hispanic population a 62 percent growth rate. It is predicted by the year 2000 that 30 percent of our population will be from today's minority and racial groups. This segment of our population will seek alternative medicine modalities.

Accessibility to health care will continue to be a problem. Despite escalating health care costs, a large percentage of our population continues to be without adequate health care. Growing poverty among our nation's rural population, ethnic groups, and at-risk elderly is not likely to improve and will place additional demands on the health care system. The gap between the "haves" and "have nots" will continue to broaden.

A third characteristic of the US health care market is mobility. Women moving into the work force are no longer available to care for aging parents. Extended family members have relocated to distances too far to provide support to loved ones with acute and chronic diseases. Even those individuals within a geographic region are mobile. Of the 37 million American professionals employed outside of the home, 75 percent are away from their offices at least one day per week. These individuals will buy time and convenience, along with health products and services, and will demand "on-the-go" services.

Growing Globalization

As we move toward a global society and as free trade becomes a reality, so too should there be a free exchange of ideas and information between dietetic communities.[1] Globalization will revolutionize the current profession of dietetics. The profession will draw clients, employees, materials, and strategic partners from a single global marketplace. Many members of the profession currently lack the language skills and knowledge of cultural differences necessary to network with food and nutrition partners from around the world. Internationalization of dietetic education and practice will be a priority in the coming decade.

Increasing Consumer Expectations

In the twenty-first century, the focus on tailoring health products and services to individual consumers will continue to grow. A more affluent and better educated consumer, with better access to information, will place new demands on providers to ensure the best care. They will place a high priority on health promotion and expect greater accountability for desired outcomes. At the same time they will be questioning the value of services. Telecommunications experts predict that new integrated circuits will become more powerful and give computer-literate health providers and clients easy access to the same information. These innovations will challenge food and nutrition communicators to distinguish their messages from misinformation, also available on the Internet.

Emerging Knowledge Economy

Over the past two millenniums, the world population has experienced a 50-fold increase. We have recognized this human growth explosion. During this same time, it has been estimated that information has exploded over 250,000 times faster than our population growth. Somehow, we have overlooked the significance of these data. In our profession, our scientific underpinnings have provided us with encyclopedic amounts of new information, and the application of knowledge in the practice arena has accelerated the specialized growth of our profession. To provide state-of-the-art information to our clients requires staying current, avoiding knowledge obsolescence, and a commitment to lifelong learning. Even though the information economy is maturing, we have yet to develop the models to reorganize the dietetic profession.

Technological Revolution

Technology to produce, store, and use information will continue to expand and will dramatically change how professionals interact with clients, colleagues, and competitors. As we approach the next decade, these changes in technology will have an enormous impact on health care. Although technology will be a mechanism to deliver health services and education in remote areas, it will also depersonalize care.

Information technology will affect dietetic professionals in two ways: It will remove routine tasks and allow them to become full partners on medical, management, and consumer teams; and it will redefine dietetic practice roles.[2] Members of the profession will have to rethink old career assumptions, abandon obsolete practice roles, and create new opportunities. The dietetic professional of the year 2010 will work more easily to address complex health problems as information technology connects scientists, practitioners, and consumers from around the world.

Restructured Work Force

With an aging population growing at a rate much faster than younger peers, there will be fewer people to take care of the nation's health care needs. Technology may provide a partial answer. Although technology may decrease the number of traditional job openings, an entire new set of opportunities will be available to those developing computer and information management skills. Technology will also facilitate cross-disciplinary interventions and will help the profession to experiment with new types of health care teams. Interactive video conferencing, counseling, long-distance diagnostic and treatment interventions, and electronic patient records will be ways to increase access to care, as a partial answer to the work force issue and to stretch the system's scarce resources.

CHANGING ROLES IN THE HEALTH CARE SYSTEM

In addition to these six macro trends, the early 1990s brought about fundamental changes in the American health care system. Mergers, consolidations, downsizing, and outsourcing have transformed the entire way in which health services are delivered. New managed care and integrated health systems, organized along a complete continuum of care, replaced more traditional organizational structures. These systems were designed to respond to the need for cost reduction in the health care industry, to improve access to quality care, and to enhance client outcomes.

Restructuring of the health care industry has led a recent Pew Health Professions Commission to predict changes and opportunities for some health care providers.[3] For example, the report suggests that half of America's hospitals will close by the turn of the century; that there will be a loss of almost 60 percent of existing hospital beds; that enormous increases will occur in primary care and community-based services and for individuals with the knowledge and skills needed to provide these services; that the need for medical specialists, nurses, pharmacists, and allied health professionals will decrease; that many allied health professions, such as dietetics, will be consolidated into new multiskilled professions; and that the demand for public health professionals to meet population-based needs will increase.

Along with challenges the dietetics profession faces as a result of the restructuring of the health care industry, there are also opportunities. Naisbitt predicts that health care will remain one of the fastest growing sectors in our economy.[4] Naisbitt suggests that annual spending for health care will reach $142 billion by 1995. This growth is driven by the Baby Boomers' desire to look and feel better and the elderly's desire to live longer. In particular, Naisbitt predicts continued growth in the diet and fitness industry.

The other good news for the profession is that in the new market-driven health care delivery system, allied health professionals provide a cost-effective alternative to the more expensive services of physicians and nurses. To be competitive in new practice roles, allied health professionals will have to develop new roles and responsibilities. The Pew Health Commission has made strong recommendations about the competencies needed for these future roles: ability to work on interdisciplinary teams, reliance on health and information technologies, strongly grounded in science and critical thinking, and cross-functional knowledge and skills.[3] The report goes on to suggest that the "emergence of new allied health professions which fall outside the often rigid boundaries of currently recognized disciplines,"[3(p.366)] this will require innovative approaches to role definition and partnering among allied health groups.

The profession's ability to continue to deliver high-quality cost-effective care, to enter the curative and preventive market in low cost settings, and to systematically document the impact of nutrition interventions will determine its future.

Implications and Challenges for the Profession

The value of describing a possible future for the profession is to be able to address the challenges faced by members of the profession and to take advantage of the opportunities the future offers. Although it is admittedly difficult to predict where the profession will be with such huge changes as global competition, information technology, and intellectual capital, the questions to be asked are: "What challenges will the future bring for the profession?" "What new assumptions will guide planning for the future of the profession?" "What new competencies will be needed by future practitioners?" "What career opportunities exist for future dietetic professionals?"

The dietetic profession faces a number of enormous challenges as the turn of the century approaches.

- *Challenge 1: Positioning dietetic professionals in an industry dominated by managed care and integrated health systems.* Although dietetic professionals have always focused on preventive care, they now face intense competition from other health care providers, including those available via the Internet. This is particularly true if the oversupply of physicians and nurses is as great as predicted. In addition, other health professionals are also struggling for recognition in these new health systems. The profession will need to deliver a new practitioner who brings both a multidisciplinary perspective and critical thinking skills needed to solve both client and delivery system problems.

- *Challenge 2: Accepting the new world of work and redefining new practice roles.* Future dietetic professionals will be entering a new world of work where practice will continually change. The turbulence of the health care marketplace will continue to experience downsizing and dramatic restructuring, all of which affects the delivery of nutrition services. Two fundamental changes will occur: Jobs will evolve from being very narrow and task-oriented to more multidisciplinary and multidimensional roles; and nothing will be permanent. Members of the profession will have to bring a generalist mind-set to the practice arena. Job insecurity will be a reality as professionals move in and out of careers and organizations many times throughout their lives.

- *Challenge 3: Demonstrating that dietetic professionals can provide high-quality cost-effective care that is measurable.* The importance of this challenge should not be minimized. In the future, there is general agreement that credentialing will become less important as the sole criterion for hiring in the future. Managed care organizations will use the ability to produce outcomes, cost-effectively, as their major employment criterion.

- *Challenge 4: Keeping our knowledge base current and obtaining a commitment to lifelong learning.* By definition, a professional is mandated to use the latest science in developing interventions and to keep practice standards current. With the rapid change in the knowledge that we bring to solve today's nutrition and eating problems, the issue of managing our continuing professional education becomes a survival strategy. It has been suggested that half of what we learn as we enter the profession is obsolete within three years. This presents a tremendous need to develop lifelong learning models refocusing on continuing professional education.

- *Challenge 5: Developing a sense of urgency in restructuring education for the profession.* The Commission on Dietetic Registration recently conducted two surveys, one with dietetic practitioners and a second with employers.[5,6,7] A new set of competencies were identified for practitioners, many of which are not included in today's educational programs. Similarly, the Pew Health Commission made strong recommendations to develop new allied health roles that are multidisciplinary and multifunctional.[3] These recommendations mandate new and comprehensive interventions in the design and delivery of dietetic educational programs.

- *Challenge 6: Keeping pace with the reengineering occurring in the industries employing dietetic professionals.* Although most of our members are employed in health care, there will continue to be a significant number employed in the food industry. Like the health care industry, the food industry is experiencing similar downsizing, outsourcing, mergers, and acquisitions, as a result of intense competition. These changes have major implications for food and nutrition specialists, some positive and others that could be highly destructive. Continuous and overlapping change is occurring in industries and organizations in which dietetic professionals are employed, making it difficult to monitor trends shaping new practice roles.

Despite our many challenges, the profession puts together an impressive number of winning combinations. We continue to be a highly respected profession, recognized worldwide as the leading organization of food and nutrition experts. With the aging population and the maturing Baby Boomers, the demand for dietetic professionals will increase. Additionally, we are already a generalist profession with the capability of easily moving into multidisciplinary and multifunctional careers. Finally, the profession has a long history of encouraging the growth and development of diversity.

The profession is likely to address these changes, in part, by restructuring itself around the technology of "connectivity" and in the way its members will deliver services to consumers. If downsizing and outsourcing continues in both the health care and food industries, individuals will be working in small ad hoc work groups, taking on specific tasks, and then moving on to yet another work task. Relationships will not be permanent and employee-company loyalty will not be valued.

With continuous and overlapping change in both practice settings and in our interactions with others, what we bring to these new work groups will be cutting-edge knowledge. To avoid obsolescence and to keep current with the research, learning and work will occur simultaneously. Technology-based self-directed learning will occupy a large portion of our work day. What an exciting time to be part of the dietetic profession!

Competition and Collaboration with Other Professions

Competition in the future will be different from the present and past. Driven by the information revolution, the past few years have seen entirely new professions emerging and consequently new competitive products and services. Virtual "meeting and dining" rooms will allow consumers, across the nation and around the world, to meet without leaving home or work. Microrobotics will allow more aging individuals to remain independent and in their own homes as mechanical maids "sense" and "fetch" for those unable to do so on their own. Health organizations, linked electronically, will provide access to experts around the world at the time the attending physician is in need of consultation. Digital highways will provide immediate access to the world's retail marketplace for information, programs, services, and entertainment. Technology will change the nature of competition in ways we would never expect.

There will continue to be more intensive competition among traditional sources: other health professionals, proprietary business, alternative health providers, and the media, to name a few. The more important question to ask, however, is "Should we be viewing these groups as competitors or collaborators?" In some cases, it will be both.

The future portends a profoundly different playing field for members of our profession. The impact of changes in the health care system has been discussed earlier. Mergers of education and information technology have produced electronic books and newsletters; personally tailored multimedia educational programs that can be accessed on demand; interactive learning programs for "at home use"; and with the projected mergers of telephone, television, and computer technologies, there are unlimited capabilities to connect teacher and learner from around the world. Similarly, the food and lodging industries have opened markets in virtually every part of the world.

Probably the greatest "competitor" or "collaborator" is the rapid growth of information technology. It is the advent of the information age that is driving changes in business, government, professions, and social institutions. Future dietetic professionals will have a new set of leadership skills with a small specialty core of food, nutrition, and health. To compete, they will be experts at discovering, evaluating, and disseminating information and other resources, and they will need such futures-related leadership skills as visioning, persuasive communication, and the ability to form strategic partnerships.

COMPETENCIES OF THE FUTURE DIETETIC PROFESSIONAL

In his book, *The Knowledge Executive,* Harlan Cleveland summarizes one of the most important critical skills of future professionals in the following statement:[7] "People who do not educate themselves, and keep re-educating themselves, to participate in the new knowledge environment will be the peasants of the information society."[7(p. 190)] Cleveland presents a strong case for not only understanding the power of being a "knowledge worker" in the twenty-first century but also for being technologically literate, being able to use existing or new technology to access and to manage the proliferation of knowledge. Others, within and external to the profession, also concur with the need for this competency.[5,8,9]

There is general agreement among employers, educators, and practitioners that the following competencies will be needed in the future:

- *leadership skills*—having the the ability to see and create new opportunities; to create new visions for the profession; and to lead others through the milieu of change that will continue to be part of our professional lives
- *professional and organizational awareness*—understanding the mission, vision, and goals of the dietetic profession; having the ability to link food and nutrition interventions to the overall health of the individual; seeing how nutrition care fits into the goals of employment sites; and appreciating organizations as dynamic political, economic, and social systems
- *problem-definition and problem-solving skills*—identifying gaps between where a situation is and should be and helping others to see how to fill these gaps
- *general business skills*—knowing the economic impacts of food and nutrition interventions; understanding strategic management, marketing, finance, logistics, accounting, and how these business functions work together
- *team building and interpersonal skills*—because of the increasing use of outsourcing and the use of temporary personnel having strong team-building skills; similarly, having persuasive communication skills to sell new ideas and to obtain support for change
- *entrepreneuralism*—having an ability to see new career opportunities, to combine that ability with necessary business skills, and to be a risk taker because of short life cycles of most careers; implies a need to challenge traditional roles and prevailing approaches to delivering food and nutrition services
- *multicultural, multidiversity competence*—having an openness to other cultural values; a global understanding and perspective; and the attitudes, skills, and knowledge needed to apply a global perspective to clients, colleagues, and employees' needs

In addition, the Commission on Dietetic Registration's recent survey of dietetic practitioners and employers identifies three major categories of competencies: conceptual, interpersonal, and technical/clinical.[5,6] The conceptual and interpersonal competencies identified in this study are similar to those discussed above. Balch emphasized the need for stronger food competencies: the biochemical and physiologic processes used to metabolize food; the environmental and behavioral influences on eating; and food safety, food science, and food production as important knowledge and skills for the future, as well as all aspects of food service management.

The Pew Health Commission report presents a mandate for multiskilling among allied health professionals.[8] Specific competencies recommended in this report, and in the 1993 Pew Health Commission report, include an ability to work on interdisciplinary teams, to rely on health and information technology, to understand legal and financial aspects of health care, and to relate knowledge at the boundaries of our profession to our own interventions.

The 1993 Pew report suggests a need for more "contemporary clinical skills" to meet the current health needs of the nation's population.[10(p. 8)] This report further identifies the ability to ensure cost-effective interventions, to encourage healthy lifestyles, and to manage information as additional competencies for the future.

On a whole, the profession must rethink its educational strategies to meet the practice needs of a rapidly changing marketplace. There is a critique by employers that incoming dietetic professionals lack certain key competencies: technology, systems-thinking, information management, interpersonal relations, and cost-effective use of resources. Because employers are no longer hiring for today, we must look to tomorrow as we "educate and re-educate" ourselves.

FROM CAREER STABILITY TO CAREER INNOVATION: FUTURE ROLES FOR THE PROFESSIONAL

The future will present many new opportunities for those who assume the responsibility for their own careers; for those who are entrepreneurial and willing to broaden their vision of the profession; and for those willing to pursue international opportunities.

Opportunities in Health Care

In summarizing the Department of Labor's Bureau of Labor Statistics latest employment projections for the US work force, a recent *ADA Courier* reported continued growth in the health care industry through the year 2005.[11] The Department of Labor predicts that employment will increase from 9 million health care jobs in 1994 to 12.1 million in 2005. Employment sites will follow the aging demographics and the restructured health care industry. Hospitals will be the slowest growing, and long-term care and community-based programs will have employment growth rates of 3 percent or more.

Specifically, this same *ADA Courier* predicts that the demand for dietetic professionals will grow as fast as the average for all industries in our nation's economy. There will be a need for increased meals and nutrition programs in long-term care, schools, correctional institutions, residential care, community health, home health care, and health and fitness clubs, to name a few. Traditional professional roles (e.g., food service administrator or clinical practitioner) will almost become obsolete in the future. The new health care environment will see dietetic professionals managing multiple departments or providing transdisciplinary health services, in which nutrition is only part of the practice role. In the future, it will not be uncommon to see food and nutrition experts earn dual degrees in medicine, pharmacy, nursing, physical therapy, or hotel and restaurant management.

Additionally, there will be some executive-level positions in managed care organizations and integrated health systems and in traditional health care organizations. These positions will require a new set of competencies in such areas as strategic planning, information management, marketing, finance, and cost-benefit analysis.

Edutainment

In a special report, Naisbitt examined future growth opportunities on an industry-by-industry basis.[4] Those growth industries of greatest interest to dietetic professionals include travel and entertainment, food, health care, children's services, and the mature market. In the travel and entertainment industry, Naisbitt suggests growth in international travel, cruise line travel, interactive television, bed and breakfast lodging facilities, and customized music. Although dietetic career opportunities in these industries may not appear readily apparent, the future entrepreneurial professional will combine educational programs and services at the same time consumers are having fun. "Edutainment" is a rapidly growing consumer trend that dietetic professionals have only recently begun to explore. Given the prediction of increased leisure travel, focusing opportunities around the entertainment industry could be a lucrative business venture.

Food

Naisbitt also predicts continued growth in the food industry. In particular, he suggests growth in roasted chicken restaurants, new varieties of microwave foods, prepared take-out meals in supermarkets, ice cream alternatives, low-cholesterol and low-fat foods, home food delivery services, and healthy food snacks in theaters, bookstores, and video stores. For the career innovator, these industries present opportunities in new product development, marketing research, food sales, food distribution, and catering, to name a few.

In addition to the Naisbitt report, Technomic, Inc., conducted a study of the casual theme restaurant industry for The American Dietetic Association (ADA). That report concluded that dietitians have been employed, either full time or as a consultant, in commercial food service for 10 years or less.[12] Most food and nutrition professionals work for the organization's marketing department and provide such services as marketing, nutrition information, menu analysis and planning, quality control, and food service management. Food service managers responding to the study suggested expanded opportunities if dietetic professionals obtained stronger business skills and a more strategic understanding of how "nutrition and health" can be used to position food products in the marketplace.

The commercial food service industry will continue to provide careers for those interested in combining an interest in foods, international cuisine, and business administration. Restaurant and in-home catering will continue to grow as consumers entertain more and cook less. Resorts hire large numbers of food professionals; food manufacturers and food distributors look to members of the profession who can provide marketing support, sales training, new product development, and food photography support. Many hotels are setting up educational/child care centers for parents traveling with kids; they need help with nutrition education programming, health and fitness programs, and developmentally appropriate feeding strategies. Associations, representing health professions, are also employing food and nutrition consultants to help develop transdisciplinary education programs.

Information Technology and Management

Varian predicts more information specialists will be needed in the future "to rescue managers from the proliferation of knowledge" surrounding a profession.[13] He suggests the following new career opportunities: organizers of user-friendly information on the Internet; database designers and managers; electronic writers and editors; instructional system designers; distance learning programmers and evaluators; and information entrepreneurs who can develop innovative ways for professionals and clients to connect and to work together. Noam, writing about the future of universities, predicts that within a decade a significant share of higher education will be offered commercially and electronically.[14] There will be a need for experts, in such subspecialties as food and nutrition, to develop, deliver, and evaluate these new and innovative educational programs. Library scientists, with a food and nutrition specialty, will be a critical future practitioner needed to organize and structure electronic data in a usable format.

Multimedia education and developing and selling electronic books, tapes, seminars, and speeches will be in great demand. Computer-related skills in any profession will translate into an average 15 percent increase in income. This gap will broaden in the future.

Opportunities for innovative software development in K–12 will exist for those who develop learning programs that are also entertaining. Cerf has commented on virtual reality as a mechanism for expanded learning:[15] "One of the things that excites me in the K–12 area is the use of simulated environments, creating classrooms that have facilities in them that we might not ever be able to build in the real world."[15(p. 46)]

Halal suggests that many traditional jobs will disappear and that knowledge entrepreneurs will replace current factory, secretarial, and other service workers.[16] He reports that Travelers Insurance has automated two-thirds of its office, replacing clerks with registered nurses who are problem solvers. Similar opportunities, in many organizations, surely are available for the creative food and nutrition experts.

As the world advances toward a new century and a new millennium, the electronic revolution will dramatically change our profession. To succeed we will need to draw on a new set of assumptions about the profession and develop a new set of competencies and a new vision for the future. E. Neige Todhunter, ADA's 1957–1958 president, best summarizes the challenge in the following:[17] "Imagination is what keeps industry going in this country—Without it we will not survive, but be relegated to the museum along with the horse and buggy—This is a world of change, very different in philosophies, values and method . . . ."

Research

With the advent of the information society, new opportunities will exist for those interested in the discovery of knowledge. There is a need for those interested in studying both nutrition science and nutrition intervention issues and problems. New and emerging clinical protocols, intervention trials, and cost-benefit studies must be tested. Similarly, there is a need for food researchers who want to develop new products or who want to understand consumer satisfaction and service quality factors; marketing research has tremendous growth potential. Advances in the food delivery system must be modeled, simulated, and tested for quality, efficiency, cost-effectiveness, and consumer acceptance. A critical business challenge is the need to significantly improve the productivity of knowledge around all our key resources.[18] Research provides the foundation for addressing this issue.

Private Practice

The latter half of the 1990s and early into the next century will be characterized by entrepreneuralism. Because women start most small businesses in the United States, this bodes well for dietetic practitioners who want to set up private practices. The list of opportunities is too great to fully elaborate on in this book. However, here are but a few: television, communication, radio, public relations, client counseling, food innovations, human resources, career placement, layout and design, lifestyle management, and customer service.

The days of climbing the corporate ladder with a single company will no longer exist. Creative practitioners, who want to work for themselves and have more quality time with their families, will find a receptive marketplace. Balch suggests that "the most valued (dietetic) members are those with a global view of health and a proficiency in a greater number of competencies."[6(p. 11)] This is especially true for those individuals working in their own practices.

Once again, Harlan Cleveland provides guidance as we explore future career opportunities:[7] "In a society of increasing information-richness, the content of many, perhaps most, jobs a generation hence is unknowable today . . . just as the generation of yesteryear was unable, through the ignorance of parents and guidance counselors, to aspire to service as astronauts, nuclear physicists, ecologists, computer programmers, television repairers, or managers of retrieval systems."[7(p. 188)]

PLANNING FOR YOUR FUTURE

In addressing the future, dietetic practitioners must meet the challenges brought about as a result of reengineering both the health delivery system and the food industry. Those individuals who can capitalize on future trends, who understand how basic assumptions will change dietetic practice, and who proactively search out new career opportunities will be well poised for the future. Others who naively believe the future is "more of the same" will find their positions going away—even after many years of dedicated service.

In analyzing the future, one thing is certain—we must always expect the unexpected, and we must assume the future is not an extension of the past. There are several assumptions, however, that can be made about the future that will guide your career decision making:

- The ability to connect electronically will revolutionize how, when, and where dietetic professionals will practice.

- Professionals, not the organization's management, will emerge as primary players in multidisciplinary teams; managers will become facilitators, coaches, and mentors.
- The concept of the organization will expand to include links to all external partners, including consumers.
- Most people will be connected, worldwide, forming new professional opportunities and risks.
- Services and products that dietetic professionals offer to clients will be "informationalized"—databases will be built into most products, programs, and services offered to consumers.
- Competition will no longer be limited to local, regional, or national audiences; it will be worldwide.
- Continual and "just-in-time" learning will be the rule for health providers and their clients.
- The model for temporary project-based organizations will be the norm.
- Most individuals will study and live with multiple cultures and languages.
- Professionals will become more entrepreneurial and innovative in their approach to career design.

As we have discussed, turbulent times create both threats and opportunities for members of the profession. How should individual members shape their careers to fit into future scenarios? What steps can be taken now to secure a position in the future?

- Be visionary and manage your own career. Make a conscious shift of mind so as not to rely on traditional practice roles. Be open to future opportunities.
- Build a portfolio of skills that will position you for future career changes. There will be a need for people who can increase productivity of resources and who can develop cost-effective solutions to problems.
- If you are not already techno-literate, you should quickly move in that direction. Be able to design organizational and consumer programs that use multiple multimedia approaches and formats. Since 1984, the numbers of workers who use a computer in their jobs has risen from 25 percent to more than 50 percent.
- Be adept at building relationships, both internal and external, to the profession. A distinct competitive advantage will come to those who know how to network and connect with consumers, experts, and information.
- Become an expert at accessing, acquiring, disseminating, and evaluating knowledge. It is our key strategic resource.

- Consider working at the periphery of our profession and related professions. Develop multi- and transdisciplinary skills. Seek out areas in nursing, physical therapy, therapeutic recreation, and medicine, to name a few, and assume personal responsibility for developing entry-level skills to add to your portfolio.

Our entire professional infrastructure is changing at a rate unequaled in the past. We must shift our minds individually and collectively to move with changes in our environment. The future belongs to those who can dream and then translate those dreams into reality.

CONCLUSION

The dietetic profession is changing and becoming increasingly responsive to the needs of consumers and the marketplace. Because of changes in population demographics, increasing globalization, and changes in the health care system, the profession is faced with challenges but also great opportunities. Planning toward and preparing for the future through developing technical and personal skills, such as acquisition and dissemination of knowledge, leadership qualities, and willingness to change, will serve the dietitian well into the next century.

DEFINITIONS

Allied Health Professions Health care practitioners providing services that supplement and assist those in direct health care.

Demographics Population statistics relating to characteristics of those making up the population such as births, deaths, and ages that are used in scientific studies.

Globalization Process of becoming worldwide in scope or business or practice.

Multicultural Term pertaining to different cultures as among countries, and populations.

Multidisciplinary Describing a collection of several disciplines either similar or diverse in nature.

REFERENCES

1. Parks S, Bajus B. President's page: challenging the future—an evolving global perspective for the profession. *J Am Diet Assoc.* 1994;94:782–784.
2. Parks S. Challenging the future: impact of information technology on dietetic practice, education, and research. *J Am Diet Assoc.* 1994;94:202–204.

3. Pew Health Professions Commission. *Critical Challenges: Revitalizing the Health Professions for the Twenty-First Century.* San Francisco: USFS Center for Health Professions; 1995.

4. *223 Hot, New Future Business Trends for the 1990s.* A special report prepared exclusively for subscribers to John Naisbitt's Trend Letter. Washington, DC: The Global Network; 1993.

5. Kane M, Cohen A, Smith E, Lewis C, et al. 1995 commission on dietetic registration dietetics practice audit. *J Am Diet Assoc.* 1996;96:1292–1301.

6. Balch G. Employers' perceptions of the roles of dietetic practitioners: challenges to service and opportunities to thrive. *J Am Diet Assoc.* 1996;96:1301–1305.

7. Cleveland H. *The Knowledge Executive.* New York: Truman Talley Books/EP Dutton; 1989.

8. Pew Health Professions Commission. *Healthy America: Practitioners for 2005.* Durham, NC: Pew Health Professions Commission; 1991.

9. Finn S. Opportunities for dietitians—1996 and beyond. *Diet Curr.* 1996;23:11–14.

10. Pew Health Professions Commission: *Health Professions Education for the Future: Schools in Service to the Nation.* San Francisco: Pew Health Professions Commission; 1993.

11. Career management: exploring the options. *ADA Courier.* 1996;35(6):3–4.

12. Technomic, Inc. *Executive Summary Foodservice Opportunity Assessment for Registered Dietitians and Dietetic Technicians Registered.* Report to The American Dietetic Association; 1994.

13. Varian H. The next generation information manager. *Educom Rev.* 1997:12–14.

14. Noam E. On the future of the university. *Educom Rev.* July/August 1996:38–41.

15. Cerf V. Opportunities for innovation—Vint Cerf on the World Wide Web: part II. *Educom Rev.* 1996:42–77.

16. Halal W. Rise of the knowledge entrepreneur. *Futurist.* November/December 1996: 13–16.

17. Todhunter EN. Our profession moves ahead. *J Am Diet Assoc.* 1957;33:681–684.

18. Joyce P, Voytek K. Navigating the new workplace. *Voc Educ J.* 1996.

Code of Ethics for the Profession of Dietetics

(Adopted by House of Delegates,
The American Dietetic Association, October 1987)

Preamble

The American Dietetic Association and its credentialing agency, the Commission on Dietetic Registration, believe it is in the best interests of the profession and the public it serves that a Code of Ethics provide guidance to dietetic practitioners in their professional practice and conduct. Dietetic practitioners have voluntarily developed a Code of Ethics to reflect the ethical principles guiding the dietetic profession and to outline commitments and obligations of the dietetic practitioner to self, client, society, and the profession.

The purpose of the Commission on Dietetic Registration is to assist in protecting the nutritional health, safety, and welfare of the public by establishing and enforcing qualifications for dietetic registration and for issuing voluntary credentials to individuals who have attained those qualifications. The Commission has adopted this Code to apply to individuals who hold these credentials.

The Ethics Code applies in its entirety to members of The American Dietetic Association who are Registered Dietitians (RDs) or Dietetic Technicians Registered (DTRs). Except for sections solely dealing with the credential, the Code applies to all American Dietetic Association members who are not RDs or DTRs. Except for aspects solely dealing with membership, the Code applies to all RDs and DTRs who are not ADA members. All of the aforementioned are referred to in the Code as "dietetic practitioners."

Principles

1. The dietetic practitioner provides professional services with objectivity and with respect for the unique needs and values of individuals.
2. The dietetic practitioner avoids discrimination against other individuals on the basis of race, creed, religion, sex, age, and national origin.

3. The dietetic practitioner fulfills professional commitments in good faith.
4. The dietetic practitioner conducts himself/herself with honesty, integrity, and fairness.
5. The dietetic practitioner remains free of conflict of interest while fulfilling the objectives and maintaining the integrity of the dietetic profession.
6. The dietetic practitioner maintains confidentiality of information.
7. The dietetic practitioner practices dietetics based on scientific principles and current information.
8. The dietetic practitioner assumes responsibility and accountability for personal competence in practice.
9. The dietetic practitioner recognizes and exercises professional judgment within the limits of his/her qualifications and seeks counsel or makes referrals as appropriate.
10. The dietetic practitioner provides sufficient information to enable clients to make their own informed decisions.
11. The dietetic practitioner who wishes to inform the public and colleagues of his/her services does so by using factual information. The dietetic practitioner does not advertise in a false or misleading manner.
12. The dietetic practitioner promotes or endorses products in a manner that is neither false nor misleading.
13. The dietetic practitioner permits use of his/her name for the purpose of certifying that dietetic services have been rendered only if he/she has provided or supervised the provision of those services.
14. The dietetic practitioner accurately presents professional qualifications and credentials.
    a. The dietetic practitioner uses "RD" or "registered dietitian" only when registration is current and authorized by the Commission on Dietetic Registration.
    b. The dietetic practitioner provides accurate information and complies with all requirements of the Commission on Dietetic Registration program in which he/she is seeking initial or continued credentials from the Commission on Dietetic Registration.
    c. The dietetic practitioner is subject to disciplinary action for aiding another person in violating any Commission on Dietetic Registration requirements or aiding another person in representing himself/herself as an RD or DTR when he/she is not.
15. The dietetic practitioner presents substantiated information and interprets controversial information without personal bias, recognizing that legitimate differences of opinion exist.
16. The dietetic practitioner makes all reasonable effort to avoid bias in any kind of professional evaluation. The dietetic practitioner provides objec-

tive evaluation of candidates for professional association memberships, awards, scholarships, or job advancements.

17. The dietetic practitioner voluntarily withdraws from professional practice under the following circumstances:

    a. The dietetic practitioner has engaged in any substance abuse that could affect his/her practice.

    b. The dietetic practitioner has been adjudged by a court to be mentally incompetent.

    c. The dietetic practitioner has an emotional or mental disability that affects his/her practice in a manner that could harm the client.

18. The dietetic practitioner complies with all applicable laws and regulations concerning the profession. The dietetic practitioner is subject to disciplinary action under the following circumstances:

    a. The dietetic practitioner has been convicted of a crime under the laws of the United States which is a felony or a misdemeanor, an essential element of which is dishonesty and which is related to the practice of the profession.

    b. The dietetic practitioner has been disciplined by a state and at least one of the grounds for the discipline is the same or subtantially equivalent to these principles.

    c. The dietetic practitioner has committed an act of misfeasance or malfeasance which is directly related to the practice of the profession as determined by a court of competent jurisdiction, a licensing board, or an agency of a governmental body.

19. The dietetic practitioner accepts the obligation to protect society and the profession by upholding the Code of Ethics for the Profession of Dietetics and by reporting alleged violations of the Code through the defined review process of The American Dietetic Association and its credentialing agency, the Commission on Dietetic Registration.

(Refer to the following reference for the full text of the "Procedures for Review Process"): *J Am Diet Assoc*. 1988;88:1592–1596.

Standards of Education (1997)

Standard One: The mission statement or philosophy and measurable goals for the program shall provide guidance to the program.

Principle: Philosophical premises underlie the establishment and nature of any planned program. This philosophical basis determines the goals to which a program is directed. Identification, articulation, and ongoing re-examination of the philosophy and goals of an educational program enable the program faculty to progress, and the program to develop in an efficient, planned manner.
Criterion:

1. The mission statement or philosophy of the program shall reflect the environment in which the program exists and be compatible with the mission statement or philosophy of the sponsoring institution and the Standards of Practice of the American Dietetic Association.
2. Measurable goals for the program shall reflect the mission statement or philosophy and are the basis for evaluation of program effectiveness.

Standard Two: A program shall be accountable to its students.

Principle: Fair, equitable, and considerate treatment of both prospective students and those enrolled in an educational program will be incorporated into all aspects of the program.
Criterion:

1. A current and accurate description of the program shall be available to prospective students.
2. A current and accurate description of the program shall be available to enrolled students in a bulletin, catalog, manual, or other program materials.

3. Admission requirements and procedures shall protect student civil rights and comply with institutional equal opportunity programs.
4. Written program policies and procedures shall be available to students enrolled in the program, protect the rights of students, and be consistent with current institutional practice.
5. Program length and tuition and fees shall be based on the program goals, conform to commonly accepted practice in higher education, and be consistent with the competence students are expected to achieve.

Standard Three. Resources available to the program shall be identified and their contribution to the program described.

Principle: Resources are necessary for effective education to occur in a dietetics education program. Resources include competent and sufficient administrators and faculty, support personnel, and adequate services to provide for the planned education of students.

Criterion:

1. The program shall provide evidence that the administrative and financial support, learning resources, physical facilities, and support services needed to accomplish the measurable goals for the program are available.
2. The program shall seek advice on an ongoing basis from individuals or groups outside the program.
3. Each accredited/approved program shall designate a Program Director, who is employed by the sponsoring institution.
4. Documented qualifications for a Program Director shall include credentialing as a Registered Dietitian by the Commission on Dietetic Registration and a minimum of a Master's Degree.
5. Individual faculty shall demonstrate competence appropriate to their teaching responsibilities. In addition, faculty in regionally accredited colleges and universities shall meet the institution's criteria for appointment. Faculty/ preceptors in supervised practice programs shall be credentialed or licensed as appropriate for the area they are supervising students or demonstrate equivalent education and experience.
6. Faculty/student ratio for the supervised practice component of a program shall reflect the need for individualized instruction. A program shall justify its faculty/student ratio by demonstrating where, how, and to what extent individualized instruction takes place.
7. Facilities used for supervised practice shall provide learning experiences compatible with the competencies students are expected to achieve.
8. Written agreements signed by administration with appropriate authority shall be in effect and on file which delineate the responsibility between the sponsoring institution and affiliating institutions, organizations, and/or agencies.

Standard Four. The curriculum shall provide for attainment of the expected competence of the program graduate.

Principle: An entry-level dietetics education program is based on expected knowledge, skills, and competencies required to practice dietetics as defined by The American Dietetic Association. The curriculum sequentially builds knowledge, skills, and competencies for each student. The curriculum will vary with the program environment, the type of program, measurable goals and outcomes for the program, and student needs.
Criterion:

1. The curriculum shall be consistent with the mission statement or philosophy and measurable goals for the program.
2. The curriculum shall be based upon the required Foundation Knowledge and Skills and/or Competency Statements for credentialing eligibility as a Dietetic Technician Registered or Registered Dietitian.
3. For the supervised practice component of dietitians education programs, the curriculum shall include a minimum of one emphasis area in addition to the core competencies.
4. Both didactic and practice-related learning experiences shall be included in the curriculum in accordance with the type of program to develop communication, collaboration, problem solving, and critical thinking skills.
5. Planned learning experiences shall be offered in a logical progression from introductory to the expected competence of program graduates.
6. The program shall document that planned learning experiences provide for attainment of the expected competence described in measurable goals for the program.
7. Students in supervised practice programs shall not routinely replace employees except for planned professional staff experiences.
8. A minimum of 900 clock hours for dietitians programs including program emphasis areas and 450 clock hours for technician programs is required for supervised practice.
9. The curriculum for all programs shall include experiences with other disciplines and exposure to a variety of settings, individuals, and groups.

Standard Five. A systematic approach shall be used in managing and evaluating the program.

Principle: An education program requires the application of sound management principles. Systematic and continuous internal and external evaluation provides necessary feedback to ensure that program goals continue to be appropriate and that goals are attained.

Criterion:

1. The sponsoring institution and/or program shall have policies that support effective program management.
2. The program shall be integrated within the administrative structure of the sponsoring institution.
3. The responsibilities of the Program Director shall include the assessment, planning, implementation, and evaluation critical to an effective program. The Program Director shall have the authority to effectively manage the program.
4. Administrators, faculty, students, and other appropriate constituencies shall participate in systematic planning, implementation, and evaluation of the program on a regular and continuing basis.
5. Student progress shall be measured using a variety of strategies during and at the conclusion of the program to verify competence.
6. Outcome measures for program graduates shall be developed and evaluated for achievement of measurable goals. One outcome measure shall be the pass rate of first-time test takers on the Registration Examination. If the pass rate is less than 89% for first-time test takers, a plan of action for improvement shall be provided.
7. Continuous program evaluation shall address achievement of measurable goals for the program. Data shall be analyzed to identify the extent to which measurable goals for the program are being achieved. Appropriate corrective action shall be taken when measurable goals for the program are not being achieved.
8. Short- and long-term plans for management of the program shall be delineated based on evaluation of the program.
9. Dietetic Internship Programs certified by USDE for Title IV, Higher Education Act of 1965 as amended (HEA) funding shall document compliance with Title IV, HEA responsibilities, including audits, program reviews, monitoring default rates, and other requirements as necessary. If the program's default rate exceeds the federal threshold (currently 20%), a default reduction plan as required by USDE shall be provided.

Source: Reprinted with permission from *Accreditation/Approval Manual for Dietetics Education Programs,* 4th edition, © 1997, American Dietetic Association.

Didactic Component of Dietetic Education Programs

Foundation Knowledge and Skills for Didactic Component of Entry-Level Dietitian Education Programs

The entry-level dietitian is knowledgeable in the eight areas listed below. The foundation knowledge and skills precede achievement of the core and emphasis area(s) competencies, which identify the performance level expected upon completion of the supervised practice program

Foundation learning is divided as follows: basic knowledge of a topic, working or indepth knowledge of a topic as it applies to the profession of dietetics, and ability to demonstrate the skill at a level that can be developed further. To successfully achieve the foundation knowledge and skills, graduates must have demonstrated the ability to communicate and collaborate, solve problems, and apply critical thinking skills.

A. COMMUNICATIONS

Graduates will have *basic knowledge about:*
A.1.1. Negotiation techniques
A.1.2. Lay and technical writing
A.1.3. Media presentations

Graduates will have *working knowledge of:*
A.2.1. Interpersonal communication skills
A.2.2. Counseling theory and methods
A.2.3. Interviewing techniques
A.2.4. Educational theory and techniques
A.2.5. Concepts of human and group dynamics

A.2.6.   Public speaking
A.2.7.   Educational materials development

Graduates will have *demonstrated the ability to:*
A.3.1.   Present an educational session for a group
A.3.2.   Counsel individuals on nutrition
A.3.3   Demonstrate a variety of documentation methods
A.3.4.   Explain a public policy position regarding dietetics
A.3.5.   Use current information technologies
A.3.6.   Work effectively as a team member

B.   PHYSICAL AND BIOLOGICAL SCIENCES

Graduates will have *basic knowledge about:*
B.1.1.   Exercise physiology

Graduates will have *working knowledge of:*
B.2.1.   Organic chemistry
B.2.2.   Biochemistry
B.2.3.   Physiology
B.2.4.   Microbiology
B.2.5.   Nutrient metabolism
B.2.6.   Pathophysiology related to nutrition care
B.2.7.   Fluid and electrolyte requirements
B.2.8.   Pharmacology: Nutrient-nutrient and drug-nutrient interaction

Graduates will have *demonstrated the ability to:*
B.3.1.   Interpret medical terminology
B.3.2.   Interpret laboratory parameters relating to nutrition
B.3.3.   Apply microbiological and chemical considerations to process controls

C.   SOCIAL SCIENCES

Graduates will *basic knowledge about:*
C.1.1.   Public policy development

Graduates will have *working knowledge of:*
C.2.1.   Psychology
C.2.2.   Health behaviors and educational needs
C.2.3.   Economics and nutrition

D. RESEARCH

Graduates will have *basic knowledge about:*
D.1.1.   Research methodologies
D.1.2.   Needs assessments
D.1.3.   Outcomes based research

Graduates will have *working knowledge of:*
D.2.1.   Scientific method
D.2.2.   Quality improvement methods

Graduates will have *demonstrated the ability to:*
D.3.1.   Interpret current research
D.3.2.   Interpret basic statistics

E. FOOD

Graduates will have *basic knowledge about:*
E.1.1.   Food technology
E.1.2.   Biotechnology
E.1.3.   Culinary techniques

Graduates will have *working knowledge of:*
E.2.1.   Sociocultural and ethnic food consumption issues and trends for various consumers
E.2.2.   Food safety and sanitation
E.2.3.   Food delivery systems
E.2.4.   Food and non-food procurement
E.2.5.   Availability of nutrition programs in the community
E.2.6.   Formulation of local, state, and national food security policy
E.2.7.   Food production systems
E.2.8.   Environmental issues related to food
E.2.9.   Role of food in promotion of a healthy lifestyle
E.2.10. Promotion of pleasurable eating
E.2.11. Food and nutrition laws/regulations/policies
E.2.12. Food availability and access for the individual, family, and community
E.2.13. Applied sensory evaluation of food

Graduates will have *demonstrated the ability to:*
E.3.1.   Calculate and interpret nutrient composition of foods
E.3.2.   Translate nutrition needs into menus for individuals and groups

E.3.3.   Determine recipe/formula proportions and modifications for volume food production

E.3.4.   Write specifications for food and foodservice equipment

E.3.5.   Apply food science knowledge to functions of ingredients in food

E.3.6.   Demonstrate basic food preparation and presentation skills

E.3.7.   Modify recipe/formula for individual or group dietary needs

F. NUTRITION

Graduates will have *basic knowledge about:*

F.1.1.   Alternative nutrition and herbal therapies

F.1.2.   Evolving methods of assessing health status

Graduates will have *working knowledge of:*

F.2.1.   Influence of age, growth, and normal development on nutritional requirements

F.2.2.   Nutrition and metabolism

F.2.3.   Assessment and treatment of nutritional health risks

F.2.4.   Medical nutrition therapy, including alternative feeding modalities, chronic diseases, dental health, mental health, and eating disorders

F.2.5.   Strategies to assess need for adaptive feeding techniques and equipment

F.2.6.   Health promotion and disease prevention theories and guidelines

F.2.7.   Influence of socioeconomic, cultural, and psychological factors on food and nutrition behavior

Graduates will have *demonstrated the ability to:*

F.3.1.   Calculate and/or define diets for common conditions, i.e., health conditions addressed by health promotion/disease prevention activities or chronic diseases of the general population, e.g., hypertension, obesity, diabetes, diverticular disease

F.3.2.   Screen individuals for nutritional risk

F.3.3.   Collect pertinent information for comprehensive nutrition assessments

F.3.4.   Determine nutrient requirements across the lifespan, i.e., infants through geriatrics and a diversity of people, culture, and religions

F.3.5.   Measure, calculate, and interpret body composition data

F.3.6.   Calculate enteral and parenteral nutrition formulations

G. MANAGEMENT

Graduates will have *basic knowledge about:*

G.1.1.   Program planning, monitoring, and evaluation

G.1.2.   Strategic management

G.1.3. Facility management
G.1.4. Organizational change theory
G.1.5. Risk management

Graduates will have *working knowledge of:*
G.2.1. Management theories
G.2.2. Human resource management, including labor relations
G.2.3. Materials management
G.2.4. Financial management, including accounting principles
G.2.5. Quality improvement
G.2.6. Information management
G.2.7. Systems theory
G.2.8. Marketing theory and techniques
G.2.9. Diversity issues

Graduates will have *demonstrated the ability to:*
G.3.1. Determine costs of services/operation
G.3.2. Prepare a budget
G.3.3. Interpret financial data
G.3.4. Apply marketing principles

H. HEALTH CARE SYSTEMS

Graduates will have *basic knowledge about:*
H.1.1. Health care policy and administration
H.1.2. Health care delivery systems

Graduates will have *working knowledge of:*
H.2.1. Current reimbursement issues
H.2.2. Ethics of care

Foundation Knowledge and Skills for Didactic Component of Entry-Level Dietetic Technician Education Programs

The entry-level dietetic technician is knowledgeable in the eight areas listed below. The foundation knowledge and skills may be integrated with achievement of the competencies, which identify the performance level expected upon completion of the supervised practice component of the program.

Foundation learning is divided as follows: basic knowledge of a topic, working or indepth knowledge of a topic as it applies to the profession of dietetics, and ability to demonstrate the skill at a level that can be developed further. To successfully achieve the foundation knowledge and skills, graduates must have demonstrated the ability to communicate and collaborate, solve problems, and apply critical thinking skills.

A.   COMMUNICATIONS

Graduates will have *basic knowledge about:*
A.1.1.   Counseling theory and methods
A.1.2.   Methods of teaching
A.1.3.   Concepts of human and group dynamics
A.1.4.   Educational materials development

Graduates will have *working knowledge of:*
A.2.1.   Interpersonal communication skills
A.2.2.   Interviewing techniques
A.2.3.   Basic mathematics
A.2.4.   Written communication

Graduates will have *demonstrated the ability to:*
A.3.1.   Present an educational session for target groups
A.3.2.   Counsel individuals on nutrition for common conditions, i.e., health conditions addressed by health promotion/disease prevention activities or chronic diseases of the general population, e.g., hypertension, obesity, diabetes, diverticular disease
A.3.3.   Speak in front of a group
A.3.4.   Demonstrate a variety of documentation methods
A.3.5.   Use current information technologies
A.3.6.   Work effectively as a team member

B.   PHYSICAL AND BIOLOGICAL SCIENCES

Graduates will have *basic knowledge about:*
B.1.1.   Applied concepts of chemistry

B.1.2. Applied concepts of physiology
B.1.3. Applied concepts of microbiology
B.1.4. Nutrient-nutrient and drug-nutrient interactions

Graduates will have *demonstrated the ability to:*
B.3.1. Interpret medical terminology
B.3.2. Interpret laboratory parameters relating to nutrition
B.3.3. Apply microbiological and chemical considerations to recipe development

C. SOCIAL SCIENCES

Graduates will have *basic knowledge about:*
C.1.1. Psychology/sociology
C.1.2. Health behaviors and educational needs
C.1.3. Economics and nutrition
C.1.4. Public policy issues

D. RESEARCH

Graduates will have *basic knowledge about:*
D.1.1. Interpretation of current research
D.1.2. Needs assessment
D.1.3. Basic statistics
D.1.4. Quality improvement

E. FOOD

Graduates will have *basic knowledge about:*
E.1.1. Sociocultural and ethnic food consumption issues and trends for various consumers
E.1.2. Food technology issues
E.1.3. Availability of nutrition programs in the community
E.1.4. Environmental issues related to food
E.1.5. Promotion of pleasurable eating
E.1.6. Food availability and access for the individual, the family, and the community
E.1.7. Food and nutrition laws/regulations/policies
E.1.8. Role of food in promotion of a healthy lifestyle

Graduates will have *working knowledge of:*
E.2.1. Basic concepts and techniques of food preparation

E.2.2. Applied sensory evaluation of food
E.2.3. Food production systems
E.2.4. Food delivery systems
E.2.5. Food and non-food procurement

Graduates will have *demonstrated the ability to:*
E.3.1. Calculate and analyze nutrient composition of foods
E.3.2. Translate nutrition needs into means for individuals and groups
E.3.3. Determine recipe/formula proportions and modifications for volume food production
E.3.4. Apply functions of ingredients in food preparation
E.3.5. Write specifications for food and equipment
E.3.6. Assist with food demonstrations
E.3.7. Apply food safety and sanitation techniques

F. NUTRITION

Graduates will have *basic knowledge about:*
F.1.1. Fundamentals of nutrition and metabolism
F.1.2. Assessment of health risks
F.1.3. Influence of socioeconomic, cultural, and psychological factors on food and nutrition behavior
F.1.4. Health promotion and disease prevention theories
F.1.5. Strategies to assess need for adaptive feeding techniques and equipment

Graduates will have *working knowledge of:*
F.2.1. Influence of age, growth, and normal development on nutrition requirements
F.2.2. Applied clinical nutrition

Graduates will have *demonstrated the ability to:*
F.3.1. Calculate diets for common conditions, i.e., health conditions addressed by health promotion/disease prevention activities for chronic diseases of the general population, e.g., hypertension, obesity, diabetes, diverticular disease
F.3.2. Screen individuals for nutritional risk
F.3.3. Determine nutrient requirements across the lifespan, i.e., infants through geriatrics and a diversity of people, culture, and religions
F.3.4. Measure and calculate body composition
F.3.5. Calculate basic enteral and parenteral nutrition formulas

G. MANAGEMENT

Graduates will have *basic knowledge about:*
G.1.1.   Program planning, monitoring, and evaluation
G.1.2.   Marketing theory and techniques
G.1.3.   Systems theory
G.1.4.   Labor relations
G.1.5.   Materials management
G.1.6.   Financial management
G.1.7.   Facility management
G.1.8.   Quality improvement
G.1.9.   Risk management
G.1.10. Diversity issues

Graduates will have *working knowledge of:*
G.2.1.   Applied management theories
G.2.2.   Applied human resources management
G.2.3.   Information management

Graduates will have *demonstrated the ability to:*
G.3.1.   Collect and interpret information
G.3.2.   Determine costs of services/operations

H. HEALTH CARE SYSTEMS

Graduates will have *basic knowledge about:*
H.1.1.   Current reimbursement issues
H.1.2.   Health care policy
H.1.3.   Health care delivery systems

Graduates will have *working knowledge of:*
H.2.1.   Ethics of care

Source: Reprinted with permission from *Accreditation/Approval Manual for Dietetics Education Programs,* 4th edition, pp. 45–48 and 55–47, © 1997, American Dietetic Association.

Supervised Practice Component of Dietetic Education Programs

Competency Statements for the Supervised Practice Component of Entry-Level Dietitian Education Programs

Competency statements specify what every dietitian should be able to do at the beginning of his or her practice career. The core competency statements build on appropriate knowledge and skills necessary for the entry-level practitioner to perform reliably at the verb level indicated. One or more of the emphasis areas should be added to the core competencies so that a supervised practice program can prepare graduates for identified market needs. Thus, all entry-level dietitians will have the core competencies and additional competencies according to the emphasis area(s) completed.

The minimum performance level for the competency is indicated by the action verb used at the beginning of the statement. The action verbs reflect four levels of performance. The higher level of performance assumes the ability to perform at the lower level:

1. *assist*—independent performance under supervision, or
   participate—take part in team activities;
2. *perform*—able to initiate activities without direct supervision, or
   conduct—activities performed independently;
3. *consult*—able to perform specialized functions that are discrete delegated activities intended to improve the work of others, or
   supervise—able to oversee daily operation of a unit including personnel, resource utilization, and environmental issues; or, coordinate and direct the activities of a team or project workgroup;
4. *manage*—able to play, organize, and direct an organization unit through actual or simulated experiences, including knowing what questions to ask.

If the verb "manage" is used, it assumes that the student will progress from "supervise" or "perform/do" the activity while in the program. (Note: the perform level is indicated in parentheses at the end of the statement to which it applies.) Students may demonstrate that they can manage or supervise through such activities as quality improvement audits, systems review, or directing an activity coordinating others.

Core Competencies for Dietitians (CD)

Upon completion of the supervised practice component of dietitian education, all graduates will be able to do the following:

CD1.   Perform ethically in accordance with the values of The American Dietetic Association

CD2.   Refer clients/patients to other dietetics professionals or disciplines when a situation is beyond one's level of area of competence (perform)

CD3.   Participate in professional activities

CD4.   Perform self-assessment and participate in professional development

CD5.   Participate in legislative and public policy processes as they affect food, food security, and nutrition

CD6.   Use current technologies for information and communication activities (perform)

CD7.   Supervise documentation of nutrition assessment and interventions

CD8.   Provide dietetics education in supervised practice settings (perform)

CD9.   Supervise counseling, education, and/or other interventions in health promotion/disease prevention for patient/clients needing medical nutrition therapy for common conditions, e.g., hypertension, obesity, diabetes, and diverticular disease

CD10.   Supervise education and training for target groups

CD11.   Develop and review educational materials for target populations (perform)

CD12.   Participate in the use of mass media for community-based food and nutrition programs

CD13.   Interpret and incorporate new scientific knowledge into practice (perform)

CD14.   Supervise quality improvement, including systems and customer satisfaction, for dietetics service and/or practice

CD15.   Develop and measure outcomes for food and nutrition services and practice (perform)

CD16. Participate in organizational change and planning and goal-setting processes

CD17. Participate in business or operating plan development

CD18. Supervise the collection and processing of financial data

CD19. Perform marketing functions

CD20. Participate in human resources functions

CD21. Participate in facility management, including equipment selection and design/redesign of work units

CD22. Supervise the integration of financial, human, physical, and material resources and services

CD23. Supervise production of food that meets nutrition guidelines, cost parameters, and consumer acceptance

CD24. Supervise development and/or modification of recipes/formulas

CD25. Supervise translation of nutrition into foods/menus for target populations

CD26. Supervise design of menus as indicated by the patient's/client's health status

CD27. Participate in applied sensory evaluation of food and nutrition products

CD28. Supervise procurement, distribution, and service within delivery systems

CD29. Manage safety and sanitation issues related to food and nutrition

CD30. Supervise nutrition screening of individual patients/clients

CD31. Supervise nutrition assessment of individual patients/clients with common medical conditions, e.g., hypertension, obesity, diabetes, diverticular disease

CD32. Assess nutritional status of individual patients/clients with complex medical conditions, i.e., more complicated health conditions in select populations, e.g., renal disease, multi-system organ failure, trauma

CD33. Manage the normal nutrition needs of individuals across the lifespan, i.e., infants through geriatrics and a diversity of people, cultures, and religions

CD34. Design and implement nutrition care plans as indicated by the patient's/client's health status (perform)

CD35. Manage monitoring of patient's/client's food and/or nutrient intake

CD36. Select, implement, and evaluate standard enteral and parenteral nutrition regimens, i.e., in a medically stable patient to meet nutritional requirements where recommendations/adjustments involve primarily macronutrients (perform)

CD37.   Develop and implement transitional feeding plans, i.e., conversion from one form of nutrition support to another, e.g., total parenteral nutrition to tube feeding to oral diet (perform)

CD38.   Coordinate and modify nutrition care activities among caregivers (perform)

CD39.   Conduct nutrition care component of interdisciplinary team conferences to discuss patient/client treatment and discharge planning

CD40.   Refer patients/clients to appropriate community services for general health and nutrition needs and to other primary care providers as appropriate (perform)

CD41.   Conduct general health assessment, e.g., blood pressure, vital signs (perform)

CD42.   Supervise screening of the nutritional status of the population and/or community groups

CD43.   Conduct assessment of the nutritional status of the population and/or community groups

CD44.   Provide nutrition care for population across the lifespan, i.e., infants through geriatrics, and a diversity of people, cultures, and religions (perform)

CD45.   Conduct community-based health promotion/disease prevention programs

CD46.   Participate in community-based food and nutrition program development and evaluation

CD47.   Supervise community-based food and nutrition programs

Competency Statements for Entry-Level Dietitian Education Programs Emphasis Areas

The core competencies ensure that everyone enrolled in a coordinated program or dietetic internship program has learning experiences reflecting the breadth of dietetics practice. The core provides the broad base of diverse experiences necessary for the future career mobility illustrated in the model for dietetics practice.

All dietitian education supervised practice programs must offer at least one emphasis area. The emphasis areas are not intended to prepare specialists or advanced level practitioners as defined for credentialing purposes. Competencies for each emphasis area build on the core competencies and are designed to begin to develop the depth necessary for future proficiency in that area of dietetics practice. More experience in at least one area provides a model for learning throughout one's professional life.

For establishing an emphasis area, the program has the following options:

- Use one or more of the four defined emphasis areas; or,
- Develop a general emphasis by selecting a minimum of seven competency statements, relevant to program mission and goals, with at least one from each of the four defined emphasis areas. The selected competencies should build on the core competencies. General emphasis does not mean achievement of all competencies from all emphasis areas; or,
- Create a unique emphasis area with a minimum of seven competency statements, based on environmental resources and identified needs.

Four emphasis areas and corresponding competencies for each emphasis are identified below.

Nutrition Therapy Emphasis Competencies (NT)

NT1.   Supervise nutrition assessment of individual patients/clients with complex medical conditions, i.e., more complicated health conditions in select populations, e.g., renal disease, multi-system organ failure, trauma

NT2.   Integrate pathophysiology into medical nutrition therapy recommendations (perform)

NT3.   Supervise design through evaluation of nutrition care plan for patients/clients with complex medical conditions, i.e., more complicated health conditions in select populations, e.g., renal disease, multi-system organ failure, trauma

NT4.   Select, monitor, and evaluate complex enteral and parenteral nutrition regimens, i.e., more complicated health conditions in select populations, e.g., renal disease, multi-system organ failure, trauma (perform)

NT5.   Supervise development and implementation of transition feeding plans from the inpatient to home setting

NT6.   Conduct counseling and education for patients/clients with complex needs, i.e., more complicated health conditions in select populations, e.g., renal disease, multi-system organ failure, trauma

NT7.   Perform basic physical assessment

NT8.   Participate in nasoenteric feeding tube placement and care

NT9.   Participate in waivered point-of-care testing, such as blood glucose monitoring

NT10.   Participate in the care of patients/clients requiring adaptive feeding devices

NT11.   Manage clinical nutrition services

Community Emphasis Competencies (CO)

CO1.   Manage nutrition care for population groups across the lifespan

CO2.   Conduct community-based food and nutrition program outcome assessment/evaluation

CO3.   Develop community-based food and nutrition programs (perform)

CO4.   Participate in nutrition surveillance and monitoring of communities

CO5.   Participate in community-based research

CO6.   Participate in food and nutrition policy development and evaluation based on community needs and resources

CO7.   Consult with organizations regarding food access for target populations

CO8.   Develop a health promotion/disease prevention intervention project (perform)

CO9.   Participate in waivered point-of-care testing, such as hematocrit and cholesterol levels

Foodservice Systems Management Emphasis Competencies (FS)

FS1.   Manage development and/or modification of recipes/formulas

FS2.   Manage menu development for target populations

FS3.   Managed applied sensory evaluation of food and nutrition products

FS4.   Manage production of food that meets nutrition guidelines, cost parameters, and consumer acceptance

FS5.   Manage procurement, distribution, and service within delivery systems

FS6.   Manage the integration of financial, human, physical, and material resources

FS7.   Manage safety and sanitation issues related to food and nutrition

FS8.   Supervise customer satisfaction systems for dietetics services and/or practice

FS9.   Supervise marketing functions

FS10.   Supervise human resource functions

FS11.   Perform operations analysis

Business/Entrepreneur Emphasis Competencies (BE)

BE1. Perform organization and strategic planning
BE2. Develop business or operating plan (perform)
BE3. Supervise procurement of resources
BE4. Manage the integration of financial, human, physical, and material resources
BE5. Supervise organizational change process
BE6. Supervise coordination of services
BE7. Supervise marketing functions

Competency Statements for the Supervised Practice Component of Entry-Level Dietetic Technician Education Programs

Competency statements specify what every dietetic technician should be able to do at the beginning of his or her practice career. The competency statements build on appropriate knowledge and skills necessary for the entry-level practitioner to perform reliably at the level indicated.

The minimum performance level for the competency is indicated by the action verb used at the beginning of the statement. The action verbs reflect four levels of performance. The higher level of performance assumes the ability to perform at the lower level:

1. *assist*—independent performance under supervision, or
   participate—take part in team activities;
2. *perform*—able to initiate activities without direct supervision, or
   conduct—activities performed independently;
3. *consult*—able to perform specialized functions that are discrete delegated activities intended to improve the work of others, or
   supervise—able to oversee daily operation of a unit including personnel, resource utilization, and environmental issues; or, coordinate and direct the activities of a team or project workgroup;
4. *manage*—able to plan, organize, and direct an organization unit through actual or simulated experiences including knowing what questions to ask.

If the verb "supervise" is used, it assumes that the graduate will progress from "perform/do" the activity while in the program. (Note: the perform level is indicated in parentheses at the end of the statement to which it applies.) Students may demonstrate that they can supervise an activity rather than an individual, through such activities as quality improvement audits or coordinating the work of others.

Competencies for Dietetic Technicians (DT)

Upon completion of the supervised practice component of a dietetic technician education program, the graduate will be able to do the following:

DT1.   Perform ethically in accordance with the values of The American Dietetic Association

DT2.   Refer clients/patients to other dietetics professionals or disciplines when a situation is beyond one's level of competence (perform)

DT3.   Participate in professional activities

DT4.   Perform self-assessment and participate in professional development

DT5.   Participate in legislative and public policy processes as they affect food, food security, and nutrition

DT6.   Use current technologies for information and communication activities (perform)

DT7.   Document nutrition screenings, assessments, and interventions (perform)

DT8.   Provide dietetics education in supervised practice settings (perform)

DT9.   Educate patient/clients in disease prevention and health promotion and medical nutrition therapy for common conditions, e.g., hypertension, obesity, diabetes, diverticular disease (perform)

DT10. Conduct education and training for target groups

DT11. Assist with development and review of educational materials for target populations

DT12. Apply new knowledge or skills to practice (perform)

DT13. Participate in quality improvement, including systems and customer satisfaction, for dietetics service and/or practice

DT14. Participate in development and measurement of outcomes for food and nutrition services and practice

DT15. Participate in organizational change and planning and goal-setting processes

DT16. Participate in development of departmental budget/operating plan

DT17. Collect and process financial data (perform)

DT18. Assist with marketing functions

DT19.   Participate in human resources functions

DT20.   Participate in facility management, including equipment selection and design/redesign of work units

DT21.   Supervise organizational unit, including financial, human, physical, and material resources and services

DT22.   Supervise production of food that meets nutrition guidelines, cost parameters, and consumer acceptance

DT23.   Develop and/or modify recipes/formulas (perform)

DT24.   Supervise translation of nutrition into foods/menus for target populations

DT25.   Design menus as indicated by the patient's/client's health status (perform)

DT26.   Participate in applied sensory evaluation of food and nutrition products

DT27.   Supervise procurement, distribution, and service within delivery systems

DT28.   Supervise safety and sanitation issues

DT29.   Perform nutrition screening of individual patients/clients

DT30.   Assess nutritional status of individual patients/clients with common medical conditions, i.e., health conditions addressed by health promotion/disease prevention activities or chronic diseases of the general population, e.g., hypertension, obesity, diabetes, diverticular disease (perform)

DT31.   Assist with nutrition assessment of individual patients/clients with complex medical conditions, i.e., more complicated health conditions in select populations, e.g., renal disease, multi-system organ failure, trauma

DT32.   Participate in the management of the normal nutrition needs of individuals across the lifespan, i.e., infants through geriatrics and a diversity of people, cultures, and religions

DT33.   Assist with design and implementation of nutrition plans as indicated by the patient's/client's health status

DT34.   Monitor patients'/clients' food and/or nutrient intake (perform)

DT35.   Participate in the selection, monitoring, and evaluation of standard enteral nutrition regimens, i.e., in a medically stable patient to meet nutritional requirements where recommendations/adjustments involve primarily macronutrients

DT36.   Implement transition feeding plans (perform)

DT37.   Participate in interdisciplinary team conferences to discuss patient/client treatment and discharge planning

DT38.   Refer patients/clients to appropriate community services for general health and nutrition needs and to other primary care providers as appropriate (perform)

DT39.   Conduct general health assessment, e.g., blood pressure, vital signs

DT40.   Conduct screening of the nutritional status of the population and/or community groups

DT41.   Assist with assessment of the nutritional status of the population and/or community groups

DT42.   Participate in nutrition care for population groups across the lifespan, i.e., infants through geriatrics and a diversity of people, cultures, and religions

DT43.   Participate in community-based or worksite health promotion/disease prevention programs

DT44.   Participate in development and evaluation of community-based food and nutrition program

DT45.   Implement and maintain community-based food and nutrition programs (perform)

Source: Reprinted with permission from *Accreditation/Approval Manual for Dietetics Education Programs,* 4th edition, pp. 49–53 and 558–560, © 1997, American Dietetic Association.

APPENDIX E

Curricula Representative of Dietetic Education Programs

I. Coordinated Undergraduate Program in Dietetics
    Southwestern Medical Center at Dallas
    The University of Texas
    Dallas, TX
    Director: Jo Anne Carson, MS, RD, LD

II. Didactic Program in Dietetics
    Department of Nutritional Sciences
    Oklahoma State University
    Stillwater, Oklahoma
    Director: Barbara Stoecker, PhD, RD, LD

III. Dietetic Technician Two-Year Program
     Columbus State Community College
     Columbus, Ohio
     Director: Louise Conway, MS, RD

IV. Generic Curriculum for Didactic Program in Dietetics and Coordinated
    Programs

V. Generic Curriculum for a Dietetic Technician Program

The University of Texas, Southwestern Medical Center
Department of Clinical Nutrition

SUGGESTED PLAN FOR MEETING PREREQUISITE COURSE REQUIREMENTS

Freshman Year	Credits	Sophomore Year	Credits
English	6	Organic Chemistry***	4
U.S. History	6	U.S. Government	3
General Chemistry	4	Texas Government	3
College Algebra	3	Microbiology**	3
Sociology OR Cultural		Nutrition	3
Anthropology	3	Speech*	3
Introductory		Physiology**	3
Psychology	3	Economics	

Additional courses are needed to meet admission requirements of 60 semester hours credit. Physical Education and/or Military Science Courses will not be counted toward this requirement.

  *Recommended but not required.
  **Some schools require Biology as a prerequisite to Physiology and
    Microbiology. Physiology of all body systems may require 8 hours.
***Many schools require 8 hours of General Chemistry before Organic Chemistry.

Junior Summer		Credits
HCS 3101	Medical Terminology	1
HCS 3311	Biochemistry (Lecture)****	3
HCS 3244	Introduction to Computer Fundamentals****	2
HCS 4308	Human Anatomy****	3
CD 3101	Orientation to Clinical Dietetics	1
		10

Junior Fall		Credits
CD 3411	Clinical Nutrition A	4
CD 3151	Clinical Nutrition A Practicum	1
CD 3310	Nutrition in Human Metabolism	3
CD 3341	Food Science****	3
AHE 3354	Health-Care Systems****	3
HCS 4103	Teaching and Learning in the Clinical Setting	1
		15

Junior Spring   *Credits*

CD 3412	Clinical Nutrition B	4
CD 3252	Clinical Nutrition B Practicum	2
CD 3422	Management in Foodservice Operations	4
HCS 3112	Biochemistry (Lab)****	1
AHE 3396	Statistics and Epidemiology****	3
		14

Senior Fall   *Credits*

CD 4313	Clinical Nutrition C	3
CD 4653	Clinical Nutrition C Practicum	6
CD 4233	Nutrition Education	2
CD 4331	Nutrition and Growth and Development	3
CD 4161	Nutrition for the Elderly	1
		15

Senior Spring   *Credits*

CD 4214	Clinical Nutrition D	2
CD 4654	Clinical Nutrition D Practicum	6
CD 4334	Nutrition in Health Care Delivery	3
CD 4332	Nutritional Care in Pediatrics	3
		14

****Equivalent course may be completed prior to admission.

Courtesy of The University of Texas, Southwestern Medical Center, Dallas, Texas.

OKLAHOMA STATE UNIVERSITY

COLLEGE OF

BACHELOR OF

HUMAN ENVIRONMENTAL SCIENCES	
SCIENCE HUMAN ENVIRONMENTAL SCIENCE	
DEGREE	
NUTRITIONAL SCIENCES	
MAJOR 5043	
(DIETETICS)	
OPTION	

GENERAL REQUIREMENTS

For students matriculating:

Academic Year	1997–98
Total hours	128*
Minimum overall grade-point average	2.25

Other GPA requirements, see below.

General Education Requirements *62* Hours		
Area	Hrs	To Be Selected From
English Composition and Oral Communication	9	ENGL 1113 or 1313; and 1213 or 1413 or 3323. (See Academic Regulation 3.5 in Catalog.) SPCH 3733 or 3793 (or 2713)
American History and Government	6	HIST 1103 POLSC 1113
Analytical and Quantitative Thought (A)	6	MATH 1483 or 1513 STAT 2013
Humanities (H)	6	PHILO 3833 or 4013 or REL 3833 or 4013 and 3 hours from lower division course designated (H).
Natural Sciences (N)	17	BIOL 1304 CHEM 1215, 1225 (or 1314, 1515) ZOOL 3204

continues

Social and Behavior Sciences (S)	6	ECON 2013 SOC 1113
International Dimension (I)	*	(See NSCI 3543 under "Major Requirements.")
Scientific Investigation (L)	12	BIOCH 3653 CHEM 3015 MICRO 2124

College/Departmental Requirements *9* Hours		
Human Environmental Sciences**	6	2.50 GPA in the following FRCD 2113 HES 1111 HES 3002
Nutritional Sciences**	3	NSCI 4643 with minimum grade of "C"

Major Requirements *53* Hours**
NSCI Courses 2111. Professional Careers in Dietetics 2114. Principles of Human Nutrition 3133. Science of Food Preparation 3213. Management in Hospital and Foodservice Systems 3223. Nutrition in the Life Cycle 3543. Food and the Human Environment 3553. Purchasing in Hospital & Foodservice Systems 4013. Experimental Foods 4323. Human Nutrition and Metabolism 4365. Quantity Food Production Management 4373. Creative Teaching of Nutrition 4573. Institution Organization & Management 4733. Community Nutrition 4853. Medical Nutrition Therapy I 4863. Medical Nutrition Therapy II ACCTG 2103 HRAD 1114 Introduction to Food Preparation
Minimum GPA 2.50

continues

Electives *4* Hours
This degree program meets the Didactic Program in Dietetics Academic Course Requirements of the American Dietetic Association

Other Requirements:

*30 upper-division hours required

**A 2.50 Major GPA is required. This includes all courses in College Departmental and Major Requirements

A grade of "C" or better is required in all NSCI 3000- and 4000-level courses

Students will be held responsible for degree requirements in effect at the time of matriculation (date of first enrollment) and any changes that are made, so long as these changes do not result in semester credit hours being added or do not delay graduation.

————————————————   ————————————————

DEAN   DEPARTMENT HEAD

HES-11

Courtesy of Oklahoma State University, Oklahoma.

COLUMBUS STATE COMMUNITY COLLEGE PLAN OF STUDY
BUSINESS AND PUBLIC SERVICES DIVISION
Effective Autumn 1996
HOSPITALITY MANAGEMENT
DIETETIC TECHNICIAN MAJOR

Name _____

Student # _____

Date Entered _____

FIRST QUARTER		CR	LEC/LAB HR	PREREQ
HOSP102	Foodservice Equipment (T)	2	1/2	
HOSP122	Sanitation and Safety (T)	3	3/0	
DIET191	Dietetic Tech. Practicum I (T)	1	1/3	
ENGL101	Beginning Composition (G)	3	3/0	ENGL100 or Place
MLT100	Introduction to Healthcare (T)	3	2/2	Place in ENGL101
CPT101	Computer Literacy (B)	3	2/2	
	TOTAL CREDITS	15		

SECOND QUARTER		CR	LEC/LAB HR	PREREQ
HOSP107	Food Principles (T)	5	5/0	
HOSP109	Food Production (T)	3	1/7	HOSP102 & HOSP122 DIET191
DIET192	Dietetic Practicum II (T)	2	1/7	
MULT101	Medical Terminology (B)	2	2/0	
MATH102	Beginning Algebra (B)	4	4/0	DEV031 or Place
	TOTAL CREDITS	16		

continues

THIRD QUARTER		CR	LEC/LAB HR	PREREQ
HOSP121	Computer Applications in Foodservice (T)	2	1/2	CPT101
HOSP123	Food Purchasing (T)	3	3/0	DEV031
SSCI101	Cultural Diversity (G)	5	5/0	Place in ENGL101
DIET193	Dietetic Practicum III (T)	12	1/7	DIET192
HOSP153	Nutrition (T)	5	5/0	DEV030
TOTAL CREDITS		17		

FOURTH QUARTER		CR	LEC/LAB HR	PREREQ
BMGT1111	Management (B)	5	5/0	
ENGL102	Essay and Research (G)	3	3/0	ENGL101
BIO101	Intro to Anatomy and Physiology (B)	3	3/0	
COMM105	Speech (G)	3	3/0	ENGL100
TOTAL CREDITS		14		

FIFTH QUARTER		CR	LEC/LAB HR	PREREQ
DIET297	Dietetic Practicum IV (T)	3	2/7	DIET193
DIET275	Diet Therapy I (T)	5	4/2	HOSP153 & BIO101
BIO169	Human Physiology (B)	5	4/2	BIO101 or 161
HOSP205	Records and Cost Controls (T)	4	3/2	
TOTAL CREDITS		17		

continues

SIXTH QUARTER		CR	LEC/LAB HR	PREREQ
HOSP225	Menu Planning (T)	3	3/0	HOSP153 & HOSP107
DIET298	Dietetic Practicum V (T)	2	1/7	DIET297
DIET276	Diet Therapy II (T)	5	4/2	DIET275 & BIO169
ENGL202	Writing for Health & Human Services (G)	3	3/0	ENGL102 & Prac. Enrollment
HOSP224	Hosp. Personnel Mgmt. (T)	5	5/0	BMGT111
	TOTAL CREDITS	16		

SEVENTH QUARTER		CR	LEC/LAB HR	PREREQ
DIET265	Dietetic Tech. Seminar (T)	1	1/0	DIET298
DIET299	Dietetic Practicum VI (T)	3	1/10	DIET298
HOSP219	Food Production Mgmt. (T)	4	1/8	Final Quarter
HUM1XX	HUM111, 112, 113, 151 or 152 (G)	5	5/0	PLACE IN ENGL101
	TOTAL CREDITS	13		

GRADUATION REQUIREMENTS

(G) = General Education
(B) = Basic Education
(T) = Technical Education

Total General Education	22 hours
Basic Education	22 hours
Total Non-Technical	44 hours
Total Technical	66 hours
TOTAL CREDITS	110 hours

Courtesy of Columbus State Community College, Columbus, Ohio.

GENERIC CURRICULUM FOR A DIDACTIC PROGRAM IN DIETETICS AND COORDINATED PROGRAM*

(Based on the 1997 Foundation Knowledge and Skills for Didactic Component of Entry-Level Dietitian Education Programs)

A. Communications
    Educational methods
    Speech
    Learning theory
    Computer science/usage
    Counseling/interviewing

B. Physical and Biological Sciences
    General Chemistry
    Organic Chemistry
    Biochemistry
    Physiology or Anatomy
    Microbiology

C. Social Sciences
    Sociology
    Psychology
    Economics
    Ethics (or in Humanities)
    Public Policy

D. Research
    Research methodology
    Statistics

E. Food
    Food production and service
    Food science/technology
    Sociocultural aspects of foods

F. Nutrition
    Basic and advanced nutrition
    Medical Nutrition Therapy
    Community nutrition
    Nutrition in the life cycle

*The Coordinated Program curriculum will further include supervised practice totaling a minimum of 900 clock hours.

G. Management
   Management theory and human resource management
   Mathematics/Accounting and financial management

H. Health Care Systems
    Health care policy and delivery
    Ethics

General Education
   English composition
   History
   U.S. Government
   Humanities

Supporting and Elective Courses
   Business, Languages, Health and Wellness, other

GENERIC CURRICULUM FOR A DIETETIC
TECHNICIAN PROGRAM*

(Based on the 1997 Foundation Knowledge and Skills for Didactic Component of Entry-Level Dietetic Technician Education Programs)

A. Communications
    Mathematics
    English composition
    Computer science/usage
    Speech
    Counseling/interviewing
    Educational techniques

B. Physical and Biological Sciences
    General Chemistry
    Physiology
    Microbiology

C. Social Sciences
    Psychology
    Sociology

D. Research
    Research methodology

E. Food
    Food production and service

F. Nutrition
    Basic nutrition
    Medical Nutrition Therapy
    Nutrition in the life cycle
    Community nutrition

G. Management
    Management theory and human resource management
    Financial management

H. Health Care
    Health care policy and delivery
    Ethics

General Education
    History
    U.S. Government
    Humanities

*The curriculum will further include supervised practice totaling a minimum of 450 clock hours.

Membership Categories in The American Dietetic Association

Classification and Dues	Qualifications
Active—Route (A) $140.00	Any person who has earned a baccalaureate degree, meets academic requirements specified by ADA, and meets one or more of the following criteria: • is a Registered Dietitian (RD) or has established eligibility to take the Registration Examination for Dietitians • has completed a preprofessional practice experience program (dietetic internship, coordinated or AP4 program) accredited or approved by CAADE, or • has earned a master's or doctoral degree conferred by a regionally accredited college or university
Route (B) $140.00	Any person who has earned either a master's or doctoral degree and who holds one degree in one of the following areas: dietetics, foods and nutrition, nutrition, community public health nutrition, food science, food service systems management. Degree used to satisfy membership qualifications must be conferred by a regionally accredited college or university.
Route (C) $98.00	Any person who meets one of the following: • is a Dietetic Technician, Registered (DTR), or has established eligibility to take the Registration Examination for Dietetic Technicians, or • has completed an associate degree program for dietetic technicians accredited/approved by CAADE

Classification and Dues	Qualifications
Retired: from Active (A+B) $70.00 and former active (C) $49.00	Any current Active member who is: • no longer employed in dietetics practice or education and is at least 62 years of age, or • is retired on total (permanent) disability

Returning Student: former Active (A+B) $70.00, former active (C) $49.00	Any current Active (Route A or B) member who is:
	• returning to school on a full-time basis or any current Active (Route C) member who is:
	  – returning to school on a full-time basis for a baccalaureate degree or
	  – returning to complete an CAADE accredited/approved preprofessional practice program
	(Members must apply annually.)

Associate $40.50	Any person who meets one of the following:
Category 1	• is a graduate of a baccalaureate degree program who has completed CAADE-approved academic requirements but is not yet eligible for Active membership
Category 2	• is a student enrolled in an CAADE-accredited/approved program or a preprofessional experience program accredited/approved by CAADE who does not meet requirements for Active membership
Category 3	• is a student enrolled in a regionally accredited, postsecondary education program that is non-CAADE accredited/approved. This classification is available to students who state their intent to enter a CAADE-accredited/approved program.

Source: © 1996, The American Dietetic Association, *"Directory of Dietetic Programs."* Used by permission.

Position Papers Issued by The American Dietetic Association

Child food and nutrition programs. *J Am Diet Assoc*. 1996;96:913–917. (Expires 2001)

Competitive foods in schools. *J Am Diet Assoc*. 1991;91:1123–1125. (Expires 1997)

Nutrition services for children with special health needs. *J Am Diet Assoc*. 1995;95:809–812. (Expires 1998)

Nutrition standards for child care programs. *J Am Diet Assoc*. 1994;94:323–328. (Expires 1998)

Promotion and support of breast feeding. *J Am Diet Assoc*. 1993;93:467–469. (Reaffirmed)

School-based nutrition programs and services (joint position with the Society of Nutrition Education and the American School Food Service Association). *J Am Diet Assoc*. 1995;95:367–369. (Expires 2000)

Vegetarian diets. *J Am Diet Assoc*. 1993;93:1317–1319. (Reaffirmed)

Nutrition intervention in the treatment of anorexia nervosa, bulimia nervosa, and binge eating. *J Am Diet Assoc*. 1994;94:902–907. (Expires 1999)

American Diabetes Association: nutrition recommendations and principles for people with diabetes mellitus. *J Am Diet Assoc*. 1994;94:504–506.

Nutrition in comprehensive program planning for persons with developmental disabilities. *J Am Diet Assoc*. 1992;92:613–615. (Reaffirmed)

Domestic hunger and inadequate access to food. *J Am Diet Assoc*. 1990;90:1437–1441. (Reaffirmed)

World hunger. *J Am Diet Assoc*. 1995;95:1160–1162. (Expires 2000)

The impact of fluoride on dental health. *J Am Diet Assoc*. 1994;94:1428–1430. (Expires 1999)

Nutrition intervention in the care of persons with human immunodeficiency virus infection. (Jointly developed with the Canadian Dietetic Association.) *J Am Diet Assoc*. 1994;94:1042–1045. (Expires 1999)

Second Report of the National Cholesterol Education Program Expert Panel. Not reprinted in the *Journal;* copies are available from ADA. The original report was published in *JAMA.* 1993;269:3015–3023.

Nutrition care for pregnant adolescents. *J Am Diet Assoc.* 1994;94:449–450. (Expires 1998)

Health implications of dietary fiber. *J Am Diet Assoc.* 1993;93:1446–1447. (Reaffirmed)

Nutrition for physical fitness and athletic performance for adults. (Jointly developed with the Canadian Dietetic Association.) *J Am Diet Assoc.* 1993;93:691–696. (Expires 1998)

Environmental issues. *J Am Diet Assoc* 1993;93:589. (Reaffirmed)

Enrichment and fortification of foods and dietary supplements. *J Am Diet Assoc.* 1994;94:661–663. (Expires 1999)

Women's health and nutrition. (Jointly developed with the Canadian Dietetic Association.) *J Am Diet Assoc* 1995;95:362–366. (Expires 1998)

Phytochemicals and functional foods. *J Am Diet Assoc* 1995;95:493–496. (Expires 1998)

Vitamin and mineral supplementation. *J Am Diet Assoc.* 1996;96:73–76. (Expires 1999)

Oral health and nutrition. *J Am Diet Assoc.* 1996;96:184–189. (Expires 2001)

Food irradiation. *J Am Diet Assoc.* 1996;96:69–72. (Expires 1999)

Biotechnology and the future of food. *J Am Diet Assoc.* 1995;95:1429–1432. (Expires 1999)

Fat replacements. *J Am Diet Assoc.* 1991;91:1285–1288. (Reaffirmed)

Appropriate use of nutritive and nonnutritive sweeteners. *J Am Diet Assoc.* 1993;93:816–821. (Reaffirmed)

Cost-effectiveness of medical nutrition therapy. *J Am Diet Assoc.* 1995;95:88–91. (Reaffirmed)

Affordable and accessible health care services. *J Am Diet Assoc.* 1992;92:746–748. (Reaffirmed)

Nutrition services in managed care. *J Am Diet Assoc.* 1992;92:391–395. (Expires 2000)

Management of health care food and nutrition services. *J Am Diet Assoc.* 1993;93 914–915. (Reaffirmed)

Legal and ethical issues in feeding the permanently unconscious patient. *J Am Diet Assoc.* 1995;95:231–234. (Expires 1999)

Issues in feeding the terminally ill adult. *J Am Diet Assoc.* 1992;92:996–1002. (Reaffirmed)

The role of the registered dietitian in enteral and parenteral nutrition support. *J Am Diet Assoc.* 1991;91:1440–1441. (Reaffirmed)

Nutrition monitoring of the home parenteral and enteral patient. *J Am Diet Assoc.* 1994;94:664–666. (Expires 1998)

Nutrition, aging, and the continuum of care. *J Am Diet Assoc*. 1996;96:1048–1052. (Expires 1999)

Nutrition education of health professionals. *J Am Diet Assoc*. 1991;91:611–613. (Reaffirmed)

Nutrition—essential component of medical education. *J Am Diet Assoc*. 1994;94:555–557. (Expires 1998)

Nutrition education for the public. *J Am Diet Assoc*. 1996;96:1183–1187. (Expires 2000)

Food and nutrition misinformation. *J Am Diet Assoc*. 1995;95:705–707. (Expires 2000)

Weight management. *J Am Diet Assoc*. 1997;97:71–74. (Approved 1996)

Food and water safety. *J Am Diet Assoc*. 1997;97:184–189. (Approved 1996)

Trans fatty acids. Copy available from ADA. (Approved 1996)

Sources of Information About the Profession of Dietetics

The American Dietetic Association
  216 W. Jackson Blvd.
  Chicago, Illinois 60606-6995
  Telephone: 1-800-877-1600
      Education and Accreditation—Ext. 4811
      Registration—Ext. 4856
      Career information—Ext. 4744
      Publications—Ext. 4744 (Including the annual "Directory of Dietetics
        Programs")
      Membership—Ext. 4841
      Scholarships—Ext. 4820

The National Center for Nutrition and Dietetics of The American Dietetic
Association
  216 W. Jackson Blvd.
  Chicago, Illinois 60606-6995
      Consumer Hotline—1-800-366-1655
      Office—1-800-877-1600

Washington Office of The American Dietetic Association
  1225 Eye St. N.W., Suite 1250
  Washington, D.C. 20005-3914
  Telephone: 202-371-0500

State or District Dietetic Association
  State and/or district offices may be listed in telephone directories. Otherwise,
  contact a dietitian (see below) or a college or university.

College or university offering dietetics programs
All land-grant universities offer the dietetics major. Many other four-year and two-year colleges also offer the major including the dietetic technician major. Libraries at most colleges/universities have copies of other catalogs from all states. Also check the Internet home pages for many universities. High school counselors and public libraries will also have career information.

A Dietitian
Dietitians may be contacted from a local telephone directory, at a local hospital, a public health department or agency, a school food service program, a college/university, a cooperative extension office.

ADA website
http:www.eatright.org

INDEX

Q

Quality assurance standards, 223–225
Quality control, food services, 304
Quality management, 124

R

Radio broadcast education, 61
Ragalie, Jean, 245, 250, 252
Registered dietetic technician, 82–83. *See also* Dietetic technicians
Registered dietitian, 14, 45–46, 82–83
  employment by area of practice, 155
  nutrition care activities of, 110
  professional activities of, 107–108
  work settings for, 111
Registration, 14
  commission on, 128
  development of, 81–83
Rehearsal, 46
Reimbursement, 210–211
Research, 67, 68–69, 279, 323
  ADA practice groups, 195–196
  careers in, 194
  case study for, 198–199
  dietitians in, 190–193
  ethics in, 196–197
  importance to profession of, 194–195
  legal issues of, 196–197
  specialists, 180
Resources, 375–376
Review, 47
Rhodes, Sara, 305–306
Richards, Ellen H., 8–9
Roberts, Lydia J., 10
Role delineation studies, 18, 85–87, 102–112
  nutrition care activities, 109–110
  professional activities, 107–108
  work settings, 111
Rorer, Sarah Tyson, 8
Rose, Mary Schwartz, 9
Rosenbloom, Christine, 261
Russell, Carlene, 227–228

S

Salaries, 23–25
Saldanha, Leila, 192
Satellite technology education, 61

School nutrition programs, 158–159
Scurvy, 5
Secondary prevention, of illness, 177
Secondary school education, 186–187
Service to others, 13
Sichterman, Carol, 227
Sippy diet, 136
Skill building, 251
Skin lesions, 5
Social Security Act, Title V, 174
Social welfare, 8
Specialized areas of practice, 79, 83–88, 179–180
Sports and Cardiovascular Nutritionists, 261
Sports nutrition, 261–263
Stancik, Vi, 238–239
Standards of dietetic practice, 84, 124–125
Standards of education, 33–35
State associations, 128–129
State licensure, 88–89
State programs, 283
Storey, Rita, 250, 251, 252, 253
Stroke, 260
Supervised practice, 46–47
  education components of, 347–356
  programs for, 47–50
    application to, 51–52
    changes in, 50
    questions about, 50–51

T

Teaching, 7–8
Team, 95–96
  in clinical practice, 143–146
  meaning of, 96–101
  members, 99, 101
  roles and responsibilities of, 102
Teamwork, 99–101, 319
Technological revolution, 314
Telephone education, 61
Tertiary intervention, 177
Therapeutic dietitian, 136
Todhunter, E. Neige, 323

U

University education, 187–188
University of Texas program, 358–359